Large Scale Genome Variation in Health and Disease

Editor

Ad Geurts Van Kessel, Nijmegen

35 figures, 24 in color, and 21 tables, 2006

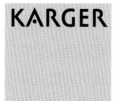

Basel · Freiburg · Paris · London · New York ·
Bangalore · Bangkok · Singapore · Tokyo · Sydney

Reprint of **Cytogenetic and Genome Research** (ISSN 1424–8581)
Vol. 115, No. 3–4, 2006

Cover illustration
Two patients who each have different single-copy duplications within the BAC clone (RP11-90K7) would have indistinguishable aCGH resulta. See article by Cho et al., this issue, p. 262.

S. Karger
Medical and Scientific Publishers
Basel · Freiburg · Paris · London
New York · Bangalore · Bangkok
Singapore · Tokyo · Sydney

Disclaimer
The statements, options and data contained in this publication are solely those of the individual authors and contributors and not of the publisher and the editor(s). The appearance of advertisements in the journal is not a warranty, endorsement, or approval of the products or services advertised or of their effectiveness, quality or safety. The publisher and the editor(s) disclaim responsibility for any injury to persons or property resulting from any ideas, methods, instructions or products referred to in the content or advertisements.

Drug Dosage
The authors and the publisher have exerted every effort to ensure that drug selection and dosage set forth in this text are in accord with current recommendations and practice at the time of publication. However, in view of ongoing research, changes in government regulations, and the constant flow of information relating to drug therapy and drug reactions, the reader is urged to check the package insert for each drug for any change in indications and dosage and for added warnings and precautions. This is particularly important when the recommended agent is a new and/or infrequently employed drug.

KARGER   Fax +41 61 306 12 34
E-Mail karger@karger.ch
www.karger.com

Contents

Contents

Cytogenet Genome Res 115:197 (2006)
DOI: 10.1159/000095914

Preface

Until recently it was thought that variation in the human genome was, except for some large scale variants encountered in both tumor cells and normal cells, mostly restricted to so-called single nucleotide polymorphisms (SNPs). However, with the development of novel genome-wide technologies emanating from the human genome project such as microarray-based genomic profiling, it has become clear that large-scale DNA copy number variations (CNVs), ranging from single kilobases to several megabases, are much more common than expected before (current estimate $>3 \times 10^8$ bases of DNA in the human genome). This novel information, which may have a profound impact on a wide range of disciplines ranging from molecular genetics to clinical genetics, is currently being stored and catalogued in comprehensive data bases. Depending on the platform used, CNVs can be detected with varying degrees of accuracy and resolution, and additional information on loss of heterozygosity and/ or uniparental disomy can be retrieved. It is widely assumed now that (cryptic) CNVs may be associated with disease, particularly when arising de novo. In case of congenital malformation, neurocognitive and/or mental retardation syndromes, several CNVs could be linked to specific subsets of these disorders and, in some cases, these links have indeed led to the identification of (candidate) disease genes. Additionally, in various malignant disorders (cancer), cryptic and/or large-scale genomic deletions and/or amplifications have pointed at the location and involvement of specific tumor suppressor genes and proto-oncogenes, respectively.

In this special issue of *Cytogenetic and Genome Research* several aspects of these newly identified large-scale genome variations are discussed, including their etiology and the putative role of flanking low copy repeats therein, questions on to what extent CNVs may act as harmless bystanders or not, and suggestions on how to employ this novel information for the delineation of genotype-phenotype associations, disease gene identification and, ultimately, clinical practice including diagnosis, prognosis and treatment.

With special thanks to all of those who contributed,

Ad Geurts van Kessel
Nijmegen, August 2006

KARGER

Fax +41 61 306 12 34
E-Mail karger@karger.ch
www.karger.com

© 2006 S. Karger AG, Basel
1424–8581/06/1154–0197$23.50/0

Accessible online at:
www.karger.com/cgr

Cytogenet Genome Res 115:198–204 (2006)
DOI: 10.1159/000095915

Historical development of analysing large-scale changes in the human genome

P.L. Pearson

Department of Genetics and Evolutionary Biology, University of Sao Paulo, Sao Paulo (Brazil)

Manuscript received 4 June 2006; accepted in revised form for publication by A. Geurts van Kessel, 5 June 2006.

Abstract. A widely held belief today is that genomics really only started with the DNA sequence information emanating from the genome programs for various organisms, with the human genome playing the leading role. In fact there is a discernable trail stretching for more than a 100 years from the observations of Boveri on tissue instability involving polyploidy in sea urchin embryos and human tumours to the present day. This historical review follows that trail and shows that many theoretical and technical advantages taken for granted in today's genomics era rely heavily on earlier cytogenetic and gene mapping discoveries. Three specific examples of technical developmental paths involving in situ hybridisation, flow-sorting and DNA reassociation kinetics will be explored. In the mid-1980s the two former approaches merged to give rise to several applications of which chromosome painting and chromosome CGH are arguably the most important. The latter developed into array CGH which has now become the pre-eminent method for detecting micro-imbalances in a large number of targets. A competing emerging technology is that of genome-wide SNP typing, which itself is a product of the much earlier RFLP approach linked to DNA sequence information. Do such approaches spell the final demise of the microscope? Perhaps for narrowly defined activities this may occur, but for addressing general questions, microscopic examination will remain pre-eminent.

Copyright © 2006 S. Karger AG, Basel

As a direct result of the information and technical advances emanating from the human genome program, many innovative approaches have been proposed and developed in recent years for tracking both large- and small-scale changes in the human genome. These methods are now being extensively employed in many areas of biological and medical investigation and include identifying cryptic genome changes in cancer, neural disorders with special reference to mental deficiency and autism, comparative evolutionary studies, to mention but a few. This special issue of *Cytogenetic and Genome Research* is replete with extensive descriptions of these techniques and their applications. I do not wish to go into the fine nuances of the methods, these are amply covered by other contributors, but to trace the historical developments that have led to our current situation and, occasionally to comment on some of the advantages and shortcomings of the different approaches.

When, why and how did genome analysis start?

Genomics is an ugly Americanised term, coined in the mid-1980s at a rump meeting of scientists at one of the Cold Spring Harbour Symposia to discuss the forming of a new journal on genome variation. The publisher thought '*Genomics*' would make a cute and catchy title for the journal and to the eternal devaluation of the English language the term has now become common parlance and the suffix 'omics' widely extended to other related areas, such as proteomics. We now seem to be in the middle of the 'omics' era. Whatever the grammatical correctness of the term, genomics is commonly regarded as the study of genome variation at the molecular level. The archetypically correct journal Nature has recently accepted the inevitable reluctantly and now also uses '-omics' in the title of its genome web site. There is a naïve belief amongst many young scientists that

Request reprints from P.L. Pearson
    Department of Genetics and Evolutionary Biology
    Institute for Biological Sciences, University City, University of Sao Paulo
    05508-090 Sao Paulo (Brazil)
    telephone: +55 1 9978 0929; e-mail: peterlpearson@uol.com.br

screening for changes on a genome scale only seriously commenced with the initiation of the respective genome programs for humans and other species some 15 years ago, culminating in the so-called completion of sequencing the human genome 3, 4 or 5 years ago, depending on which completion announcement one chooses to take as the base line. I argue that this is a narrow and misleading view giving scant consideration to the impressive amount of information on genome variation at the chromosome and DNA level gathered before the advent of the genome programs. While it is true that the genome program has led to an immense intensification of activities aided by screening methods with true genome-wide coverage, genome screening first started at the chromosome level more than 100 years ago and later moved down to the molecular level some 50 years ago.

The first genome pioneers

Early cytogeneticists studying chromosome variation within and between species at the turn of the 20th century can be legitimately regarded as the first genome pioneers. Foremost among these was Theodore Boveri, who described tissue instability involving polyploidy derived from polyspermy in sea urchin embryos (1907) and in human tumours (1914). Nettie Stevens (1905) was one of the first to distinguish sex chromosomes, in this case in males of the beetle *Tenebrio* and shortly afterwards in *Drosophila*. With Edmund Wilson (Wilson, 1905) she is credited with providing the first observational evidence supporting the theory of chromosome inheritance, all prior proposals being inferential. An interesting anecdote is that the term 'X' for X chromosome derives from observations of Henking (1890) who observed an extra body in the spermatogenesis of the plant bug *Pyrrochus apterus*, later determined to have a single sex chromosome in males, did not know what it was and referred to the mysterious object as 'X'. The subsequent derivation of the name given to the Y chromosome now becomes obvious. Nettie Stevens had the extreme good fortune to study with both Theodore Boveri and Thomas Hunt Morgan. The latter had for more than a decade resisted the theories on the role of chromosomes and nucleus in inheritance. Ironically, following Steven's observations it took Morgan a further six years (Morgan, 1911) to finally draw the correct conclusion that it was the nucleus (chromosomes) and not the cytoplasm that predominantly determined the development and form of an organism. Morgan's reluctant conversion stemmed from his own observations on sex linkage in *Drosophila* and to the irrefutable conclusion that several phenotypic features were inherited stably with the X chromosome and therefore *must* be carried on the X chromosome. There are none so fervent as reformed sinners and Morgan carried on for the rest of his life as a passionate protagonist of the central dogma of the gene and chromosome theory of inheritance. With his students Sturtevant, Bridges and Muller, he constructed genetic linkage maps for all *Drosophila* chromosomes and these studies laid the foundation of gene mapping by meiotic recombination in all organisms including man, for which Morgan and colleagues received the Nobel Prize in Physiology or Medicine in 1934. The method is just as relevant today as it was then, and is still the only way of deriving an initial map location for the genes determining human genetic diseases where a phenotype segregating in a family is the only starting point, all modern molecular technology not withstanding.

There is a discernable trail stretching from the observations of Boveri to the present day. In particular, Boveri's results stimulated the study of genome (chromosome) changes in tumour cells. As with several later developments in genetics, a discovery of such importance to medical science guarantees an increase of funding and resources that can rarely be matched in other areas. Many cytogenetic studies on tumour cells were initiated which showed that a large number of tumours were grossly aneuploid, mainly with increases in chromosome number. Prior to 1956, the year in which the human chromosome count of 46 was established by Tjio and Levan (1956) it was believed that man had 48 chromosomes similar to the great apes. The technical improvements in chromosome preparation (hypotonic treatment and colcemid) that permitted Tjio and Levan to make their observations also enabled oncologists to perform more accurate chromosome observations in tumours. This led to describing the Philadelphia chromosome in chronic myeloid leukaemia by Nowell and Hungerford (1960). However, it was realized that DNA measurements on the nuclei of tumour cells would also provide a measure of the level of ploidy. Since the DNA quantity differences between G1, S and G2 cell cycle phases could be recognised, it was also possible to calculate the proportion of cells that were in active division. Early observations used UV absorption pioneered by Caspersson (1940), who 30 years later was to become much more widely known for his contributions to chromosome banding. The development of bright field, two wavelength, micro densitometry of Feulgen-stained specimens was more or less contemporary with the UV approach and was a solid but extremely slow screening method, which went on for some 20 years (for review see Hardie et al., 2002). Importantly, these methods were used to accurately determine genome sizes and the same values were used some 35 years later in the calculations on how much DNA would have to be sequenced in the genome programs of different organisms. While estimates of the number of genes in man have varied between >100,000 and 25,000 over that period of time, the estimates of the amount of DNA have remained constant, an enormous compliment to the accuracy of those early genome pioneers. Towards the end of the 1960s flow cytometry became commercially available (Herzenberg et al., 2002), and overnight more or less blew away the use of previous methods, because of its high speed and accuracy in measuring the DNA quantity of individual cells. In a matter of minutes the ploidy level and replication characteristics of many thousands of cancer cells could be determined. Even after 35 years this method still remains important in determining variability in DNA quantity in tumour cell populations. Nearly 100,000 oncology articles in which flow cytometry plays a central role have been published in the intervening period and without doubt this approach to studying genome variation has had the largest impact to date. The ability of flow cytometers to also sort objects based on DNA quantity and composition opened up possibilities of separating chromosomes of different size and base composition. This approach will be addressed later.

From the point of view of defining the ways in which constitutive chromosome changes can affect the phenotype, an important early way station on the genome trail involved the observations of Blakeslee (1924) on the Jimson weed; he discovered that the individual trisomies for all chromosomes were each associated with a unique seed phenotype. The Dutch ophthalmologist Waardenburg (1932) was aware of large phenotypic changes induced by chromosome changes in *Drososphila* from the work of Morgan and colleagues and speculated that the human condition of Down syndrome was caused by a specific trisomy, thereby predating the ultimate discovery of trisomy 21 in Down syndrome by 27 years. The publications of Lejeune on the discovery of trisomy 21 in Down syndrome (Lejeune et al., 1959) and others on sex chromosome abnormalities were a major wake-up call that changed human genetics overnight from a cottage to a major industry. Within ten years more humans were karyotyped than for the total of all other organisms ever examined. In 1970 a major development on the genome trail occurred, namely the development of human chromosome banding patterns permitting individual chromosome recognition subsequently enshrined in a standardised nomenclature in 1971. It is amazing that this banding description has remained largely unchanged and has been the *lingua franca* for human geneticists the world over for more than 35 years. Although now that a raster based on DNA sequence is available for all human chromosomes, as long as visual analysis of chromosomes through a microscope takes place, banding nomenclature will continue to be used indefinitely. This ability to determine chromosome location by a banding pattern mirrored the polytene chromosomes of *Drosophila* so successfully used for the physical location of genes by Morgan and colleagues. The human chromosome banding patterns provided the primary mapping scaffold on which the highly successful gene mapping workshops from 1973 to 1992 were based. These were the direct forerunners of the human genome program.

The gene mapping workshops

From this point onwards the genome trail splits into several tracks, which occasionally recombine or end in box canyons. Please forgive the lack of chronological continuity in the following.

Essentially, three major approaches were considered in the mapping workshops, namely: mapping markers and phenotypes by meiotic segregation in families, co-segregation of human markers and entire chromosomes or chromosome fragments (radiation hybrids) in human/rodent somatic cell hybrids and the direct physical mapping of gene

sequences to individual chromosomes by in situ hybridisation. Later workshops from about 1986 onwards also considered the physical mapping of individual chromosome regions by contig mapping; that is defining contiguous clones that overlapped each other so that chromosome regions were reconstructed. The first attempts were made using λ-phage and cosmid clones, but the use of much larger insert cloning vectors, including YACs (Little et al., 1989) and BACs (Wang et al., 1994), speeded up the process enormously. As it turned out BACs eventually won the day and were adopted as the global vehicle for reconstructing and sequencing the entire human genome, because of their far greater insert stability and despite the fact that the inserts were much shorter (~150 kb) than in YACs (>1 Mb).

In situ hybridisation

At the time of the first mapping workshop in 1973, in situ hybridisation was still in its infancy and was based on probe labelling by radioactive tracers and detection by autoradiography. There was much heated debate at the first workshop on the levels of incorporated radioactivity required to get specific localisation of gene sequences to a chromosome region. While it was obvious that loci with highly repetitive DNA such as the ribosomal cistrons (Henderson et al., 1972) or satellite DNAs (Jones and Corneo, 1971) could be mapped comparatively easily, the same was not true for loci comprised of single copy DNA. One group claimed to have mapped the haemoglobin beta gene using directly in vivo labelled mRNA extracted from reticulocytes (Price et al., 1972). One of the in situ hybridisation aficionados at the meeting caused great hilarity with his remark that he had just determined on his pocket calculator, that with the probable specificity and radioactive levels of the probe used in mapping the haemoglobin locus, the investigators would had to have started their autoradiographic exposures some time in the Pleistocene. This scepticism was well founded and the gene was remapped correctly some time later. A combination of small technical improvements occurred over the following years to permit radioactive single copy sequences to be localised to chromosomes, albeit involving a lot of grain counting and statistical analysis to make a specific localisation.

FISH approaches

From about 1980 onwards the power of in situ hybridisation to map genes increased enormously, principally through the availability of highly specific DNA probes produced by recombinant DNA techniques, biotin labelling of probes using fluorochromes as tracers (Langer-Safer et al., 1982), suppression of cross-reacting repeat sequences (Lichter et al., 1988) and vastly improved fluorescent microscopy and image processing to permit multi-probe and multi-fluor labelling. The whole process was faster, more accurate and *much* prettier to look at than previous autoradiographic procedures. The procedure was called FISH, an abbreviation for Fluorescent In Situ Hybridisation, and for the next two decades program organizers frequently named sessions or whole conferences with what they thought were catchy titles such as 'FISHing for diseases' or 'FISH and CHIPS' when both in situ hybridisation and DNA chip technology were on the program together. However, like three-day-old fish, after the third recurrence, the naming lost most of its charm. In any case, the net result was that FISH analysis started to make a tremendous impact on cytogenetic diagnosis. From about 1995 onwards, as probes became available for many known microdeletion and (sub)telomere regions, FISH provided a remarkably accurate diagnosis for many commonly encountered cryptic rearrangements and identification of markers and additional material. However, the main problem with the standard FISH approach is that each hybridisation is restricted to a single locus or maximally to several if hybridised simultaneously in the same reaction mixture. However, this also involves the use of several fluorochromes simultaneously, a complexity that was, and still is, beyond the scope of most screening laboratories. This means that screening all telomeres and known microdeletion regions in each patient involves many separate hybridisations.

Comparative genome hybridisation

Enter Dan Pinkel and colleagues. In 1992 they published a method that revolutionised screening for chromosome abnormalities and provided the means of total genome screening for duplications or deletions at the metaphase chromosome level of resolution (Kallioniemi et al., 1992). The technique proved extremely useful for studying tumours with complex rearrangements and where availability of dividing cells was at a premium. Chromosome preparations from the tumour itself were not required, just the DNA. This was labelled with a red fluorochrome and hybridised to normal human chromosome preparations with an equal amount of green-labelled normal DNA. The chromosome preparations were subsequently examined under a fluorescent microscope and regions where there was duplication or amplification of tumour DNA showed up as red, normal amount of tumour DNA as yellow and deleted tumour DNA as green. The method was called chromosome Comparative Genome Hybridisation or chromosome CGH and more than 1,000 publications have appeared since its initiation, mainly on tumours but also on standard cytogenetic screening (Kirchhoff et al., 2001) and pre-implantation genetic diagnosis (Wells and Delhanty, 2000). The four main disadvantages of the method are: that sophisticated microscopic and image analysis equipment is required, that the hybridisations can take up to several days, that the analysis of the results is time-consuming and that the method provides no information on the structure of the chromosome. In patient care situations where time is of the essence, such as in pre-implantation genetic diagnosis, the time factor can be a serious limitation.

Microarray approaches

Enter Dan Pinkel and colleagues once again. In a new CGH approach (Snijders et al., 2001) they replaced the chromosome template used in chromosome CGH with an array of BAC probes spotted onto slides. This variant had the distinct advantage of offering a much higher resolution than that offered by metaphase chromosomes. Not surprisingly, the method is called array CGH and is available for whole genome scanning either as a 1-Mb raster comprising up to 3,500 BACs or a complete tiling path raster with about 35,000 BACs. Several other articles in this special issue describe the use of array CGH for detecting cryptic chromosome unbalances. In broad terms it appears that over 15% of mentally retarded patients possess causative deletions or duplications not detected by classical chromosome analysis and the technique offers a sensitive method of screening imbalances in other congenital abnormalities and tumours. Construction of CGH arrays would not have been possible without information on the chromosome location of all the BAC clones. Although the chromosome location was initially established by FISH, now that the DNA sequence information is available for all human chromosomes, the chromosome location of the BACs can also be confirmed by their position relative to the standardized DNA sequence of each chromosome. Unlike the chromosome banding pattern nomenclature in which the bands are numbered outwards from the centromere to the telomeres, the current convention with DNA sequence is to start numbering nucleotides from pter through the centromere to qter. Given that many chromosome regions including telomeres, centromeres and other regions contain highly repetitive DNA sequences present in variable copy number in different individuals, the absolute size of each chromosome varies from person to person and the BAC contigs used to generate the sequence data have to be anchored to arbitrary points on a raster. The raster chosen is that of the nucleotide sequence position on an average length chromosome for a given chromosome. This means that the sequence coordinates of many mapped objects are going to change as the map is refined. So for example, inserting or removing a contig and its associated DNA sequence upstream changes all the sequence coordinates of the rest of the chromosome downstream. On a personal historical note, I proposed using an arbitrary reference point coordinate system (ARP map) at the gene mapping workshop in 1988 to take into account exactly some of the problems that are arising with the integrated genome maps, namely to bridge regions which could not be analyzed or still remained to be done and to prevent changes in the map coordinates of one part of a chromosome also causing changes in the coordinates of other parts of the same chromosome. The proposal was not taken up at the time, but it gives me some satisfaction that the principle is now embodied in the integrated map and sequence browsers of the NCBI and Ensembl, albeit in an incomplete form.

Sorting chromosomes

In the early 1980s FACS machines were starting to be employed for isolating human metaphase chromosomes which were then used for creating chromosome-specific libraries, first by cloning in vectors and, following the discovery of PCR by Kary Mullis in 1986 (Mullis et al., 1992), by directly amplifying the DNA from the isolated chromosomes by DOP-PCR (Telenius et al., 1992) or priming from interspersed repeats (Ledbetter et al., 1990). [Note; it is intriguing that although Mullis received the Nobel Prize for medicine in 1993 for his monumental discovery, he only has 17 cited publications. Is he the least published Nobel laureate for medicine ever?]. Many chromosome-specific libraries were produced in this way and used for extensive mapping of many human chromosomes. The DOE laboratories at Los Alamos and Lawrence Livermore developed especially dedicated high-speed cell sorters and were gradually making chromosome-specific libraries available to the mapping community. However, several groups including those of Sam Latt (Disteche et al., 1982), Malcom Ferguson-Smith (Harris et al., 1985) and Bryan Young (Davies et al., 1981) successfully sorted human metaphase chromosomes and made chromosome-specific libraries by cloning in λ-phage vectors using much slower, commercially available FACS machines than those at the DOE laboratories. It was subsequently discovered that the libraries could be used for painting human chromosomes (Lichter et al., 1988; Gray et al., 1992; Telenius et al., 1992) and, by adjusting the stringency of the hybridisation, also in cross-species hybridisation even between species which are evolutionarily very distant from each other. This latter method pioneered by the group of Ferguson-Smith has permitted studies on the evolution of mammalian karyotypes using the human karyotype as the principle starting point. Recent results support DNA sequence homology (Yang et al., 2003) showing that the eutherians are phylogenetically very different from the classification based on classical morphology and give credence to an out of Africa origin for many eutherian phyla. The relationship of marsupials and monotremes to the other mammals is still under investigation. The method represents an extremely powerful tool to demonstrate the variability between the genomes of species at the chromosomal level. The intriguing question is how does such cross-species hybridisation work, given that nearly all the signal involves non-coding sequences. Does this mean that non-coding sequences are much more conserved than originally believed? For example, what is the average sequence homology of non-coding sequences between mice and men, by comparison to rabbits and men? On a practical note, Ferguson-Smith's group provides a unique and extremely useful service on request to sort the chromosomes of any vertebrate species to permit similar studies to be performed in other phyla. The Welcome Trust subsidizes the service and the only requirement is for the group making the request to provide a cell line from which chromosomes can be sorted (Cambridge Resource Centre for Comparative Genomics: http://www.vet.cam.ac.uk/genomics/).

Replacing the microscope?

In the mid-1970s, the benefits of the recombinant DNA revolution were just starting to appear and the first human gene sequences became available for analysis in the form of cDNAs derived from isolating individual types of messenger RNA; cDNA libraries only became available later. Two of the first gene sequences that became available in this way were those of the alpha- and beta-globin genes. Several groups developed strategies for hybridizing a radiolabelled cDNA of a given gene with total human DNA in solution and studying the rate of association of the cDNA with the total DNA (Muto, 1977). This method derived many of its features from the Cot curve analyses developed by Britten and Kohne in the late 1960s for calculating the proportion of repeat sequences in genomic DNA (Britten and Kohne, 1968) by the rate of renaturation. The rate of association was equivalent to the number of copies of the relevant gene or DNA type in the genomic DNA. In an epic publication, Kan and colleagues demonstrated that they could distinguish the number of copies of alpha-globin between normal individuals (4 copies) and various forms of alpha-thalassemia with 3, 2, 1 or 0 copies. The only variant that they failed to uniquely recognize was the 3-copy form, which they could not distinguish from the normal (Kan et al., 1976). Some time later I came across this publication and realised that counting genes in this way was the same as counting chromosomes if you had at least one sequence for each chromosome *and* it was not even necessary to look down a microscope! The biggest problem was that in 1978, the number of cloned genes was very small and that most chromosomes did not yet have at least one DNA marker assigned to them. However, I was very enthusiastic to develop a molecular approach to detect copy number changes and undaunted set out with my technician (now Professor Bert Bakker) to isolate our own chromosome-specific clones by shotgun cloning of placental DNA in a plasmid vector, and mapping each insert with somatic cell hybrids to specific chromosomes using Southern blotting. We immediately saw that about 20% of probes exhibited fragment length variation following cutting with a limited number of restriction enzymes, now called Restriction Fragment Length Polymorphisms (RFLPs), quickly lost sight of the original aim of developing 'chromosome analysis without microscopy' and instead developed probes for mapping disease genes and phenotypes which we used ourselves in many mapping studies and also made freely available to others. Many groups, including our own, used the RFLPs for tracing regions of loss of heterozygosity in tumours (Devilee et al., 1989) and established the basis for deletion screening, which is now an integral part of modern screening in both cancer and idiopathic congenital abnormalities. Although the slow speed and tedium of Southern blotting was replaced by the analytically more accurate use of Short Tandem Repeat Sequences (STRs) combined with automated DNA sequence analysis, these methods have now been replaced by rapid genome wide SNP screening using a multiplicity of ingenious detection methods. However, the analytical principle remains the same as

Cytogenet Genome Res 115:198–204 (2006)

RFLP screening 30 years earlier, including some of the problems. When screening tumours, it is standard practise to compare the tumour results of a given set of RFLPs or SNPs with the pattern seen in normal tissues from the same individual. However, given the low heterozygosity frequency of SNPs and RFLPs, by definition always less than 50% and generally less than 30%, the majority of loci are going to be homozygous and not informative for loss of heterozygosity (LOH). In a tumour–normal tissue comparison, one knows from the normal tissue which loci will be informative in the tumour of a given individual and which not.

The same is not true for constitutive abnormalities where there is no way of knowing a priori with a 100% certainty whether loci are heterozygous and therefore informative; there is only a probability based on the frequency of the minor allele. The response of the SNP equipment producers to this complication has been to produce detection systems with a SNP density as high as one SNP per 10 kb across the whole genome. Even at this high density and an average minor allele frequency of 20% and average heterozygote frequency of 32%, this means that only deletions of 150 kb or larger would be detected with >99% certainty based on LOH and that the rate of detection would decrease rapidly with decreases in deletion size (100 kb with 98% certainty, 50 kb with 86% certainty, 20 kb with 46% certainty, etc.). Duplication detection depends on whether the SNP equipment concerned is capable of quantitative measurements and accurately distinguishing two copies of one allele from a single copy of the other. This brings into doubt the strategy of looking for LOH as against simply looking at oligonucleotide signal levels irrespective of whether or not there is an SNP present in the sequence. Currently, many SNP detection systems are purely qualitative and those that have the theoretical capacity for quantitative detection, such as the Affymetrix GeneChip, have not yet been exhaustively tested for the sensitivity and reproducibility of their quantitative measurements. Although approaches have been used detecting lack of Mendelian segregation for given SNPs to identify potential deletion regions, this only works for large samples (Conrad et al., 2006) and is not suitable for the majority of patient care situations. At this moment, deletion and duplication detection using the SNP approach has to rely on an extremely high SNP density to be certain of detection and involves a concomitant exponential increase in cost. A re-emphasis on quantitative measurement rather than on LOH would permit much lower SNP densities to be used than at present.

The massive conversion to using SNPs for mapping studies is a current fashion fed by the DNA sequence information from the genome program and the marketing ability of the SNP chip manufacturers to package their goods in attractive ways with claims of up to hundreds of thousands of SNP typings per day per machine. So if it is new, fast and easy to use, it *must* save time and money, right? Wrong! Genome wide screens using high-density SNPs generate an enormous amount of information, but because of low information content per SNP combined with extensive linkage disequilibrium most of the information is noise. Take a case in point. Prior to 1980, human linkage maps hardly existed

in any extended form due to lack of polymorphic markers. The introduction of molecular markers in the form of RFLPs (Botstein et al., 1980) changed that overnight and led to the production of linkage maps at a 10-cM resolution for all chromosomes within six years. It took the discovery of microsatellites with much higher levels of heterozygosity than RFLPs and a further ten years of active research by several well funded groups to increase the map resolution to 2 cM or lower (Dib et al., 1996). The argument stating that using SNPs in large quantities will compensate for their lower information content is theoretically true in linkage studies, but still has to be rigorously demonstrated in practice; few total genome linkage scans with SNPs have been published to date. However, the cost of genotyping with such large volumes of SNP markers comes at an increased financial burden that few centres can afford. In the context of deletion mapping SNPs offer one major advantage over CGH approaches, namely that they provide information on whether it is the paternally or maternally derived chromosome that is deleted in phase known situations.

Do the technical advances in defining copy number changes mean we can now jettison the microscope? Despite my enthusiasm to do so 25 years ago, maybe at that time I was pretty jaundiced by having to run a large clinical cytogenetics service, the answer is clearly no. All techniques have their advantages and disadvantages and while molecular approaches have the virtue of a much higher resolution than the microscope, they are generally myopic and only good at doing a limited number of things. The microscope is the broad, blunt instrument needed to focus the molecular approaches in the right direction. In situations where it is known a priori what has to be looked for, such as specific aneuploidies in pre-implantation and prenatal screening, then a direct molecular approach without microscopic intervention is technically justified. This begs the question of why such direct molecular approaches have not become more widely used than at present. There are several sociological reasons to explain this reluctance, including conservatism in not changing an already long-established protocol of microscopic investigation, that introduction of a new method usually increases the cost because the old method is still being used as well so why bother with a new one, worries that a pure molecular analysis will fail to pick up occasional other types of aberrations such as translocations, and the ever-increasing fear of litigation for not having detected something even if the method used was not capable of doing so and this had been explained to the patient before hand. However, the evidence is now clear, also from several of the articles published in this special issue, that causative regional copy number changes are turning up in clinical phenotypes (craniosynastosis and obesity are two such examples; Krepischi-Santos et al., this issue), that only one year ago would never have been expected to be associated with such structural changes. Without doubt, the major block of widely introducing the genome-wide methods of array CGH and SNP analyses is not their technical difficulty but their high price. By comparison between my present country of residence, Brazil, and my previous, the Netherlands, I see this financial gulf very clearly and it is this factor alone which will limit their wide spread penetration in developing countries unless international price structures change radically and quickly. One particularly worrying aspect in Brazil, and many other developing countries for that matter, is that importation duties nearly double the price, making the situation even more untenable.

Final remarks

In this personalised historical review of tracing changes in the genome, I have argued that most of what we do now, in the so-called post genome era (what ever that means), was being done before and for some techniques up to 100 years ago. In all that time, microscopic investigation has been central and will remain so, and although the new molecular approaches have become extremely important, generally they will remain an adjunct to the microscope. One of the sad things about attending large genetic congresses these days for an old-timer like myself, is that the lecture halls are full of young people whose genetic horizons are limited to molecular analysis and have never experienced the joy of looking down a microscope at their own or other peoples chromosomes in glorious fluorescent colours. At least I can say: 'Been there – done that'.

References

Blakeslee A: Distinction between primary and secondary chromosomal mutants in Datura. Proc Natl Acad Sci USA 10:109–116 (1924).

Botstein D, White RL, Skolnick M, Davis RW: Construction of a genetic linkage map in man using restriction fragment length polymorphisms. Am J Hum Genet 32:314–331 (1980).

Boveri T: Zellenstudien VI. Die Entwicklung dispermer Seeigeleier. Ein Beitrag zur Befruchtungslehre und zur Theorie des Kernes. Jena Z Naturwiss 43:1–292 (1907).

Boveri T: Zur Frage der Entstehung maligner Tumoren. (Gustav Fischer, Jena 1914).

Britten RJ, Kohne DE: Repeated sequences in DNA. Hundreds of thousands of copies of DNA sequences have been incorporated into the genomes of higher organisms. Science 161:529–540 (1968).

Caspersson T: Nukleinsäureketten und Genvermehrung. Chromosoma 1:605 (1940).

Conrad DF, Andrews TD, Carter NP, Hurles ME, Pritchard JK: A high-resolution survey of deletion polymorphism in the human genome. Nat Genet 38:75–81 (2006).

Davies KE, Young BD, Elles RG, Hill ME, Williamson R: Cloning of a representative genomic library of the human X chromosome after sorting by flow cytometry. Nature 293:374–376 (1981).

Devilee P, van den Broek M, Kuipers-Dijkshoorn N, Kolluri R, Khan PM, et al: At least four different chromosomal regions are involved in loss of heterozygosity in human breast carcinoma. Genomics 5:554–560 (1989).

Dib C, Faure S, Fizames C, Samson D, Drouot N, et al: A comprehensive genetic map of the human genome based on 5,264 microsatellites. Nature 380:152–154 (1996).

Disteche CM, Kunkel LM, Lojewski A, Orkin SH, Eisenhard M, et al: Isolation of mouse X-chromosome specific DNA from an X-enriched lambda phage library derived from flow sorted chromosomes. Cytometry 2:282–286 (1982).

Gray JW, Lucas JN, Pinkel D, Awa A: Structural chromosome analysis by whole chromosome painting for assessment of radiation-induced genetic damage. J Radiat Res (Tokyo) 33 Suppl:80–86 (1992).

Hardie DC, Gregory TR, Hebert PD: From pixels to picograms: a beginners' guide to genome quantification by Feulgen image analysis densitometry. J Histochem Cytochem 50:735–749 (2002).

Harris P, Boyd E, Ferguson-Smith MA: Optimising human chromosome separation for the production of chromosome-specific DNA libraries by flow sorting. Hum Genet 70:59–65 (1985).

Henderson AS, Warburton D, Atwood KC: Location of ribosomal DNA in the human chromosome complement. Proc Natl Acad Sci USA 69:3394–3398 (1972).

Henking H: in McClung CE (1902) 'The accessory Chromosome: Sex Determinant?'. Biol Bull 3:43–84 (1890).

Herzenberg LA, Parks D, Sahaf B, Perez O, Roederer M, Herzenberg LA: The history and future of the fluorescence activated cell sorter and flow cytometry: a view from Stanford. Clin Chem 48:1819–1827 (2002).

Jones KW, Corneo G: Location of satellite and homogeneous DNA sequences on human chromosomes. Nat New Biol 233:268–271 (1971).

Kallioniemi A, Kallioniemi OP, Sudar D, Rutovitz D, Gray JW, et al: Comparative genomic hybridization for molecular cytogenetic analysis of solid tumors. Science 258:818–821 (1992).

Kan YW, Golbus MS, Dozy AM: Prenatal diagnosis of alpha-thalassemia. Clinical application of molecular hybridization. N Engl J Med 295:1165–1167 (1976).

Kirchhoff M, Rose H, Lundsteen C: High resolution comparative genomic hybridisation in clinical cytogenetics. J Med Genet 38:740–744 (2001).

Krepischi-Santos ACV, Vianna-Morgante AM, Jehee FS, Passos-Bueno MR, Knijnenburg J, et al: Whole-genome array-CGH screening in undiagnosed syndromic patients: old syndromes revisited and new alterations. Cytogenet Genome Res 115:254–261 (2006).

Langer-Safer PR, Levine M, Ward DC: Immunological method for mapping genes on Drosophila polytene chromosomes. Proc Natl Acad Sci USA 79:4381–4385 (1982).

Ledbetter SA, Nelson DL, Warren ST, Ledbetter DH: Rapid isolation of DNA probes within specific chromosome regions by interspersed repetitive sequence polymerase chain reaction. Genomics 6:475–481 (1990).

Lejeune J, Gautier M, Turpin R: [Study of somatic chromosomes from 9 mongoloid children]. C R Hebd Seances Acad Sci 248:1721–1722 (1959).

Lichter P, Cremer T, Borden J, Manuelidis L, Ward DC: Delineation of individual human chromosomes in metaphase and interphase cells by in situ suppression hybridization using recombinant DNA libraries. Hum Genet 80:224–234 (1988).

Little RD, Porta G, Carle GF, Schlessinger D, D'Urso M: Yeast artificial chromosomes with 200- to 800-kilobase inserts of human DNA containing HLA, V kappa, 5S, and Xq24-Xq28 sequences. Proc Natl Acad Sci USA 86:1598–1602 (1989).

Morgan T: An attempt to analyze the constitution of the chromosomes on the basis of sex-limited inheritance in Drosophila. J Exp Zool 11:365–412 (1911).

Mullis K, Faloona F, Scharf S, Saiki R, Horn G, Erlich H: Specific enzymatic amplification of DNA in vitro: the polymerase chain reaction. 1986. Biotechnology 24:17–27 (1992).

Muto M: Estimation of gene reiteration from hybridization kinetics in moderate deoxyribonucleic acid excess. Biochem J 165:19–25 (1977).

Nowell P, Hungerford D: A minute chromosome in human chronic granulocytic leukemia. Science 132:1497–1501 (1960).

Price PM, Conover JH, Hirschhorn K: Chromosomal localization of human haemoglobin structural genes. Nature 237:340–342 (1972).

Snijders AM, Nowak N, Segraves R, Blackwood S, Brown N, et al: Assembly of microarrays for genome-wide measurement of DNA copy number. Nat Genet 29:263–264 (2001).

Stevens N: Studies in spermatogenesis with especial reference to the 'Accessory Chromosome'. (Carnegie Institute of Washington, Washington 1905).

Telenius H, Pelmear AH, Tunnacliffe A, Carter NP, Behmel A, et al: Cytogenetic analysis by chromosome painting using DOP-PCR amplified flow-sorted chromosomes. Genes Chromosomes Cancer 4:257–263 (1992).

Tjio H, Levan A: The chromosome numbers of man. Hereditas 42:1–6 (1956).

Waardenburg P: Das menschliche Auge und seine Erbanlangen, p 44 (The Hague: Martinus Nijhoff, 1932).

Wang M, Chen XN, Shouse S, Manson J, Wu Q, et al: Construction and characterization of a human chromosome 2-specific BAC library. Genomics 24:527–534 (1994).

Wells D, Delhanty JD: Comprehensive chromosomal analysis of human preimplantation embryos using whole genome amplification and single cell comparative genomic hybridization. Mol Hum Reprod 6:1055–1062 (2000).

Wilson E: The chromosomes in relation to the determination of sex in insects. Science 22:500–502 (1905).

Yang F, Alkalaeva EZ, Perelman PL, Pardini AT, Harrison WR, et al: Reciprocal chromosome painting among human, aardvark, and elephant (superorder Afrotheria) reveals the likely eutherian ancestral karyotype. Proc Natl Acad Sci USA 100:1062–1066 (2003).

Cytogenet Genome Res 115:205–214 (2006)
DOI: 10.1159/000095916

Development of bioinformatics resources for display and analysis of copy number and other structural variants in the human genome

J. Zhang[a]   L. Feuk[a]   G.E. Duggan[a]   R. Khaja[a]   S.W. Scherer[a, b]

[a]The Centre for Applied Genomics and the Program in Genetics and Genomic Biology, The Hospital for Sick Children and [b]Department of Molecular and Medical Genetics, University of Toronto, Toronto, Ontario (Canada)

Manuscript received 23 March 2006; accepted in revised form for publication by A. Geurts van Kessel, 15 May 2006.

Abstract. The discovery of an abundance of copy number variants (CNVs; gains and losses of DNA sequences >1 kb) and other structural variants in the human genome is influencing the way research and diagnostic analyses are being designed and interpreted. As such, comprehensive databases with the most relevant information will be critical to fully understand the results and have impact in a diverse range of disciplines ranging from molecular biology to clinical genetics. Here, we describe the development of bioinformatics resources to facilitate these studies. The Database of Genomic Variants (http://projects.tcag.ca/variation/) is a comprehensive catalogue of structural variation in the human genome. The database currently contains 1,267 regions reported to contain copy number variation or inversions in apparently healthy human cases. We describe the current contents of the database and how it can serve as a resource for interpretation of array comparative genomic hybridization (array CGH) and other DNA copy imbalance data. We also present the structure of the database, which was built using a new data modeling methodology termed Cross-Referenced Tables (XRT). This is a generic and easy-to-use platform, which is strong in handling textual data and complex relationships. Web-based presentation tools have been built allowing publication of XRT data to the web immediately along with rapid sharing of files with other databases and genome browsers. We also describe a novel tool named eFISH (electronic fluorescence in situ hybridization) (http://projects.tcag.ca/efish/), a BLAST-based program that was developed to facilitate the choice of appropriate clones for FISH and CGH experiments, as well as interpretation of results in which genomic DNA probes are used in hybridization-based experiments.

Copyright © 2006 S. Karger AG, Basel

During the last few years numerous studies have identified a large number of copy-number variants (CNVs) and other structural variants in the human genome (Iafrate et al., 2004; Sebat et al., 2004; Sharp et al., 2005; Tuzun et al., 2005; Conrad et al., 2006; Hinds et al., 2006; McCarroll et al., 2006). A CNV is a term collectively used to describe gains and losses of DNA sequences >1 kb in length (reviewed in Feuk et al., 2006a) and the relative high frequency of CNVs in the human genome has generated considerable excitement in the field (Carter, 2004; Check, 2005; Lee, 2005; Eichler, 2006). Since these changes can be hundreds of kilobases in size they can have a direct effect on transcription and transcriptional regulation, which in turn may be a cause for disease susceptibility and phenotypic variation. There are currently more than 1,000 CNVs described in literature, but this represents only a small fraction of all CNVs expected to exist in the human population.

The main approach used to identify CNVs to date has been array-based comparative genomic hybridization (CGH) (Kallioniemi et al., 1992; Pinkel et al., 1998). The

Supported by Genome Canada, the McLaughlin Centre for Molecular Medicine, and the Hospital for Sick Children Foundation. L.F. is supported by the Swedish Medical Research Council. S.W.S. is an investigator of the Canadian Institutes of Health Research and an International Scholar of the Howard Hughes Medical Institute.

Request reprints from Stephen W. Scherer
   The Centre for Applied Genomics
   Program in Genetics and Genomic Biology
   The Hospital for Sick Children
   MaRS Centre – East Tower, 101 College Street, Room 14-701
   Toronto, Ontario, M5G 1L7 (Canada)
   telephone: +1-416-813-7613; fax: +1-416-813-8319
   e-mail: steve@genet.sickkids.on.ca

J.Z. and L.F. contributed equally to this work.

development of the array-CGH technology and other oligo-nucleotide-based platforms (Feuk et al., 2006a) has important implications for both research and clinical diagnostics laboratories. Specific arrays targeting the micro-deletion and duplication syndrome regions are now commercially available for diagnostic purposes, alongside whole-genome coverage arrays which give a global view of genome imbalances. The introduction of these high-throughput technologies into diagnostic and clinical settings, and possibly all genetic research studies (Feuk et al., 2006b), allows scanning for rearrangements at an unprecedented resolution, but at the same time creates challenges in terms of data handling, interpretation, and validation.

For each sample screened using a whole-genome coverage array-based platform, anywhere between 5 and 300 variants might be found (depending on which of the currently available platforms was used and the stringency of cutoffs applied). This data must then be stored in an appropriate way, and regions should be validated in some way and then prioritized for further analysis. In order to deal with some of these issues we have developed new bioinformatics resources. The first is the public database called 'The Database of Genomic Variants', with the aim of cataloguing all CNVs described in the literature in a format accessible to medical geneticists and molecular biologists alike. The database was built using a new platform for data handling and sharing called BioXRT, which in turn is based on the Cross-Referenced Tables (XRT) data model. For maximum translational impact, it is necessary to establish online databases to facilitate information sharing within a research community. For example, for collections of locus-specific disease mutations alone, there were 262 databases as of 2002 (Claustres et al., 2002); and the 2005 updated Nucleic Acids Research online Molecular Biology Database Collection included 719 databases, an increase of 171 over the previous year, and this listing was far from exhaustive (Galperin, 2005). Online databases provide many advantages, such as wide-accessibility, advanced querying, fast retrieval and persistent referencing. Despite varied content and architectures, most of these databases are functionally similar; instead of in-house development of such databases, if a generic and easy-to-use platform could be used a significant amount of duplicate effort would be avoided. The BioXRT platform was developed with the aim to provide a lightweight generic solution for housing and publishing biological data. Besides the prototypic Database of Genomic Variants described here, BioXRT has now been adapted to many other online databases that are widely utilized by the genetics community.

Lastly, we present a tool named eFISH (electronic fluorescent in situ hybridization), which is a BLAST-based approach to predict the results of FISH and other hybridization-based assays. The eFISH program was created to facilitate the selection of genomic probes and analysis of results for FISH experiments, but can be used in the interpretation of results from any DNA hybridization-based approaches.

Results and discussion

The Database of Genomic Variants

Following the initial reports on global distribution of CNVs in the human genome (Iafrate et al., 2004; Sebat et al., 2004), it was apparent that the ~300 regions described represented only a small fraction of all the CNVs in the human genome. Clearly, there was demand for a database where information on structural variants in general, and CNVs in particular, could be stored and accessed by the research community. Not only would this simplify the comparison of new datasets to what has already been published, but would also allow the compilation of up to date summary statistics and analysis of this type of variation. There are currently two existing databases which focus on collecting data on submicroscopic structural variation; The Database of Genomic Variants (http://projects.tcag.ca/variation/) (Iafrate et al., 2004) described for the first time in detail here, and the Human Structural Variation Database (http://humanparalogy.gs.washington.edu/structuralvariation/) (Sharp et al., 2005).

The Database of Genomic Variants currently has the aim of cataloguing all submicroscopic structural variants >1 kb in size identified in control individuals that have been documented in peer-reviewed literature. The majority of these are CNVs, but there are also inversion breakpoint regions. The main goal of the database is to provide a user-friendly resource for the scientific and medical genetics community. The DECIPHER (DatabasE of Chromosomal Imbalances and Phenotype in Human using Ensembl Resources; see http://www.sanger.ac.uk/PostGenomics/decipher/) initiative, for example, uses this as the source of its genomic variant data track.

The database can be searched by a genomic feature, such as gene name, clone name or DNA sequence (Fig. 1). Alternatively, the contents of the database can be browsed in either table format or in a genome browser displaying relevant information (e.g. gene, cytogenetic location, segmental duplication, genomic clone, etc). Each entry in the table is linked to a page that contains more detailed information about the locus in question (Fig. 2). One recent update to the database is that for any variant identified in the HapMap sample set, we also include information on which samples that were found to carry a specific variant. This serves two purposes; first, knowing that a specific sample carries a specific variant makes it useful as a control sample when testing new methods or trying to find the sensitivity and accuracy of a certain method, and second, it facilitates further analysis of structural variants in relation to other data available for the HapMap samples, including SNP data and gene expression data.

Data currently in The Database of Genomic Variants

There are currently 1,267 regions of structural variation in the database. Of these, 1,207 have been reported as CNVs, 37 as inversion breakpoints and the remaining 23 as regions containing both CNVs and inversion breakpoints. In total, the 1,267 variants cover 143 Mb of genomic sequence. The

Database of Genomic Variants

A curated catalogue of large-scale variation in the human genome

About This Project | Genome Browser | Download | Links | Email us

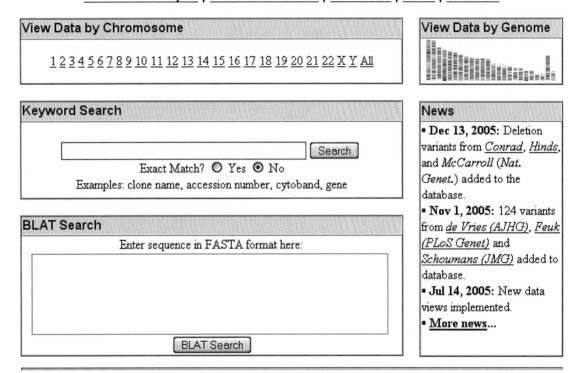

View Data by Chromosome

1 2 3 4 5 6 7 8 9 10 11 12 13 14 15 16 17 18 19 20 21 22 X Y All

View Data by Genome

Keyword Search

[   ] [Search]

Exact Match? ○ Yes ● No

Examples: clone name, accession number, cytoband, gene

News

- **Dec 13, 2005:** Deletion variants from *Conrad*, *Hinds*, and *McCarroll* (*Nat. Genet.*) added to the database.
- **Nov 1, 2005:** 124 variants from *de Vries (AJHG)*, *Feuk (PLoS Genet)* and *Schoumans (JMG)* added to database.
- **Jul 14, 2005:** New data views implemented.
- **More news...**

BLAT Search

Enter sequence in FASTA format here:

[   ]

[BLAT Search]

Contact us: Department of Genetics and Genomic Biology, MaRS Centre - East Tower, 101 College Street, Toronto, Ontario, M5G 1L7, Canada

Fig. 1. The Database of Genomic Variants. The home page of the Database of Genomic Variants is shown. The data can be viewed in table format by clicking on a chromosome of interest. Alternatively, the database can be searched using a keyword, which could be a gene name, clone name, or cytogenetic band. If the region entered overlaps with a genomic variant, it can be viewed in a genome browser or in the context of CNVs overlapping the region. The database can also be queried using DNA sequence. The search is based on BLAT to identify matching regions. In the top right corner a genome-wide overview of structural variants in the genome can be viewed. The 'download' link can be used for downloading the entire contents of the database for incorporation into other browsers.

average size of entries is 118 kb. This is likely not a reflection of the true size distribution of CNVs, as it is currently influenced by the bias in how they were assessed. The majority of the variants in the database have been identified by either CGH arrays or by using SNP data to detect deletions by identifying regions showing Mendelian inconsistencies, null genotypes or Hardy-Weinberg disequilibrium. The highest resolution of the array-CGH studies published to date is ~35 kb, but most arrays do not reach that level of resolution. Looking specifically at regions in the database identified by array-CGH, the average size of regions is 289 kb. The use of SNP data is less biased in terms of the size of regions that can be detected, but instead is biased in that

only deletions can be detected (and not duplications). At present, the database contains data from 36 research papers. It is important to point out that the database only reports on the regions described in each study, regardless of whether they have been validated by independent approaches. All methods currently used for identification of structural variation will generate some false-positive regions, and since these are included in the published datasets some regions represented in the database are not true structural variants. As more data is published, it will become more clear which of the variants are common polymorphisms and which regions are rare mutations or false positives. Of all 1,267 regions, 280 have been reported by two or more separate stud-

Locus: Locus0157

Genome context (see the graphic below):

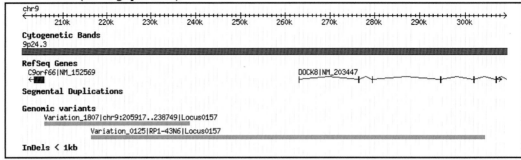

Variation: Variation 0125

    Landmark: RP1-43N6 (Genome Browsers: TCAG Segmental Duplication , UCSC , Ensembl)

    Variation Type: CopyNumber

    Overlap with TCAG Segmental Duplication: No

    Gap within 100k: No

    Known Genes: DOCK8

    Method: Array CGH

    Reference: Iafrate et al. (2004)

    Pub Med ID: 15286789

    Frequency Information:

        Subject Cohort: Control

        Sample Size: 55 in total (39 unrelated healthy individuals and 16 individuals with previously characterized chromosomal imbalances)

        Normal Gain: 1

        Normal Loss: 1

        Total Gain/Loss: 2

Variation: Variation 1807

    Landmark: chr9:205,917..238,749 (Genome Browsers: TCAG Segmental Duplication , UCSC , Ensembl)

    Variation Type: CopyNumber

    Overlap with TCAG Segmental Duplication: No

    Gap within 100k: No

    Method: Null genotypes

    Individual: NA18576

    Reference: McCarroll et al. (2005)

    Frequency Information:

        Subject Cohort: Control

        Sample Size: 269 HapMap individuals

Fig. 2. Detailed information about a specific variant. An example of a page displaying detailed information for a locus harboring a CNV is shown. A simple graphical overview is provided for genomic context information. This includes chromosomal position, genes and segmental duplications. If the same region has been identified in several studies, each finding is assigned a unique variation ID. For each entry, there is a link to Pubmed to see the abstract of the article from which the information is extracted. There is also detailed information about study cohort, sample size and methodology.

ies. The region reported in most papers is the *defensin* gene cluster on chromosome 8, which has been identified as polymorphic in nine different studies.

The most obvious link between copy number changes and their effect on gene expression is when the CNV directly overlaps a gene. The 1,267 CNVs currently in the database overlap with a total of 1,298 genes, and of these 846 are contained entirely within the boundaries of the regions reported to contain CNVs. It is important to point out that in cases where genomic clones on array-CGH experiments are reported to show copy number variation, it is impossible to determine the exact boundaries of the variant without

performing further experiments. A more detailed analysis of the genes present in CNV regions shows that certain gene ontology categories are found at higher frequencies than expected by chance. The biological processes most significantly overrepresented in CNV regions are shown in Table 1. Genes important for interaction with the environment and defense against pathogens seem to be very variable in copy number between individuals. These genes may be amenable to copy number variation as a means to quickly adapt to external threat and changing surroundings. There are several examples where gene copy number affects response to exposure to common drugs, e.g. increased copy

Table 1. GO terms describing biological processes for genes within CNVs

GO ID	GO term	Observed	All gene	Expected	Ratio
GO:0007565	pregnancy	13	43	1.1	11.881
GO:0006805	xenobiotic metabolism	8	28	0.7	11.228
GO:0009613	response to pest, pathogen or parasite	5	25	0.6	7.859
GO:0006952	defense response	12	77	2.0	6.124
GO:0007600	sensory perception	38	486	12.4	3.073
GO:0006968	cellular defense response	5	67	1.7	2.933
GO:0008152	metabolism	15	371	9.4	1.589
GO:0005975	carbohydrate metabolism	9	224	5.7	1.579
GO:0006955	immune response	12	308	7.8	1.531

GO terms for biological processes that are significantly overrepresented for genes in CNV regions are shown. Only categories with more than five genes observed and GO level 2–5 are included.

number pf CYP2D6 leads to faster metabolizing of debrisoquine (Ingelman-Sundberg, 2002). A more recent example shows how CNVs can play important roles in defense against pathogens, as exemplified by carriers of extra copies of *CCL3L1* having increased resistance against HIV (Gonzalez et al., 2005).

Scanning for copy number changes will become a routine part of many monogenic disease studies, as well as part of the study design to identify complex disease genes (Feuk et al., 2006b). The number of CNVs identified will therefore increase on a regular basis. There are also on-going efforts to identify all large CNVs in the HapMap samples, using multiple array-based platforms (Freeman et al., 2006). Once a good dataset exists for control samples, it will facilitate interpretation of data from studies in patient cohorts. The Database of Genomic Variants will continue to be updated as new studies are published, and will aim to provide the best possible resource for researchers working in the field of structural variation. All data will also continue to be made available in standardized files for incorporation into other genome databases.

The Cross-Referenced Tables (XRT) data model
The Database of Genomic Variants is based on an open source database platform called BioXRT (http://projects.tcag.ca/bioxrt). It was designed to be a generally applicable platform for databases in the biomedical research field. Although the content and the architecture among most databases in biomedicine are quite different, many of them do share a common cycle of tasks including: (i) collecting and curating data from different sources such as public databases, scientific literature and internal laboratory results; (ii) integrating this information using an appropriate model; (iii) loading data into a relational database, and (iv) providing a web-based interface for users to query and browse the data in a read-only fashion. When updating with new data, they follow a repetitive cycling pattern. These common tasks make it practically feasible to build and maintain a biology database using a generic platform. By avoiding in-house development, a generic approach can prevent unnecessary duplication of effort.

A data model is a description of the data for a particular subject area, how they are defined and organized, and how they relate to one another. It includes the data items and their relationship. Taking the large diversity and fast emerging pace of biological data (in this case structural variation data) into account, a broadly applicable and extensible data model is essential for a generic approach to build biological databases. With this in mind, we developed a data modeling system termed Cross-Referenced Tables (XRT). For simplicity, the XRT model uses tab-delimited flat files (i.e. text tables) as a basic modeling unit to keep data items. A text table structured by a field/value convention is the most natural format and is commonly used in many public biological data sources. It is capable of storing arbitrary data items by simply adding new fields, and is generally applicable to any textual information. Additionally, no special tool is needed to prepare or parse a text table. However, it also has some caveats, such as lack of referencing and constraints, and difficulty in modeling complex data with a single table. To overcome these limitations, we applied several rules to the text tables, basically, injecting mechanisms to handle relationships among data items.

XRT is a simple file schema, which encapsulates data in an object hierarchy with arbitrary attributes and relationships. It organizes data into different classes according to its biological meaning (e.g. gene, Gene Ontology term and OMIM entry). Each class has as many attributes as necessary to describe the properties of its elements, and its attributes can be settled in one or more XRT tables. An XRT table is a tab-delimited flat file. The first line specifies the attribute names, while the following lines contain the actual attribute values for elements with each element having a unique identifier (ID, primary key in database terminology). Special attributes called P_ID for parent ID and C_ID for child ID keep track of references between data elements (in database terms, these relationships are known as foreign keys). The relationship can be one to one, one to many, many to one, or many to many. The XRT class name is defined as the string before the first dot (.) of the XRT table file name, for example, the class name of XRT table Transcript.main.xrt is Transcript. Online documentation on de-

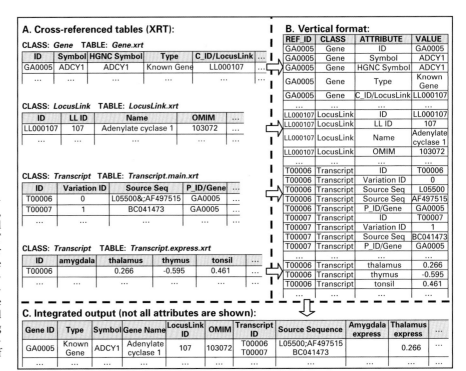

A. Cross-referenced tables (XRT):

CLASS: *Gene*   TABLE: *Gene.xrt*

ID	Symbol	HGNC Symbol	Type	C_ID/LocusLink	...
GA0005	ADCY1	ADCY1	Known Gene	LL000107	...
...	...	...	...	...	...

CLASS: *LocusLink*   TABLE: *LocusLink.xrt*

ID	LL ID	Name	OMIM	...
LL000107	107	Adenylate cyclase 1	103072	...
...	...	...	...	...

CLASS: *Transcript*   TABLE: *Transcript.main.xrt*

ID	Variation ID	Source Seq	P_ID/Gene	...
T00006	0	L05500&;AF497515	GA0005	...
T00007	1	BC041473	GA0005	...
...	...	...	...	...

CLASS: *Transcript*   TABLE: *Transcript.express.xrt*

ID	amygdala	thalamus	thymus	tonsil	...
T00006		0.266	-0.595	0.461	...

B. Vertical format:

REF_ID	CLASS	ATTRIBUTE	VALUE
GA0005	Gene	ID	GA0005
GA0005	Gene	Symbol	ADCY1
GA0005	Gene	HGNC Symbol	ADCY1
GA0005	Gene	Type	Known Gene
GA0005	Gene	C_ID/LocusLink	LL000107
...	...	...	...
LL000107	LocusLink	ID	LL000107
LL000107	LocusLink	LL ID	107
LL000107	LocusLink	Name	Adenylate cyclase 1
LL000107	LocusLink	OMIM	103072
...	...	...	...
T00006	Transcript	ID	T00006
T00006	Transcript	Variation ID	0
T00006	Transcript	Source Seq	L05500
T00006	Transcript	Source Seq	AF497515
T00006	Transcript	P_ID/Gene	GA0005
T00007	Transcript	ID	T00007
T00007	Transcript	Variation ID	1
T00007	Transcript	Source Seq	BC041473
T00007	Transcript	P_ID/Gene	GA0005
...	...	...	...
T00006	Transcript	thalamus	0.266
T00006	Transcript	thymus	-0.595
T00006	Transcript	tonsil	0.461
...	...	...	...

C. Integrated output (not all attributes are shown):

Gene ID	Type	Symbol	Gene Name	LocusLink ID	OMIM	Transcript ID	Source Sequence	Amygdala express	Thalamus express	...
GA0005	Known Gene	ADCY1	Adenylate cyclase 1	107	103072	T00006 T00007	L05500;AF497515 BC041473		0.266	...
...	...	...	...	...	...	...	...	...	...	...

Fig. 3. XRT example and its format transformation. (**A**) Four cross-referenced tables, XRTs; (**B**) the vertical format of the original XRTs; (**C**) integrated output of the source XRT tables. The XRT model is very flexible for changes and adding new data types. New table (with new attributes) can be added to an existing class later on without touching any existing table(s), and different tables (even for the same class) can be generated and maintained separately as long as appropriate referencing is kept. This feature allows database expansion of new data and facilitates integration of data from scattered sources.

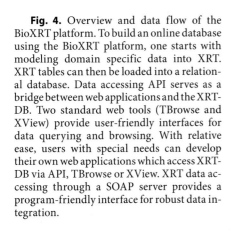
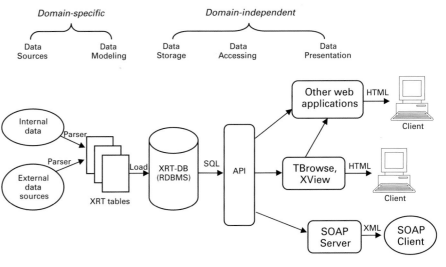

Fig. 4. Overview and data flow of the BioXRT platform. To build an online database using the BioXRT platform, one starts with modeling domain specific data into XRT. XRT tables can then be loaded into a relational database. Data accessing API serves as a bridge between web applications and the XRT-DB. Two standard web tools (TBrowse and XView) provide user-friendly interfaces for data querying and browsing. With relative ease, users with special needs can develop their own web applications which access XRT-DB via API, TBrowse or XView. XRT data accessing through a SOAP server provides a program-friendly interface for robust data integration.

tailed XRT specification is available at http://projects.tcag.ca/bioxrt/xrt_spec.html. An example XRT model of the gene-centric data is shown in Fig. 3A, where data is organized into three classes, and is physically contained in four XRT tables. Figure 3 also illustrates how XRT tables can be transformed into a unified vertical format (Fig. 3B) for easier data storage and manipulation, and data in this vertical format can later be converted back to a human readable table (Fig. 3C), which integrates the original XRT tables. The XRT model used in the Database of Genomic Variants is available at http://projects.tcag.ca/variation/download.html.

Implementation of the BioXRT platform. While having data modeled in XRT, we developed the BioXRT platform to provide XRT data storage and web presentation. An overview of the BioXRT platform is shown in Fig. 4. It is implemented in Perl, and is built exclusively upon open source components such as MySQL and BioPerl (http://www.bioperl.org). These choices reflect the easiest configuration to install, however, the schema and configuration are applicable to any permutation of platform factors and support will be provided to labs choosing to implement it in a different setup. To build a particular online database using

BioXRT, first of all, we needed to model the data in XRT, i.e. define classes and their relationships, such as the example model shown in Fig. 3. Then, data from either internal results or external sources is converted into XRT tables. A Perl script named 'bulk_load_xrt.pl' can later transform all XRT tables to the vertical format, and load them into the database and build the requisite indices. For the default implementation, the MySQL database management system was used to host XRT data because of its open source status, and its superior performance in read-mostly environments. Any SQL92 compliant database engine could be used with relative ease.

In order to provide an efficient, user-friendly and widely accessible interface to an XRT database, we have implemented a web application called TBrowse. The browser accesses the XRT database via a standard connection such as the Perl DBI, with an XRT-specific API which translates the data requests into appropriate SQL queries, and converts results into HTML tables. Several options can be customized to the output table (e.g. table title, column headers, and hyperlinks). For additional details about the table configuration, an online tutorial is provided at http://projects.tcag.ca/bioxrt/tutorial. In addition to browsing pre-defined tables, TBrowse also functions as a data retrieval tool, users can perform keyword searches, select columns to show and filter records on certain column(s) to obtain their data of interest. Output of TBrowse can be exported and downloaded in several formats: tab-delimited flat file, XML and Microsoft Excel file. Besides the interactive web interface, URL-based access to the XRT database is also supported in TBrowse. Due to the simplicity of a two-dimensional table, TBrowse is not entirely ideal in displaying data of complex structure. Another web application called XView was implemented, which can recursively handle (theoretically) unlimited levels of XRT relationship in a hierarchical structure. XView presents data in an easy-to-understand hierarchical tree reflecting the logical relationship of XRT data items (an example of XView output is shown in Fig. 2). Similar to TBrowse, the tree structure is defined in a user-managed configuration file.

BioXRT sample and proof of concept databases. Besides The Database of Genomic Variants mentioned above, BioXRT has also been successfully applied in several of our online projects in a wide range including: the Human Chromosome 7 Annotation Project (Scherer et al., 2003) (http://www.chr7.org), the Genome Segmental Duplication Project (Cheung et al., 2003) (http://projects.tcag.ca/humandup), the Autism Chromosome Rearrangement Database (Xu et al., 2004) (http://projects.tcag.ca/autism/), the Genomic Clone Database (http://projects.tcag.ca/gcd/, Zhang et al., unpublished), and the Lafora Progressive Myoclonus Epilepsy Mutation Database (Ianzano et al., 2005) (http://projects.tcag.ca/lafora/). Within the chromosome 7 database, BioXRT is the primary harness for gene-centric data that are derived from diverse sources. There are currently 21 XRT tables representing 18 classes. Each table can be maintained individually, even by different curators. When new data needs to be integrated, it is simply converted into XRT

format while referencing existing data correctly, and the configuration file is updated. After being uploaded, the new data gets integrated automatically, with no need for database structure changes or program modifications.

With the BioXRT platform available, setting up an online biological database becomes significantly easier, with solutions for database schema design programs for data query and presentation already built in. The only thing users need to do is to model their data in XRT, which is like a simplified version of the relational database schema design, since only the logical design phase is involved, and no normalization or other physical design concerns are required.

Biological data is rarely static due to the fast pace of new data emergence, change is unavoidable no matter which modeling tool has been used. This means that considerable effort is needed for data re-modeling. The advantages of XRT's simplicity stand out while handling data model changes, which actually was the initial motivation of the BioXRT project. Modification (adding, changing and deleting) of the XRT classes and/or their attributes can be easily done through the updating of XRT tables. More importantly, due to the content-independency of the BioXRT platform, no effort is needed for database or program re-engineering to accommodate the updated XRT model. Thus, the XRT model is highly flexible and broadly applicable, and the reusability of the BioXRT platform is maximized.

We believe the light-weight approach presented here is an attractive solution for biological data sharing. This open source initiative was developed with two missions; first, to allow biologists the ability to quickly bring their research data online, where data is widely accessible throughout the world, and secondly, to provide outside developers the opportunity to contribute their own ideas and requirements to enhance BioXRT's ability to accomplish biological goals.

eFISH

With the exception for regions commonly interrogated by FISH in diagnostic labs and in targeted research studies, the majority of genomic clones including those used in the sequencing and assembly of the human genome reference sequence, have not been mapped in a standardized way. Choosing suitable clones for FISH experiments can therefore be problematic, as many clones give rise to multiple hybridization signals, making the FISH results difficult or impossible to interpret. One of the problems with the large amounts of data being generated using array-CGH is validation of the results. FISH is one common approach for validation of clone based array results, and ideally the same clone as the one giving rise to a signal on the array should be used. The fact that many CNVs overlap regions of segmental duplications (low copy repeats) (Fredman et al., 2004; Iafrate et al., 2004; Sharp et al., 2005) further complicates analysis of FISH results for these regions.

In order to simplify the choice of clones for FISH experiments and facilitate the interpretation of results where multiple hybridization signals appear, we have developed an in silico FISH simulation program called eFISH. The input sequence can be any clone or region that can be anchored to

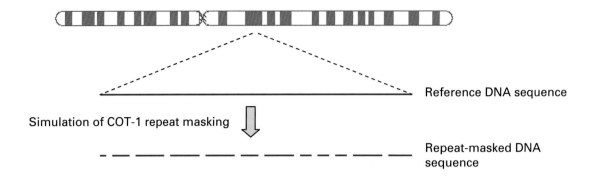

Reference DNA sequence

Simulation of COT-1 repeat masking

Repeat-masked DNA
sequence

Scoring: scan the chromosome window by
window to get probe coverage (window size:
100 kb, step: 50 kb)

BLAST

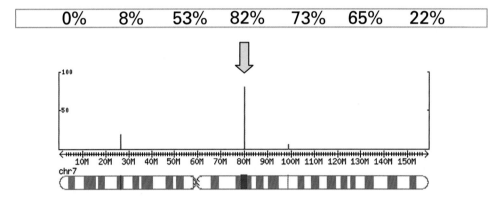

0%   8%   53%   82%   73%   65%   22%

chr7

Regions that have a score that is higher than a certain threshold (2%) will each show a peak

Fig. 5. Overview of the eFISH analysis process. Input sequences are first repeat-masked and then BLASTed against the genome in 100-kb sliding windows. When significant alignment is found (>2 kb of sequence within a window) it will be indicated by a peak in the result output. The height of the peak is relative to the amount of matched sequence within the 100-kb window.

specific coordinates in the human genome reference assembly, e.g. a BAC clone, a fosmid or chromosomal coordinates. This sequence is first repeat masked in an effort to mimic the COT-1 blocking of repeats commonly used in FISH experiments. The repeat-masked sequence is next compared to the reference human genome sequence using Mega-BLAST (Zhang et al., 2000). A sliding-window approach is used, and the input sequence is compared to a 100-kb window from the genome at a time, sliding 50 kb per window (Fig. 5). If the BLAST results within a window show a total unique alignment length of 2% or higher (i.e. at least 2 kb in the 100-kb window), it will be shown in the output. The result would always be expected to give the best match for the region the sequence was taken from. Any additional peaks in the output represent regions of high identity in other parts of the genome, which may give rise to multiple hybridization signals in FISH experiments (Fig. 6).

In order to test how well the eFISH simulations reflect actual results, a number of test assays were designed which were run using both FISH and eFISH. In all cases where one

or two regions were indicated by eFISH, those regions were also detected in the FISH experiment. When multiple regions were indicated by eFISH, regions that gave a very low score were sometimes not seen in the actual FISH result. However, this seems to be due to variability between experiments and may to some extent depend on the composition of the underlying sequence. In certain experiments, the hybridization intensities are stronger overall, and then also the signals just above the threshold in the eFISH tool gave rise to weak signals in the FISH experiment. eFISH is implemented as a widely accessible web tool. DNA sequence BLASTing has been pre-computed, which substantially speeds up the performance. Usually it takes only one or two seconds to give the prediction for one probe. eFISH is freely accessible at http://projects.tcag.ca/efish.

In our experience, eFISH is an accurate predictor of the outcome of FISH experiments. We routinely check all potential probes in eFISH before they are ordered, and it is a helpful part of the process for choosing the optimal probe for a specific region. Applying this as a step in the experi-

eFISH Result

Back to main page

Genome:	Human Genome - May 2004 Assembly (hg17)
Mapped Probes:	RP11-365N20 (chr15:36,800,725..36,968,084|BAC_End) RP11-24O14 (chr5:69,802,531..69,966,791|BAC_End)
Show Chromosomes:	☑chr5 ☑chr6 ☑chr15 ☑chr20 ☑chr22 [Check All] [Uncheck All]
Show Probes:	☑ RP11-365N20 [c15] ☑ RP11-24O14 [c5,c6,c20,c22]
Max Score (Y axis):	⦿ 100 ○ 50 ○ 10
Image Width:	⦿ 1000 ○ 2000 ○ 4000
	[Refresh]

eFISH image

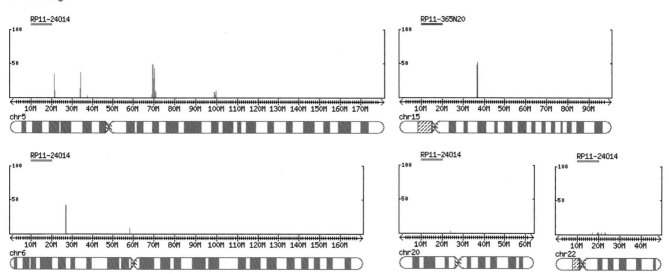

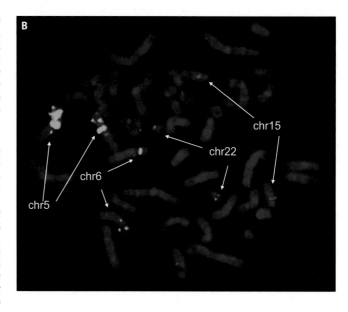

Fig. 6. Comparing eFISH to FISH. Shown in **A** is an example of the results reported from the eFISH program. In this case two probes, RP11-365N20 (clone end accession numbers are AQ543813 and AQ543816) and RP11-24O14 (clone end accession numbers are B89373 and B89383), were entered as search terms. In these two instances the entire clone sequence is not known so their end-sequences are used to identify the intervening sequence from the human genome reference assembly, and this is used for the BLAST analysis. All chromosomes where any of the two probes give a significant hit are shown. RP11-365N20, shown in red, gives a single signal on chromosome 15. RP11-24O14, shown in green, generates hits on four different chromosomes, with several signals on chromosome 5. In **B**, the results from an actual FISH experiment using the same two clones are shown. As expected, RP11-365N20 yields a single signal on chromosome 15, while RP11-24O14 shows signals on chromosomes 5, 6 and 22. All these hits, including the multiple signals detected on chromosomes 5 and 6, were predicted using the eFISH program. eFISH also predicted very weak hybridization to chromosome 20, but these cannot be seen in this experiment. The signal intensity often varies between experiments, and signals predicted by eFISH to be very low may not be detected in all experiments. Genomic clones for FISH hybridization experiments are available from several sources including BACPAC Resource Center (http://bacpac.chori.org/) and The Centre for Applied Genomics (www.tcag.ca), to name a few.

mental design also increases the success rate for our experiments and therefore decreases cost for failed or un-interpretable assays. In difficult regions containing segmental duplications, the results of eFISH are also helpful for interpretation of the data.

Summary

The complexity of genomic variation data requires the development of special databases, bioinformatics tools, and algorithms compatible to a diverse range of users, and to other databases. The resources described here provide a relevant and reliable information source for the study of structural variants in the human genome. The Database of Genomic Variants will continue to be improved including the curation and updating of new material, as it becomes available. The overall project will be considered a success when an equal number of molecular biologists, medical geneticists, physicians, and diagnostic laboratories utilize the information for a better understanding of the role of genomic variation in development and disease.

Acknowledgements

The authors would like to thank Weimin Zhu and Charles Lee of the European Bioinformatics Institute, and Jeffrey MacDonald, Cheng Qian, Terence Tang, Ying Qi, and the bioinformatics support staff of The Centre for Applied Genomics (www.tcag.ca). We also acknowledge Dr. Charles Lee of Harvard University and Brigham and Women's Hospital, Drs. Nigel Carter and Matthew Hurles (Wellcome Trust Sanger Institute), Dr. Keith Jones (Affymetrix), and Dr. Hiroyuki Aburatani (University of Tokyo) for ongoing contributions to the Copy Number and Structural Variation Project (http://www.sanger.ac.uk/humgen/cnv/).

References

Carter NP: As normal as normal can be? Nat Genet 36:931–932 (2004).

Check E: Human genome: patchwork people. Nature 437:1084–1086 (2005).

Cheung J, Estivill X, Khaja R, MacDonald JR, Lau K, et al: Genome-wide detection of segmental duplications and potential assembly errors in the human genome sequence. Genome Biol 4: R25 (2003).

Claustres M, Horaitis O, Vanevski M, Cotton RG: Time for a unified system of mutation description and reporting: a review of locus-specific mutation databases. Genome Res 12:680–688 (2002).

Conrad DF, Andrews TD, Carter NP, Hurles ME, Pritchard JK: A high-resolution survey of deletion polymorphism in the human genome. Nat Genet 38:75–81 (2006).

Eichler EE: Widening the spectrum of human genetic variation. Nat Genet 38:9–11 (2006).

Feuk L, Carson AR, Scherer SW: Structural variation in the human genome. Nat Rev Genet 7: 85–97 (2006a).

Feuk L, Marshall CR, Wintle RF, Scherer SW: Structural variants: changing the landscape of chromosomes and design of disease studies. Hum Mol Genet 15 Spec No 1:R57–66 (2006b).

Fredman D, White SJ, Potter S, Eichler EE, Dunnen JT, Brookes AJ: Complex SNP-related sequence variation in segmental genome duplications. Nat Genet 36:861–866 (2004).

Freeman JL, Perry GH, Feuk L, Redon R, McCarroll SA, et al: Copy number variation: new insights in genome diversity. Genome Res 16:949–961 (2006).

Galperin MY: The Molecular Biology Database Collection: 2005 update. Nucleic Acids Res 33: D5–24 (2005).

Gonzalez E, Kulkarni H, Bolivar H, Mangano A, Sanchez R, et al: The influence of CCL3L1 gene-containing segmental duplications on HIV-1/AIDS susceptibility. Science 307:1434–1440 (2005).

Hinds DA, Kloek AP, Jen M, Chen X, Frazer KA: Common deletions and SNPs are in linkage disequilibrium in the human genome. Nat Genet 38:82–85 (2006).

Iafrate AJ, Feuk L, Rivera MN, Listewnik ML, Donahoe PK, et al: Detection of large-scale variation in the human genome. Nat Genet 36:949–951 (2004).

Ianzano L, Zhang J, Chan EM, Zhao XC, Lohi H, et al: Lafora progressive Myoclonus Epilepsy mutation database-EPM2A and NHLRC1 (EMP2B) genes. Hum Mutat 26:397 (2005).

Ingelman-Sundberg M: Polymorphism of cytochrome P450 and xenobiotic toxicity. Toxicology 181–182:447–452 (2002).

Kallioniemi A, Kallioniemi OP, Sudar D, Rutovitz D, Gray JW, et al: Comparative genomic hybridization for molecular cytogenetic analysis of solid tumors. Science 258:818–821 (1992).

Lee C: Vive la difference! Nat Genet 37:660–661 (2005).

McCarroll SA, Hadnott TN, Perry GH, Sabeti PC, Zody MC, et al: Common deletion polymorphisms in the human genome. Nat Genet 38: 86–92 (2006).

Pinkel D, Segraves R, Sudar D, Clark S, Poole I, et al: High resolution analysis of DNA copy number variation using comparative genomic hybridization to microarrays. Nat Genet 20:207–211 (1998).

Scherer SW, Cheung J, MacDonald JR, Osborne LR, Nakabayashi K, et al: Human chromosome 7: DNA sequence and biology. Science 300:767–772 (2003).

Sebat J, Lakshmi B, Troge J, Alexander J, Young J, et al: Large-scale copy number polymorphism in the human genome. Science 305:525–528 (2004).

Sharp AJ, Locke DP, McGrath SD, Cheng Z, Bailey JA, et al: Segmental duplications and copy-number variation in the human genome. Am J Hum Genet 77:78–88 (2005).

Tuzun E, Sharp AJ, Bailey JA, Kaul R, Morrison VA, et al: Fine-scale structural variation of the human genome. Nat Genet 37:727–732 (2005).

Xu J, Zwaigenbaum L, Szatmari P, Scherer SW: Molecular cytogenetics of autism. Curr Genomics 5:347–364 (2004).

Zhang Z, Schwartz S, Wagner L, Miller W: A greedy algorithm for aligning DNA sequences. J Comput Biol 7:203–214 (2000).

Cytogenet Genome Res 115:215–224 (2006)
DOI: 10.1159/000095917

Idiopathic learning disability and genome imbalance

S.J.L. Knight   R. Regan

Oxford Genetics Knowledge Park, Wellcome Trust Centre for Human Genetics, University of Oxford, Oxford (UK)

Manuscript received 7 March 2006; accepted in original form for publication by A. Geurts van Kessel, 28 April 2006.

Abstract. Learning disability (LD) is a very common, lifelong and disabling condition, affecting about 3% of the population. Despite this, it is only over the past 10–15 years that major progress has been made towards understanding the origins of LD. In particular, genetics driven advances in technology have led to the unequivocal demonstration of the importance of genome imbalance in the aetiology of idiopathic LD (ILD). In this review we provide an overview of these advances, discussing technologies such as multi-telomere FISH and array CGH that have already emerged as well as new approaches that show diagnostic potential for the future. The advances to date have highlighted new considerations such as copy number polymorphisms (CNPs) that can complicate the interpretation of genome imbalance and its relevance to ILD. More importantly though, they have provided a remarkable ~15–20% improvement in diagnostic capability as well as facilitating genotype/phenotype correlations and providing new avenues for the identification and understanding of genes involved in neurocognitive function.

Copyright © 2006 S. Karger AG, Basel

Learning disability

Learning disability (LD), also termed mental retardation, learning difficulty, intellectual disability, developmental delay, impaired cognition or mental handicap, is an extremely common condition, affecting about 3% of the population. Patients with LD find it harder to understand and learn new things compared to other people and also have trouble understanding how new things fit into the everyday world around. Virtually all of those individuals with moderate to severe LD (intelligence quotient (IQ) under 50) need life long support and about half of those with mild LD (IQ 50–70) are significantly impaired throughout life. Although LD carries with it immense clinical, social and psychological burdens, the origins have remained poorly understood. Until recently, they have tended to be thought of in general terms, such as prenatal insult, social disadvantage and inheritance and therefore it has been impossible to provide effective therapeutic or preventive strategies. However, the past 10–15 years have brought advances in genetics research that have demonstrated unequivocally the importance of genetics, particularly genome imbalance, in the aetiology of LD such that there is now immense momentum towards furthering knowledge and technology so that we can improve diagnostic capability in this field and ultimately improve the welfare of patients and families affected.

Genome imbalance

The term genome imbalance refers to any loss or gain of DNA sequences compared with the reference DNA sequence of the genome of interest. In humans, genome imbalance may be pathogenic, confer predisposition to disease or may have no apparent clinical effect at all. Whole chromosomes may be implicated or small segments of chromosomes, even single nucleotides. The large changes can be detected using routine karyotype analysis at the 450–

Supported by the Oxford Genetics Knowledge Park (Oxford GKP) and The Health Foundation.

Request reprints from Dr Samantha J.L. Knight
    Oxford Genetics Knowledge Park
    Wellcome Trust Centre for Human Genetics, University of Oxford
    Roosevelt Drive, Headington, Oxford, OX3 7BN (UK)
    telephone: +44 1865 287 511; fax: +44 1865 287 501
    e-mail: sknight@well.ox.ac.uk

Table 1. Subtelomeric testing methods

Method used to detect subtelomeric genome imbalance	Brief description[a]
FISH-based	
Chromoprobe Multiprobe®-T System (Cytocell Ltd)	Two fluorophors detection system. Probes are mainly PACs. Allows 23 dual hybridisations on a single, customised microscope slide.
ToTel Vysion™ Multicolor FISH probe system (Vysis/Abbott, Inc.)	Three fluorophors detection system. Probes are mainly BACs. Hybridisations are split over three slides.
Modified multiplex or multi-color FISH (M-FISH): M-TEL, TM-FISH, S-COBRA FISH	More fluorophors are used in different combinations and/or ratios. Multiple probes can be hybridised to one or two target metaphases. Telomeres identified by unique color scheme and banding.
Telomere spectral karyotyping (Telomere SKY)	Similar to the M-FISH approaches except in the imaging process.
Non FISH-based	
Primed 'in situ' labelling (PRINS)	Uses metaphase chromosomes and telomere oligonucleotide primer $(CCCTAA)_7$. Primer extension reaction creates a product that can be detected by fluorescence microscopy.
High resolution chromosome analysis	Direct visualisation of telomeric regions by high resolution chromosome analysis (850 band level).
High resolution metaphase comparative genome hybridisation (CGH)	Test and reference DNAs are differentially labelled with fluorophors and co-hybridised to normal metaphase chromosomes. Deviation from the expected 1:1 fluorescence hybridisation ratio may indicate genome imbalance.
HVP analysis/scanning short tandem repeat polymorphisms (STRP) analysis	Patient and parental DNAs are genotyped by PCR across polymorphic repeats. Non-Mendelian inheritance of patient alleles indicates genome imbalance.
Locus copy number measurement by hybridization with amplifiable probes (MAPH) and multiplex ligation-dependent probe amplification (MLPA)	Telomere specific oligonucleotides give products of unique length in dosage-sensitive PCR reactions. Relative amounts of the probe amplification products reflect the copy number of the target sequences.
Telomere array CGH and comprehensive subtelomere array CGH	Test and reference DNAs are differentially labelled with fluorophors and co-hybridised to arrayed subtelomeric probes. Deviation from the expected 1:1 fluorescence hybridisation ratio may indicate genome imbalance.

[a] For full description of methodologies see Knight and Flint (2004).

500 band level, the standard test used for the detection of constitutional anomalies (present at or before birth) and cancer anomalies. However, the resolution is not sufficiently high to routinely detect rearrangements smaller than 5 Mb and even much larger abnormalities may be missed if they occur in regions where the banding pattern is not distinctive. Because these less readily detectable genome imbalances can also be clinically important, there has been a growing demand for the development of higher resolution genome-wide assays that can detect them. This is particularly the case in the field of LD where 60–80% of cases remain undiagnosed.

Cryptic genome imbalance of chromosome ends

Improved diagnosis and detection methods

The importance of cytogenetically visible regions of genome imbalance has long been recognised in syndromal conditions such as Down, Turner, Edwards, Patau, Cri du Chat, Miller Dieker, and Prader-Willi/Angelman syndromes. However, the first major advance in our ability to improve diagnostic pick-up in ILD came with the discovery that cytogenetically invisible (cryptic) genome imbalances

involving chromosome ends (telomeres) account for a significant number of moderate to severe ILD cases (Flint et al., 1995). Subsequently, subtelomeric imbalances have been identified in ILD patients using at least ten different testing strategies (Table 1). In a recent review of over 3,000 patient results, subtelomeric imbalances were noted in ~5% of cases overall, though the frequency was higher in patients with moderate to severe mental retardation (MR) (~7%) and in ~50% of cases with imbalances the rearrangements were 'de novo' whereas ~50% were familial (Knight and Flint, 2004). To date, there have been over 40 multiple case studies that, combined, have tested over 16,600 cases with ILD (Table 2). Recently, an analysis of 11,688 cases referred for subtelomere FISH in a clinical diagnostic setting gave a detection rate of ~2.6% in this comparatively unbiased population (Ravnan et al., 2006), a figure independently put forward by Yu et al. (2005).

Identifying clinical phenotypes associated with subtelomeric anomalies

Patients with ILD account for approximately 15% of all referrals passing through genetics and pediatrics clinics, but testing all individuals in this group for cryptic subtelomeric imbalance is impractical because of the cost. One less ex-

Table 2. Summary of subtelomeric studies

Reference	Method of identification[a]	Number of cases tested	Number of cases with clinically relevant subtelomeric imbalance
Flint et al., 1995	Hypervariable DNA probe analysis	99	3
Viot et al., 1998	'In house' Multi-telomere FISH and Chromoprobe Multiprobe®-T System	17	4
Vorsanova et al., 1998	Chromoprobe Multiprobe®-T System	209	8
Knight et al., 1999	Chromoprobe Multiprobe®-T System	466	22
Lamb et al., 1998	Chromoprobe Multiprobe®-T System	43	1
Slavotinek et al., 1999	Microsatellite genotyping	22	2
Bonifacio et al., 2001	PRINS	65	2
Borgione et al., 2001	Chromoprobe Multiprobe®-T System and microsatellite genotyping	60	2
Colleaux et al., 2001	Automated fluorescent microsatellite genotyping	29	4
Fan et al., 2001	Chromoprobe Multiprobe®-T System	150	6
Joyce et al., 2001	High resolution chromosome banding, modified Chromoprobe Multiprobe®-T System	200	11
Joly et al., 2001	CGH to chromosomes and Chromoprobe Multiprobe®-T System	14	5
Riegel et al., 2001	'In house' Multi-telomere FISH and Chromoprobe Multiprobe®-T System	254	13
Rosenberg et al., 2001	Microsatellite genotyping (STRPs)	120	5
Rossi et al., 2001	Chromoprobe Multiprobe®-T System	200	12
Sismani et al., 2001	Chromoprobe Multiprobe®-T System and MAPH	70	1
Anderlid et al., 2002	Chromoprobe Multiprobe®-T System, ToTel VysionTM Multicolor FISH, SKY	111	10
Baker et al., 2002a	'In house' Multi-telomere FISH	250	9
Clarkson et al., 2002	Chromoprobe Multiprobe®-T System and SKY	50	2
Dawson et al., 2002	Chromoprobe Multiprobe®-T System and ToTel VysionTM Multicolor FISH	40	3
Helias-Rodzewicz et al., 2002	Chromoprobe Multiprobe®-T System	3	3
Hollox et al., 2002	MAPH	37	6
Popp et al., 2002	M-TEL and telomere FISH	32	4
Rio et al., 2002	Microsatellite genotyping	150	15
van Karnebeek et al., 2002	High resolution chromosome banding, Chromoprobe Multiprobe®-T System	266	19
Davies et al., 2003	Chromosome analysis and MultiprobeFISH	16	3
Hulley et al., 2003	Chromoprobe Multiprobe®-T System	13	1
Jalal et al., 2003	Chromoprobe Multiprobe®-T System, TelVysion	372	24
Bocian et al., 2004	Chromoprobe Multiprobe®-T System	84	10
Koolen et al., 2004	MLPA	210	14
Pickard et al., 2004	Chromoprobe Multiprobe®-T System and MAPH	69	1
Rodriguez-Revenga et al., 2004	Chromoprobe Multiprobe®-T System	22	1
Harada et al., 2004	Subtelomeric array-CGH	69	4
Kriek et al., 2004	MAPH and telomere FISH	188	5
Rooms et al., 2004a	Microsatellite genotyping	70	0
Rooms et al., 2004b	MLPA	75	4
Novelli et al., 2004	Chromoprobe Multiprobe®-T System	92	15
Walter et al., 2004	Chromoprobe Multiprobe®-T System	50	10
Li and Zhao, 2004	Chromoprobe Multiprobe®-T System	46	2
Kok et al., 2005	Comprehensive subtelomeric array-CGH	100	8
Ravnan et al., 2006	ToTel VysionTM Multicolor FISH and Chromoprobe Multiprobe®-T System	11,688	303
Yu et al., 2005	'In house' Multi-telomere FISH	534	7
Velagaleti et al., 2005	Chromoprobe Multiprobe®-T System	18	2

[a] For abbreviations see Table 1.

pensive solution is to identify clinically a sub-group in whom small deletions occur at a much higher frequency, an approach used by de Vries et al. (2001b) who devised a five item clinical checklist. Another approach is to determine whether anomalies of particular subtelomeric regions result in an identifiable and specific phenotype, thereby directing the clinician towards the diagnosis. The most striking example of this was the elucidation of the '1p36 deletion syndrome' (Shapira et al., 1997; Knight-Jones et al., 2000). This was followed by clinically identifiable phenotypes being put

forward for a number of other subtelomeric imbalances, for example, 1qter syndrome, 2q37.3 monosomy, 3q29 microdeletion syndrome, 5q35.3 subtelomeric deletion syndrome, 6q subtelomeric deletion syndrome, subtelomeric 9q microdeletion syndrome, 14q terminal deletion syndrome, 19p13.3-pter subtelomeric deletion syndrome and 22q deletion syndrome (de Vries et al., 2001a; van Karnebeek et al., 2002; Heilstedt et al., 2003; Rauch et al., 2003; Wilson et al., 2003; Aldred et al., 2004; Stevenson et al., 2004; Stewart et al., 2004; Archer et al., 2005; Eash et al., 2005; van Bever et

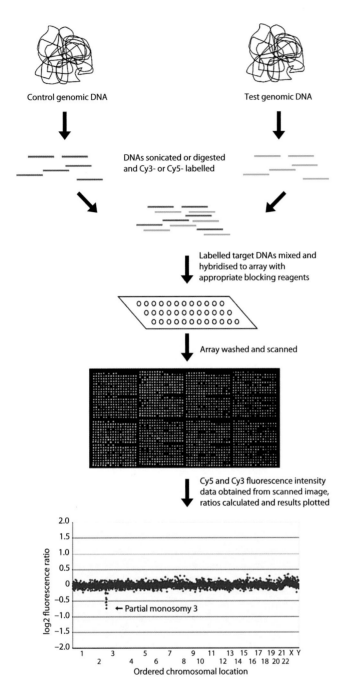

Control genomic DNA   Test genomic DNA

DNAs sonicated or digested
and Cy3- or Cy5- labelled

Labelled target DNAs mixed and
hybridised to array with
appropriate blocking reagents

Array washed and scanned

Cy5 and Cy3 fluorescence intensity
data obtained from scanned image,
ratios calculated and results plotted

← Partial monosomy 3

log2 fluorescence ratio

Ordered chromosomal location

Fig. 1. Overview of array CGH. Control and test genomic DNAs ('targets') are differentially labelled with fluorophors (e.g. Cy3-dCTP and Cy5-dCTP) and compete in a single hybridisation to a microarray containing arrayed probes of interest. The hybridised slides are scanned and the fluorescent intensity data used to determine whether there is a deviation from the expected 1:1 hybridisation ratio for any of the arrayed probes. For normal versus patient DNAs, such a deviation may indicate an increase or decrease in copy number and thereby signpost a clinically significant anomaly in the patient. In the example shown, a partial monosomy of chromosome 3 is detected in the patient sample.

al., 2005; Willatt et al., 2005). In most cases these studies were aided by the detailed phenotypic characterisation of a series of patients with similar regions of imbalance. However, accurate genotype/phenotype correlations require precise calibration of the sizes of the imbalances. For subtelomeric imbalances, this has been greatly aided by the development of a series of 'molecular rulers' (contiguous clone sets covering terminal regions) and more recently a comprehensive subtelomere array (Martin et al., 2002; Kok et al., 2005). Other aids include databases such as the European Cytogeneticists Association Register of Unbalanced Chromosome Aberrations (ECARUCA) where the entry of data from different studies provides the opportunity to compare information from rarer cases to elucidate common phenotypes.

Pathogenic versus non-pathogenic subtelomeric anomalies

For the majority of subtelomeric imbalances reported to be clinically significant, either the associated phenotypes segregate within families, the rearrangements are already known to be associated with a recognisable phenotype, or the measured sizes are so large that they are unlikely to be without phenotypic consequence. However, there are imbalances without apparent clinical effect (Knight and Flint, 2000, 2004; Martin et al., 2002; Ravnan et al., 2006). Usually, an imbalance is considered to be a benign polymorphism when one phenotypically normal parent carries the identical anomaly. However, it is possible for a patient and parent to differ in their exact breakpoints and this may be clinically relevant. Finally, there are a proportion of cases, those with small previously undocumented 'de novo' rearrangements, for whom it is impossible to determine the diagnostic implications at present. This situation will improve as the number of studies and overlapping anomalies grows and more is learned about the proportion of subtelomeric sequences that can be lost/duplicated without phenotypic effect.

LD and cryptic genome imbalance of interstitial regions

Background

The discovery that subtelomeric imbalances were an important cause of ILD naturally led to the supposition that cytogenetically invisible genome imbalance of interstitial regions might also be responsible for a significant proportion of ILD cases. Indeed, results from scanning short tandem repeat polymorphisms (STRP) suggested that a genome-wide testing strategy would be worthwhile, though this particular technique was not suited to diagnostic purposes (Rosenberg et al., 2000). Currently, the most promising technology for assaying genome imbalance of interstitial regions is CGH to microarrays (array CGH). An overview of array CGH methodology is given in Fig. 1. In the following sections we discuss different genome-wide array CGH platforms and consider both their promise and limitations for the study of ILD.

Table 3. Summary of genome-wide array CGH studies

Reference	Array 'resolution'	Selection criteria[a]	Number of samples	Clinically relevant interstitial imbalances (%)[b]	Polymorphisms/ normal variants (V), false positives (F)
Vissers et al., 2003	1 Mb	ILD and dysmorphism and suggestive phenotype	20	10	10% (V), 10% (F)
Shaw-Smith et al., 2004	1 Mb	ILD and dysmorphism	50	12	10% (V)
de Vries et al., 2005	100 kb	ILD	100	10	many (V)
Rosenberg et al., 2006	1 Mb	mentally impaired and dysmorphism	81	10	4% (V), 1.2% (F)
Schoumans et al., 2005	1 Mb	idiopathic MR and dysmorphism	41	10	many (V)
Tyson et al., 2005	1 Mb and 3 Mb	mentally impaired and suggestive phenotype	22	5	many (V)
Miyake et al., 2006	1.4 Mb	ILD and dysmorphism	30	10	many (V)
Menten et al., 2006	1 Mb	unexplained MR and suggestive features	140	8	4–6% (V)

[a] MR = mental retardation.
[b] 16–20% including subtelomeric imbalances.

'1 Mb resolution' arrays

The first genome-wide arrays to be used for the study of ILD were the '1 Mb resolution' arrays, so-called, because the arrayed probes (DNAs from large-insert clones) are spaced at approximately 1 Mb intervals throughout the genome. There have been at least seven studies to date using 1 Mb resolution arrays (Table 3). Taken together, they suggest that genome imbalances of interstitial regions account for ~10% of idiopathic learning disability cases with dysmorphism. Thus the potential utility of 1 Mb arrays in providing diagnoses in ILD is clear. However, the same studies have also highlighted limitations that must be carefully evaluated if the method is to be considered for clinical diagnostic laboratory settings. For example, issues regarding clinically benign variants/polymorphisms, resolution and false negative/false positive rates. Of these, clinically benign variants/ polymorphisms are a consideration for all array CGH platforms and are discussed separately. In terms of resolution, 50–75% of the anomalies found to date using 1 Mb arrays have been larger than 3 Mb, once again highlighting the limitations of conventional cytogenetic analysis, but also raising the question of whether these arrays achieve sufficient resolution for clinical diagnostic purposes since it is likely that a proportion of clinically relevant imbalances will pass undetected using this platform (Price et al., 2005). Furthermore, every potential imbalance indicated by only a single probe on a 1 Mb array must be followed up, hence the relatively high false positive rate. The advent of higher resolution array CGH platforms, such as tiling resolution genome-wide arrays and oligonucleotide genome-wide arrays, that achieve significantly more genome coverage, has proved timely in this respect.

Genome-wide tiling resolution arrays

The first higher resolution genome-wide array CGH platform to emerge was the tiling resolution array containing 32,447 bacterial artificial clones (BACs) with an estimated resolution of ~100 kb (Ishkanian et al., 2004). This was initially developed for cancer studies, but was later used to test 100 patients with ILD (de Vries et al., 2005). In this study, 10% of patients were found to have 'de novo' genome imbalances considered to be clinically relevant (Table 3). Of these, 77% had imbalances of <3 Mb, confirming that very small regions of genome imbalance are indeed important in ILD and that this higher resolution array may well hold more potential as a diagnostic tool than '1 Mb resolution' arrays (Table 4). Importantly, higher resolution arrays are more robust in detection; a 1 Mb duplication represented by only a single clone on a 1 Mb array will be detected by up to ten clones on a tiling path array, thereby giving a significantly lower false positive rate. The main limitation regarding tiling resolution arrays is that they are not easily accessible; purchasing arrays is cost-prohibitive and 'in house' fabrication is beyond the capabilities of most clinical diagnostic centres.

Genome-wide oligonucleotide arrays

Shortly after the development of tiling resolution arrays, high density arrays using oligonucleotides as probes emerged (Lucito et al., 2003). Oligonucleotide array CGH platforms have the potential to achieve extraordinarily high resolution that not only allows very small genome imbalances to be identified, but also allows rearrangement breakpoints to be mapped more precisely than other platforms. Their versatile design, allowing incorporation of separated exonic, intronic and non-gene sequences is also an advantage, giving them the dual capability of testing gene expression as well as genome imbalance.

The highest resolution genome-wide oligonucleotide arrays developed to date comprise 385,000 probes giving an average resolution of 30 kb throughout the genome (Lucito et al., 2003). The methodology for these, representational oligonucleotide microarray analysis (ROMA), was developed for the detection of genome imbalance in cancer and in normal individuals, but has not yet been applied to any substantial set of ILD cases, most likely due to cost of testing (http://www.nimblegen.com/). Less costly and more accessible are the 45,500 oligonucleotide probe arrays and more recently the ~185,000 and ~244,000 oligonucleotide probe arrays of Agilent Technologies that offer improved resolu-

Table 4. Clinically relevant interstitial genome imbalances in ILD cases detected by genome-wide array-CGH

Chromosome location	Deletion/duplication	Approximate size of imbalance (Mb)	Reference
1p36.23-p36.32	Deletion	4.60–8.10	Menten et al., 2006
1p36.31-p36.32	Deletion	2.80–6.00	Menten et al., 2006
1p36.11-p36.12	Duplication	5.00	Shaw-Smith et al., 2004
1p34.3-p34.2	Deletion	3.93	de Vries et al., 2005
1p31.1-p31.3	Deletion	14.00	Shaw-Smith et al., 2004
2q22.3-q23.2	Deletion	2.00	Vissers et al., 2003
2q22.3-q24.1	Deletion	14.00	Schoumans et al., 2005
2q23.1-q23.2	Deletion	0.92	de Vries et al., 2005
2q24-q31	Deletion	10.00	Schoumans et al., 2005
3p24.3-p24.1	Deletion	10.70	Rosenberg et al., 2006
3p21	Deletion	1.03	Miyake et al., 2006
3q27.1-q29	Deletion	12.37	de Vries et al., 2005
4p16.2-p16.3	Deletion	6.00	Schoumans et al., 2005
5q34-q35.1	Deletion	6.90–11.80	Menten et al., 2006
5q35.1	Deletion	0.20–2.80	Menten et al., 2006
5q35.1	Duplication	1.24	de Vries et al., 2005
6p12.3	Duplication	1.70	Rosenberg et al., 2006
7q11.21-q11.23	Deletion	8.00	Vissers et al., 2003
9q22.3	Deletion	6.50	Shaw-Smith et al., 2004
9q31.1	Deletion	2.85	de Vries et al., 2005
9q33.1	Deletion	0.54	de Vries et al., 2005
10q25.1-q26.11	Deletion	8.20–10.30	Menten et al., 2006
11q12.3-q13.1	Duplication	2.70	Tyson et al., 2005
11q14.1-q14.2	Deletion	7.49	de Vries et al., 2005
12q24.21-q24.23	Duplication	2.30	de Vries et al., 2005
13q31.3-q33.1	Duplication	12.20–13.90	Menten et al., 2006
13q32.3	Deletion	3.20	Rosenberg et al., 2006
17p13.2-p13.1, 17p13.1, 17p12, 17p11.21	Duplications	2.89	de Vries et al., 2005
17p13.1	Duplication	1.43	de Vries et al., 2005
17p12	Duplication	2.88	de Vries et al., 2005
17p11.2	Deletion	2.00	Schoumans et al., 2005
17p11.2	Deletion	5.70	Rosenberg et al., 2006
17p11.2	Duplication	1.48	de Vries et al., 2005
17q11.2	Deletion	0.10–1.90	Menten et al., 2006
17q21.31	Deletion	1.00–2.00	Shaw-Smith et al., 2004
17q23.2-q24.1	Deletion	1.10–4.20	Menten et al., 2006
18q12.3	Deletion	1.40–4.60	Menten et al., 2006
19q13.11	Deletion	1.00–2.00	Shaw-Smith et al., 2004
20q13.13-q13.2	Duplication	0.70–2.70	Menten et al., 2006
21q22	Deletion	7.00	Shaw-Smith et al., 2004
22q11.2	Duplication	2.20	Miyake et al., 2006
22q11.2, 22q11.21, 22q12.1	Deletion, Duplication, Deletion	1.10, 3.09, 3.09	Rosenberg et al., 2006
22q11.21	Duplication	3.00	Rosenberg et al., 2006
22q11.21	Deletion	2.66	de Vries et al., 2005
22q12.2	Deletion	0.70–2.20	Menten et al., 2006
Xp11.23	Deletion	1.80	Rosenberg et al., 2006
Xq28	Duplication	1.30	Rosenberg et al., 2006

tion over tiling resolution arrays (http://www.chem.agilent.com/). ILD studies using these arrays are in progress, though unpublished as yet.

Pathogenic versus non-pathogenic interstitial genome imbalance: copy number variation in the human genome

Table 4 summarises the clinically relevant interstitial genome imbalances reported to date through array CGH studies of ILD cases. However, each of these studies also noted a significant number of large-scale copy number polymorphisms (CNPs) thought to be clinically benign. CNPs contribute substantially to genomic variation between normal individuals and are therefore an important consideration when it comes to the clinical interpretation of interstitial imbalances at the genome-wide level (Iafrate et al., 2004; Sebat et al., 2004; de Vries et al., 2005; Sharp et al., 2005; Tuzun et al., 2005; Conrad et al., 2006). De Vries et al. (2005) identified a total of 258 copy number variations in 99/100 patients, thereby highlighting how crucial it is to test parental samples before drawing any conclusions regarding the pathogenicity of a genomic imbalance in ILD. Usually, a 'de novo' imbalance is implied to be clinically relevant and an inherited imbalance, clinically benign. However, without further information such assertions can never be 100% definitive because a 'de novo' imbalance can also be clinically benign whereas a combination of CNPs inherited through both parents might confer predisposition to ILD. In addition, an imbalance inherited from a clinically normal parent might confer pathogenicity through unmasking of recessive alleles. In all cases, the main aid to clinical interpretation, particularly if parental samples are unavailable, is to compare identified putative regions of genome imbalance with alterations described previously in normal individuals and also with the clinical phenotypes of patients reported to have overlapping regions of imbalance. Although this approach is currently limited (because so few studies have been done and there have been few overlapping anomalies), databases have been designed to aid in the process: (i) The Database of Genomic Variants (http://projects.tcag.ca/variation/), a curated catalogue of large-scale variation in the human genome; (ii) The Human Structural Variation database, (http://humanparalogy.gs.washington.edu/structuralvariation/), a catalogue of human genomic polymorphisms ascertained by experimental and computational analyses; (iii) ECARUCA (http://agserver01.azn.nl:8080/ecaruca/ecaruca.jsp) and (iv) the DatabasE of Chromosomal Imbalance and Phenotype in Humans using Ensembl Resources (DECIPHER, http://www.sanger.ac.uk/PostGenomics/decipher/), similar to ECARUCA but confined to submicroscopic anomalies. The use of such databases will expedite our knowledge of genome imbalance and those regions/DNA sequences that are important in the aetiology of ILD.

Future perspectives

Targeted arrays

Much of the focus of this review has been on the improving diagnostic capability in ILD through genome-wide interrogation for clinically relevant regions of imbalance. However, there have also been studies that have targeted specific chromosomes, for example the X chromosome (Veltman et al., 2004; Lugtenberg et al., 2006). In the future it is hoped that the results of these and high-resolution genome-wide studies will allow the identification of a subset of genomic regions that more commonly show genome imbalance in ILD, thereby providing identifiable targets for the development of smaller, focused arrays. Indeed, in the clinical diagnostic setting, there is already some demand for the use of array CGH in a more targeted, cost-effective way using probe sets directed towards regions already known to be involved in genetic disease, e.g. monosomy 1p36, Down syndrome critical region, DiGeorge syndome, Smith-Magenis syndrome, Williams-Beuren syndrome and subtelomeric deletion/duplication syndromes as well as many others. Indeed Bejjani et al. (2005) have already developed a targeted array for 126 medically significant and relatively common regions of chromosomal imbalance (SignatureChip,

http://www.signaturegenomics.com/). Similarly designed targeted arrays are the Spectral Genomics Constitutional Chip™ (http://www.spectralgenomics.com) and Vysis/Abbott GenoSensor Array 300 (http://www.vysis.com) that are commercially available. These are all capable of detecting genomic imbalances of clinical relevance in ILD. However, they are not pre-natal arrays because they also identify loci that neither clinicians nor patients would wish to consider during pregnancy. The format of a pre-natal array warrants more careful consideration and validation and only one such array has been developed to date (Rickman et al., 2006).

Segmental duplication arrays

Segmental duplications (SDs) are blocks of DNA that range from 1 to 400 kb in length, occur at more than one site in the genome and usually share >90% sequence identity (Eichler, 2001). Their location is associated with regions of chromosome instability or evolutionary rearrangement and they have been implicated in more than 25 genomic disorders as well as mediating normal variation in the human genome (Stankiewicz and Lupski, 2002). Therefore, it is important to consider the possibility that regions of SD might also be implicated in mediating genome imbalance in ILD. Indeed, recent array CGH studies using SD BAC arrays developed by Sharp et al. (2005) suggest that this is the case. In a study of 290 ILD cases reported with normal karyotype and normal subtelomeric results, ~5.5% genome imbalances thought to be clinically relevant were detected. Significantly, in four cases (~1.4%) the same ~478-kb critical region of deletion at 17q21.31 was identified, allowing a new and potentially common microdeletion syndrome to be described (Sharp et al., 2006). Interestingly the deleted region is flanked by SDs and in at least one case, has been found to have arisen through a paternal inversion of the region (a common European inversion recently described by Stefansson et al., 2005 and also by Cruts et al., 2005). The novel 17q21.31 microdeletion syndrome and demonstration of inheritance from a parental inversion were also reported by two other groups (Koolen et al., 2006; Shaw-Smith et al., 2006). The studies not only help to elucidate the underlying molecular mechanism for this microdeletion syndrome, but also emphasise the role of genome organisation in the mediation of genomic rearrangement.

Summary and conclusions

In this review we have focused on ILD and genomic imbalance, particularly the technological advances and associated studies that have yielded significantly improved diagnostic capability through the identification of clinically relevant genomic imbalances in this condition. We have seen how the discovery of subtelomeric imbalances in ILD provided the impetus not only for the development of alternative subtelomeric testing techniques, but also for the search for new technologies capable of detecting genome imbalances in interstitial regions throughout the genome.

Currently the most promising approach for genome-wide interrogation is array CGH. There are a number of different array CGH platforms, but it is not clear which is most suited to clinical diagnostic use for ILD. Reliability, robustness, achievable resolution, genome coverage, availability and affordability are all considerations, but currently no single platform meets all needs of all clinical diagnostic laboratories. However, it is clear that there are two main categories of demand: (i) Genome-wide 'discovery' arrays aimed towards finding new clinically relevant genomic imbalances in ILD. Available platforms range from ~1 Mb resolution arrays to very high-resolution oligonucleotide arrays. (ii) Targeted arrays for post-natal diagnosis (targeting known clinically relevant regions of imbalance) and once fully validated and ethically approved, for pre-natal diagnosis (targeting very highly selected clinically relevant regions of imbalance). Both probe sets can be added to as new clinically relevant regions of the genome are identified.

In the future, newly emerging arrays such as specialised SD arrays, high density 500K SNP arrays and PamChip three-dimensional microarrays (that can be used for array-based MAPH/MLPA) as well as new approaches such as Optical Mapping may prove useful for the genome-wide detection of imbalance in ILD (http://www.affymetrix.com/products/arrays/index.affx, http://www.pamgene.com/, http://www.opgen.com/) whereas techniques such as standard MLPA and real-time quantitative PCR may be an attractive alternative to array CGH for targeted assays of genome imbalance in LD. Importantly, alternative array and non-array based strategies that do not focus on genome imbalance remain to be explored in ILD, e.g. those that assay gene expression, transcript profiles and predisposing alleles. Also a consideration are truly balanced translocations, polyploidy, single nucleotide mutations and most inversions, that array CGH cannot detect. Though the majority of truly balanced translocations do not cause a phenotypic abnormality (Warburton, 1991) and polyploidy (usually indicated by an abnormal foetal ultrasound) is virtually always lethal in the foetus, the contribution of cryptic inversions to the aetiology of ILD remains to be elucidated.

In the meantime, there is still much to be learned from studying genome imbalance in ILD. The findings thus far have been particularly relevant in providing an impressive 15–20% more clinical diagnoses and more accurate genetic counseling, but ultimately will be important for refining genotype/phenotype correlations and identifying causative dosage-sensitive genes. This in turn will improve our understanding of cognitive development as a whole and will help pave the way for developing new therapeutic avenues that will further improve the welfare of patients and families affected by ILD.

Acknowledgements

We would like to acknowledge Dr Jenny Taylor (Oxford GKP) and Ms Kim Smith (Oxford Radcliffe Hospitals NHS Trust) for information relating to the implementation of array CGH in clinical diagnostic laboratories. We would also like to thank Dr Niki Meston (Oxford Radcliffe Hospitals NHS Trust and University of Oxford) for reading the manuscript and for valued discussion.

References

Aldred MA, Sanford RO, Thomas NS, Barrow MA, Wilson LC, et al: Molecular analysis of 20 patients with 2q37.3 monosomy: definition of minimum deletion intervals for key phenotypes. J Med Genet 41:433–439 (2004).

Anderlid BM, Schoumans J, Anneren G, Sahlen S, Kyllerman M, et al: Subtelomeric rearrangements detected in patients with idiopathic mental retardation. Am J Med Genet 107:275–284 (2002).

Archer HL, Gupta S, Enoch S, Thompson P, Rowbottom A, et al: Distinct phenotype associated with a cryptic subtelomeric deletion of 19p13.3-pter. Am J Med Genet A 136:38–44 (2005).

Baker E, Hinton L, Callen DF, Altree M, Dobbie A, et al: Study of 250 children with idiopathic mental retardation reveals nine cryptic and diverse subtelomeric chromosome anomalies. Am J Med Genet 107:285–293 (2002a).

Baker E, Hinton L, Callen DF, Haan EA, Dobbie A, Sutherland GR: A familial cryptic subtelomeric deletion 12p with variable phenotypic effect. Clin Genet 61:198–201 (2002b).

Bejjani BA, Saleki R, Ballif BC, Rorem EA, Sundin K, et al: Use of targeted array-based CGH for the clinical diagnosis of chromosomal imbalance: is less more? Am J Med Genet A 134:259–267 (2005).

Bocian E, Helias-Rodzewicz Z, Suchenek K, Obersztyn E, Kutkowska-Kazmierczak A, et al: Subtelomeric rearrangements: results from FISH studies in 84 families with idiopathic mental retardation. Med Sci Monit 10:CR143–151 (2004).

Bonifacio S, Centrone C, Da Prato L, Scordo MR, Estienne M, Torricelli F: Use of primed in situ labeling (PRINS) for the detection of telomeric deletions associated with mental retardation. Cytogenet Cell Genet 93:16–18 (2001).

Borgione E, Giudice ML, Galesi O, Castiglia L, Failla P, et al: How microsatellite analysis can be exploited for subtelomeric chromosomal rearrangement analysis in mental retardation. J Med Genet 38:E1 (2001).

Clarkson B, Pavenski K, Dupuis L, Kennedy S, Meyn S, et al: Detecting rearrangements in children using subtelomeric FISH and SKY. Am J Med Genet 107:267–274 (2002).

Colleaux L, Rio M, Heuertz S, Moindrault S, Turleau C, et al: A novel automated strategy for screening cryptic telomeric rearrangements in children with idiopathic mental retardation. Eur J Hum Genet 9:319–327 (2001).

Conrad DF, Andrews TD, Carter NP, Hurles ME, Pritchard JK: A high-resolution survey of deletion polymorphism in the human genome. Nat Genet 38:75–81 (2006).

Cruts M, Rademakers R, Gijselinck I, van der Zee J, Dermaut B, et al: Genomic architecture of human 17q21 linked to frontotemporal dementia uncovers a highly homologous family of low-copy repeats in the tau region. Hum Mol Genet 14:1753–1762 (2005).

Davies AF, Kirby TL, Docherty Z, Ogilvie CM: Characterization of terminal chromosome anomalies using multisubtelomere FISH. Am J Med Genet A 120:483–489 (2003).

Dawson AJ, Putnam S, Schultz J, Riordan D, Prasad C, et al: Cryptic chromosome rearrangements detected by subtelomere assay in patients with mental retardation and dysmorphic features. Clin Genet 62:488–494 (2002).

de Vries BB, Knight SJ, Homfray T, Smithson SF, Flint J, Winter RM: Submicroscopic subtelomeric 1qter deletions: a recognisable phenotype? J Med Genet 38:175–178 (2001a).

de Vries BB, White SM, Knight SJ, Regan R, Homfray T, et al: Clinical studies on submicroscopic subtelomeric rearrangements: a checklist. J Med Genet 38:145–150 (2001b).

de Vries BB, Pfundt R, Leisink M, Koolen DA, Vissers LE, et al: Diagnostic genome profiling in mental retardation. Am J Hum Genet 77:606–616 (2005).

Eash D, Waggoner D, Chung J, Stevenson D, Martin CL: Calibration of 6q subtelomere deletions to define genotype/phenotype correlations. Clin Genet 67:396–403 (2005).

Eichler EE: Recent duplication, domain accretion and the dynamic mutation of the human genome. Trends Genet 17:661–669 (2001).

Fan YS, Zhang Y, Speevak M, Farrell S, Jung JH, Siu VM: Detection of submicroscopic aberrations in patients with unexplained mental retardation by fluorescence in situ hybridization using multiple subtelomeric probes. Genet Med 3:416–421 (2001).

Flint J, Wilkie AO, Buckle VJ, Winter RM, Holland AJ, McDermid HE: The detection of subtelomeric chromosomal rearrangements in idiopathic mental retardation. Nat Genet 9:132–140 (1995).

Harada N, Hatchwell E, Okamoto N, Tsukahara M, Kurosawa K, et al: Subtelomere specific microarray based comparative genomic hybridisation: a rapid detection system for cryptic rearrangements in idiopathic mental retardation. J Med Genet 41:130–136 (2004).

Heilstedt HA, Ballif BC, Howard LA, Lewis RA, Stal S, et al: Physical map of 1p36, placement of breakpoints in monosomy 1p36, and clinical characterization of the syndrome. Am J Hum Genet 72:1200–1212 (2003).

Helias-Rodzewicz Z, Bocian E, Stankiewicz P, Obersztyn E, Kostyk E, et al: Subtelomeric rearrangements detected by FISH in three of 33 families with idiopathic mental retardation and minor physical anomalies. J Med Genet 39:e53 (2002).

Hollox EJ, Atia T, Cross G, Parkin T, Armour JA: High throughput screening of human subtelomeric DNA for copy number changes using multiplex amplifiable probe hybridisation (MAPH). J Med Genet 39:790–795 (2002).

Hulley BJ, Hummel M, Wenger SL: Screening for cryptic chromosomal abnormalities in patients with mental retardation and dysmorphic facial features using telomere FISH probes. Am J Med Genet 17:302–303 (2003).

Iafrate AJ, Feuk L, Rivera MN, Listewnik ML, Donahoe PK, et al: Detection of large-scale variation in the human genome. Nat Genet 36:949–951 (2004).

Ishkanian AS, Malloff CA, Watson SK, DeLeeuw RJ, Chi B, et al: A tiling resolution DNA microarray with complete coverage of the human genome. Nat Genet 36:299–303 (2004).

Jalal SM, Harwood AR, Sekhon GS, Pham Lorentz C, Ketterling RP, et al: Utility of subtelomeric fluorescent DNA probes for detection of chromosome anomalies in 425 patients. Genet Med 5:28–34 (2003).

Joly G, Lapierre JM, Ozilou C, Gosset P, Aurias A, et al: Comparative genomic hybridisation in mentally retarded patients with dysmorphic features and a normal karyotype. Clin Genet 60:212–219 (2001).

Joyce CA, Dennis NR, Cooper S, Browne CE: Subtelomeric rearrangements: results from a study of selected and unselected probands with idiopathic mental retardation and control individuals by using high-resolution G-banding and FISH. Hum Genet 109:440–451 (2001).

Knight SJ, Flint J: Perfect endings: a review of subtelomeric probes and their use in clinical diagnosis. J Med Genet 37:401–409 (2000).

Knight SJ, Flint J: The use of subtelomeric probes to study mental retardation. Methods Cell Biol 75:799–831 (2004).

Knight SJ, Regan R, Nicod A, Horsley SW, Kearney L, et al: Subtle chromosomal rearrangements in children with unexplained mental retardation. Lancet 354:1676–1681 (1999).

Knight-Jones E, Knight S, Heussler H, Regan R, Flint J, Martin K: Neurodevelopmental profile of a new dysmorphic syndrome associated with submicroscopic partial deletion of 1p36.3. Dev Med Child Neurol 42:201–206 (2000).

Kok K, Dijkhuizen T, Swart YE, Zorgdrager H, van der Vlies P, et al: Application of a comprehensive subtelomere array in clinical diagnosis of mental retardation. Eur J Med Genet 48:250–262 (2005).

Koolen DA, Nillesen WM, Versteeg MH, Merkx GF, Knoers NV, et al: Screening for subtelomeric rearrangements in 210 patients with unexplained mental retardation using multiplex ligation dependent probe amplification (MLPA). J Med Genet 41:892–899 (2004).

Koolen DA, Vissers LE, Pfundt R, de Leeuw N, Knight SJL, et al: A new chromosome 17q21.31 microdeletion syndrome associated with a common inversion polymorphism. Nat Genet 38:999–1001 (2006).

Kriek M, White SJ, Bouma MC, Dauwerse HG, Hansson KB, et al: Genomic imbalances in mental retardation. J Med Genet 41:249–255 (2004).

Lamb AN, Lytle CH, Aylsworth AS, et al: Low proportion of subtelomeric rearrangements in a population of patients with mental retardation and dysmorphic features. Am J Hum Genet 65, Suppl:A169 (1998).

Li R, Zhao ZY: Two subtelomeric chromosomal deletions in forty-six children with idiopathic mental retardation. Chin Med J (Engl) 117:1414–1417 (2004).

Lucito R, Healy J, Alexander J, Reiner A, Esposito D, et al: Representational oligonucleotide microarray analysis: a high-resolution method to detect genome copy number variation. Genome Res 13:2291–2305 (2003).

Lugtenberg D, de Brouwer AP, Kleefstra T, Oudakker AR, Frints SG, et al: Chromosomal copy number changes in patients with non-syndromic X-linked mental retardation detected by array CGH. J Med Genet 43:362–370 (2006).

Martin CL, Waggoner DJ, Wong A, Uhrig S, Roseberry JA, et al: 'Molecular rulers' for calibrating phenotypic effects of telomere imbalance. J Med Genet 39:734–740 (2002).

Menten B, Maas N, Thienpont B, Buysse K, Vandesompele J, et al: Emerging patterns of cryptic chromosomal imbalances in patients with idiopathic mental retardation and multiple congenital anomalies: a new series of 140 patients and review of the literature. J Med Genet 43:625–633 (2006).

Miyake N, Shimokawa O, Harada N, Sosonkina N, Okubo A, et al: BAC array CGH reveals genomic aberrations in idiopathic mental retardation. Am J Med Genet A 140:205–211 (2006).

Novelli A, Ceccarini C, Bernardini L, Zuccarello D, Caputo V, et al: High frequency of subtelomeric rearrangements in a cohort of 92 patients with severe mental retardation and dysmorphism. Clin Genet 66:30–38 (2004).

Pickard BS, Hollox EJ, Malloy MP, Porteous DJ, Blackwood DH, et al: A 4q35.2 subtelomeric deletion identified in a screen of patients with comorbid psychiatric illness and mental retardation. BMC Med Genet 5:21 (2004).

Popp S, Schulze B, Granzow M, Keller M, Holtgreve-Grez H, et al: Study of 30 patients with unexplained developmental delay and dysmorphic features or congenital abnormalities using conventional cytogenetics and multiplex FISH telomere (M-TEL) integrity assay. Hum Genet 111:31–39 (2002).

Price TS, Regan R, Mott R, Hedman A, Honey B, et al: SW-ARRAY: a dynamic programming solution for the identification of copy-number changes in genomic DNA using array comparative genome hybridization data. Nucleic Acids Res 33:3455–3464 (2005).

Rauch A, Beese M, Mayatepek E, Dorr HG, Wenzel D, et al: A novel 5q35.3 subtelomeric deletion syndrome: Am J Med Genet A 121:1–8 (2003).

Ravnan JB, Tepperberg JH, Papenhausen P, Lamb AN, Hedrick J, et al: Subtelomere FISH analysis of 11,688 cases: an evaluation of the frequency and pattern of subtelomere rearrangements in individuals with developmental disabilities. J Med Genet 43:478–489 (2006).

Rickman L, Fiegler H, Shaw-Smith C, Nash R, Cirigliano V, et al: Prenatal detection of unbalanced chromosomal rearrangements by array-CGH. J Med Genet 43:353–361 (2006).

Riegel M, Baumer A, Jamar M, Delbecque K, Herens C, et al: Submicroscopic terminal deletions and duplications in retarded patients with unclassified malformation syndromes. Hum Genet 109:286–294 (2001).

Rio M, Molinari F, Heuertz S, Ozilou C, Gosset P, et al: Automated fluorescent genotyping detects 10% of cryptic subtelomeric rearrangements in idiopathic syndromic mental retardation. J Med Genet 39:266–270 (2002).

Rodriguez-Revenga L, Badenas C, Sanchez A, Mallolas J, Carrio A, et al: Cryptic chromosomal rearrangement screening in 30 patients with mental retardation and dysmorphic features. Clin Genet 65:17–23 (2004).

Rooms L, Reyniers E, van Luijk R, Scheers S, Wauters J, Kooy RF: Screening for subtelomeric rearrangements using genetic markers in 70 patients with unexplained mental retardation. Ann Genet 47:53–59 (2004a).

Rooms L, Reyniers E, van Luijk R, Scheers S, Wauters J, et al: Subtelomeric deletions detected in patients with idiopathic mental retardation using multiplex ligation-dependent probe amplification (MLPA). Hum Mutat 23:17–21 (2004b).

Rosenberg C, Knijnenburg J, Bakker E, Vianna-Morgante AM, Sloos W, et al: Array-CGH detection of micro rearrangements in mentally retarded individuals: clinical significance of imbalances present both in affected children and normal parents. J Med Genet 43:180–186 (2006).

Rosenberg MJ, Vaske D, Killoran CE, Ning Y, Wargowski D, et al: Detection of chromosomal aberrations by a whole-genome microsatellite screen. Am J Hum Genet 66:419–427 (2000).

Rosenberg MJ, Killoran C, Dziadzio L, Chang S, Stone DL, et al: Scanning for telomeric deletions and duplications and uniparental disomy using genetic markers in 120 children with malformations. Hum Genet 109:311–318 (2001).

Rossi E, Piccini F, Zollino M, Neri G, Caselli D, et al: Cryptic telomeric rearrangements in subjects with mental retardation associated with dysmorphism and congenital malformations. J Med Genet 38:417–420 (2001).

Schoumans J, Ruivenkamp C, Holmberg E, Kyllerman M, Anderlid BM, Nordenskjold M: Detection of chromosomal imbalances in children with idiopathic mental retardation by array based comparative genomic hybridisation (array-CGH). J Med Genet 42:699–705 (2005).

Sebat J, Lakshmi B, Troge J, Alexander J, Young J, et al: Large-scale copy number polymorphism in the human genome. Science 305:525–528 (2004).

Shapira SK, McCaskill C, Northrup H, Spikes AS, Elder FF, et al: Chromosome 1p36 deletions: the clinical phenotype and molecular characterization of a common newly delineated syndrome. Am J Hum Genet 61:642–650 (1997).

Sharp AJ, Locke DP, McGrath SD, Cheng Z, Bailey JA, et al: Segmental duplications and copy-number variation in the human genome. Am J Hum Genet 77:78–88 (2005).

Sharp AJ, Hansen S, Selzer RR, Cheng Z, Regan R, et al: Discovery of previously unidentified genomic disorders from the duplication architecture of the human genome. Nat Genet 38:1038–1042 (2006).

Shaw-Smith C, Redon R, Rickman L, Rio M, Willatt L, et al: Microarray based comparative genomic hybridisation (array-CGH) detects submicroscopic chromosomal deletions and duplications in patients with learning disability/mental retardation and dysmorphic features. J Med Genet 41:241–248 (2004).

Shaw-Smith C, Pittman AM, Willatt L, Martin H, Rickman L, et al: Microdeletion encompassing *MAPT* at chromosome 17q21.3 is associated with developmental delay and learning disability. Nat Genet 38:1032–1037 (2006).

Sismani C, Armour JA, Flint J, Girgalli C, Regan R, Patsalis PC: Screening for subtelomeric chromosome abnormalities in children with idiopathic mental retardation using multiprobe telomeric FISH and the new MAPH telomeric assay. Eur J Hum Genet 9:527–532 (2001).

Slavotinek A, Rosenberg M, Knight S, Gaunt L, Fergusson W, et al: Screening for submicroscopic chromosome rearrangements in children with idiopathic mental retardation using microsatellite markers for the chromosome telomeres. J Med Genet 36:405–411 (1999).

Stankiewicz P, Lupski JR: Molecular-evolutionary mechanisms for genomic disorders. Curr Opin Genet Dev 12:312–319 (2002).

Stefansson H, Helgason A, Thorleifsson G, Steinthorsdottir V, Masson G, et al: A common inversion under selection in Europeans. Nat Genet 37:129–137 (2005).

Stevenson DA, Brothman AR, Carey JC, Chen Z, Dent KM, et al: 6q subtelomeric deletion: is there a recognizable syndrome? Clin Dysmorphol 13:103–106 (2004).

Stewart DR, Huang A, Faravelli F, Anderlid BM, Medne L, et al: Subtelomeric deletions of chromosome 9q: a novel microdeletion syndrome. Am J Med Genet A 128:340–351 (2004).

Tuzun E, Sharp AJ, Bailey JA, Kaul R, Morrison VA, et al: Fine-scale structural variation of the human genome. Nat Genet 37:727–732 (2005).

Tyson C, Harvard C, Locker R, Friedman JM, Langlois S, et al: Submicroscopic deletions and duplications in individuals with intellectual disability detected by array-CGH. Am J Med Genet A 139:173–185 (2005).

van Bever Y, Rooms L, Laridon A, Reyniers E, van Luijk R, et al: Clinical report of a pure subtelomeric 1qter deletion in a boy with mental retardation and multiple anomalies adds further evidence for a specific phenotype. Am J Med Genet A 135:91–95 (2005).

van Karnebeek CD, Quik S, Sluijter S, Hulsbeek MM, Hoovers JM, Hennekam RC: Further delineation of the chromosome 14q terminal deletion syndrome. Am J Med Genet 110:65–72 (2002).

Velagaleti GV, Robinson SS, Rouse BM, Tonk VS, Lockhart LH: Subtelomeric rearrangements in idiopathic mental retardation. Indian J Pediatr 72:679–685 (2005).

Veltman JA, Yntema HG, Lugtenberg D, Arts H, Briault S, et al: High resolution profiling of X chromosomal aberrations by array comparative genomic hybridisation. J Med Genet 41:425–432 (2004).

Viot G, Gosset P, Fert S, et al: Cryptic subtelomeric rearrangements detected by FISH in mentally retarded and dysmorphic patients. Am J Hum Genet 65, Suppl:A10 (1998).

Vissers LE, de Vries BB, Osoegawa K, Janssen IM, Feuth T, et al: Array-based comparative genomic hybridization for the genomewide detection of submicroscopic chromosomal abnormalities. Am J Hum Genet 73:1261–1270 (2003).

Vorsanova SG, Koloti D, Sharonin VO, Soloviev V, Yurov YB: FISH analysis of microaberrations at telomeric and subtelomeric regions in chromosomes of children with mental retardation. Am J Hum Genet 65, Suppl:A154 (1998).

Walter S, Sandig K, Hinkel GK, Mitulla B, Ounap K, et al: Subtelomere FISH in 50 children with mental retardation and minor anomalies, identified by a checklist, detects 10 rearrangements including a de novo balanced translocation of chromosomes 17p13.3 and 20q13.33. Am J Med Genet A 128:364–373 (2004).

Warburton D: De novo balanced chromosome rearrangements and extra marker chromosomes identified at prenatal diagnosis: clinical significance and distribution of breakpoints. Am J Hum Genet 49:995–1013 (1991).

Willatt L, Cox J, Barber J, Cabanas ED, Collins A, et al: 3q29 microdeletion syndrome: clinical and molecular characterization of a new syndrome. Am J Hum Genet 77:154–160 (2005).

Wilson HL, Wong AC, Shaw SR, Tse WY, Stapleton GA, et al: Molecular characterisation of the 22q13 deletion syndrome supports the role of haploinsufficiency of *SHANK3/PROSAP2* in the major neurological symptoms. J Med Genet 40:575–584 (2003).

Yu S, Baker E, Hinton L, Eyre HJ, Waters W, et al: Frequency of truly cryptic subtelomere abnormalities – a study of 534 patients and literature review. Clin Genet 68:436–441 (2005).

Cytogenet Genome Res 115:225–230 (2006)
DOI: 10.1159/000095918

Molecular karyotyping of patients with MCA/MR: the blurred boundary between normal and pathogenic variation

T.J.L. de Ravel   I. Balikova   B. Thienpont   F. Hannes   N. Maas   J.-P. Fryns
K. Devriendt   J.R. Vermeesch

Centre for Human Genetics, UZ Gasthuisberg, Leuven (Belgium)

Manuscript received 23 April 2006; accepted in original form for publication by A. Geurts van Kessel, 2 May 2006.

Abstract. Molecular karyotyping has revealed that microdeletions/duplications in the human genome are a major cause of multiple congenital anomalies associated with mental retardation (MCA/MR). The identification of a de novo chromosomal imbalance in a patient with MCA/MR is usually considered causal for the phenotype while a chromosomal imbalance inherited from a phenotypically normal parent is considered as a benign variation and not related to the disorder. Around 40% of imbalances in patients with MCA/MR in this series is inherited from a healthy parent and the majority of these appear to be (extremely) rare variants. As some of these contain known disease-causing genes and have also been found to be de novo in MCA/MR patients, this challenges the general view that such familial variants are innocent and of no major phenotypic consequence. Rather, we argue, that human genomes can be tolerant of genomic copy number variations depending on the genetic and environmental background and that different mechanisms play a role in determining whether these chromosomal imbalances manifest themselves.

Copyright © 2006 S. Karger AG, Basel

Cytogeneticists know that some chromosomes show a remarkable degree of morphological variation and common variants detected in a clinical cytogenetics laboratory are usually not reported. But sometimes it is not clear whether a particular finding is a normal variant or an abnormality. It is generally considered that if a phenotypically normal family member carries the same chromosomal anomaly, the anomaly is of no phenotypic relevance (Gardner and Sutherland, 2004; Barber et al., 2005). Some of these apparent chromosomal anomalies are deletions or duplications extending over several Mb (e.g. Bonaglia et al., 2002; Barber et al., 2005). Recently, Barber (2005) reviewed the literature on cytogenetically visible unbalanced chromosome abnormalities. In 18% of these, no phenotypic consequences were observed, in 59% of the cases the carriers of the visible chromosomal anomaly had consistently mild consequences, while in 23% of the families the affected proband had normal carrier family members. The average size of the deletions and duplications, estimated from the sizes of the bands, was close to 10 Mb (data in the chromosomal anomaly collection web site http://www.ngrl.org.uk/Wessex/collection).

In analogy with the larger cytogenetically visible imbalances, submicroscopic genomic imbalances are considered benign mainly on the grounds that they are detected in normal healthy individuals. Therefore, knowledge about these benign variations is essential to determine whether a chro-

Request reprints from Professor Dr. J.R. Vermeesch
Centre for Human Genetics
UZ Gasthuisberg, Herestraat 49
BE–3000 Leuven (Belgium);
telephone: +32 16 345 903; fax: +32 16 346 051
e-mail: Joris.Vermeesch@med.kuleuven.ac.be

mosomal imbalance detected in the DNA of individuals with either constitutional or acquired disorders could actually be causal for the observed phenotype. Array CGH analyses and other genome wide analysis tools are now uncovering a large number of benign copy number variations (CNVs) (Iafrate et al., 2004; Sebat et al., 2004; Conrad et al., 2006; Feuk et al., 2006; Hinds et al., 2006; McCarroll et al., 2006). Because knowledge about benign variation is essential for the clinical interpretation of array CGH results, a database collecting information about the benign CNVs in the human genome is being established (Iafrate et al., 2004; Feuk et al., 2006). While the available CNV information is based on the data retrieved from a relatively small number of healthy individuals using arrays with limited resolution, current large scale projects are ongoing to map this variation in a much larger number of individuals and at higher resolution (Feuk et al., 2006). It is believed that these large-scale mapping projects will serve as a reference and framework to determine whether novel detected imbalances would be benign or pathogenic. This database is already being used by human geneticists to interpret array CGH data and when a detected imbalance is part of the spectrum of benign variation, it is usually excluded as disease related (Schoumans et al., 2005; Menten et al., 2006).

While many imbalances appear benign, it is only the recurrent finding of these imbalances in normal individuals that can determine whether a certain imbalance has no phenotypic consequence. On the other hand, it is only the recurrent association of an imbalance with a disease phenotype that will allow the unequivocal association of an imbalance with a disease phenotype. In between these two extremes, array CGH analysis of patients with MCA/MR is uncovering a large number of rare imbalances inherited from apparently healthy individuals. We present the data on familial inherited variation obtained in our laboratory during the screening of 245 MCA/MR patients (100 of which were reported; Menten et al., 2006) and provide an overview of the published findings on inherited imbalances from the screening of MCA/MR patients with array CGH.

Results

General CGH array results

In this study, array CGH at 1 Mb resolution was performed on 245 selected patients with MCA/MR and normal karyotypes as described (Menten et al., 2006). Suspected microdeletions were verified by FISH and microduplications by real-time PCR, and when possible, imbalances were sought in both parents.

Sixty-two (25%) of the 245 patients had chromosomal imbalances. Microdeletions were detected in 41 patients (16.7%), microduplications in 18 patients (7.3%) and a microdeletion as well as a microduplication in three patients. Twenty-nine parent-pairs of the 62 positive patients were tested for carrier status. The origin of the chromosomal imbalance was de novo in 19/29 (65%), maternal in six and paternal in four patients.

Case reports of the imbalances inherited from normal parents

Patient 1. This 7-year-old mentally retarded boy to normal young parents had a low birth weight. He has short stature, brachycephaly, prominent ears, a thin upper lip, long nasal septum and pointed chin. He also has broad thumbs and a bifid hallux on the left foot. He has a maternally inherited deletion of chromosome 1q21.1, karyotype 46,XY, arr cgh 1q21.1(RP11-533N14→RP11-301M17)×1.

Patient 2 (Menten et al., 2006; case 6). This is the child of a non-consanguineous couple. She has mild mental retardation, is generally hirsute, has a few pigmented naevi, a coarse facies with full nares, a thick lower lip and long eyelashes. The CT scan indicated wide pontine cisterns, an arachnoid cyst/megacistena magna and cerebellar hemisphere hypoplasia. Array CGH revealed a 46,XX, arr cgh 3p12.1(RP11-474M18)×1 karyotype.

Patient 3 (Menten et al., 2006; case 5). This mentally retarded 4-year-old boy has axial hypotonia, peripheral spasticity and suffers from seizures. He has strabismus and abnormal pigmentation of the axilla and left shoulder. CT brain scan revealed gyral anomalies, agenesis of the corpus callosum and hypoplasia of the cerebellum and brainstem. His karyotype is 46,XY, arr cgh 3p12.2(RP11-425D6→RP11-359D24)×3, the duplication of chromosome 3p12.2 being of paternal origin.

Patient 4 (Menten et al., 2006; case 7). This boy with severe mental retardation, mild hypotonia, a pectus excavatum, a sandal gap and a sacral dimple also has sparse eyebrows, a high nasal bridge and narrow palpebral fissures. He has frequent otitis media. His karyotype is 46,XY, arr cgh 5q34q35.1(RP11-505G12→RP11-420L4)×1, 15q13.1 (RP11-408F10, RP11-38E12)×1. The 0.8–3.5-Mb deletion of chromosome 15q13.1 is a polymorphism based on the Toronto database of genomic variants.

Patient 5. This is the second child to a healthy, non-consanguineous couple. Her birth was complicated by a knotted umbilical cord and she initially had feeding difficulties. Examination at one year of age revealed a length and head circumference at –2SD, axial hypotonia and peripheral hypertonia. She has a mild developmental delay, is hyperactive and has problems with sleeping. Fundoscopy showed tortuous retinal blood vessels. Her karyotype is 46,XX, arr cgh 9p21.3(RP11-15P13→RP11-113D19)×1, 17p11.2(RP11-385D13→RP11-121A13)×3.

Patient 6 (Menten et al., 2006; case 17). This young adult woman has mild to moderate mental retardation, micro-brachycephaly, synophris, almond-shaped palpebral fissures, a wide nasal bridge and macrostomia. Her 46,XX, arr cgh 15q22.2(RP11-231A23)×1 karyotype revealed a 3.1-Mb deletion of chromosome 15q22.2.

Patient 7. This adult woman with an IQ of 75 has suffered from childhood failure to thrive, feeding and breathing problems. She has a paresis of the lower branch of the facial nerve with mouth asymmetry and a short neck with limited movement. Bilateral colobomata of the choroid, retina and papil, strabismus and epicanthic folds, right-sided choanal atresia, aplasia of the semicircular canals, stapes dysplasia

Table 1. Affected chromosomal segments and associated features in patients with inherited chromosomal imbalances

Chromosome segment	Number of clones	Clones del/dup[a]	Size (Mb)[a]	Parental origin[b]	Sex	Reference
del(1)(p21p21)	1	NR	<1	Pat	F	Vissers et al., 2003; case 3
del(1)(q21.1)	2	RP11-533N14, RP11-301M17	0.9–4.0	Mat	M	This report; case 1
del(2)(p12)	1[c]	RP11-89C12	1	Mat/Pat	F	Rosenberg et al., 2006; case 15
del(3)(p12.1)	1	RP11-474M18	0.1–2.5	Pat	F	Menten et al., 2006; case 6
del(5)(q34q35.1)	8	RP11-505G12→RP11-420L4	6.9–11.8	Mat	M	Menten et al., 2006; case 7
del(9)(p21.3)	2	RP11-15P13, RP11-113D19	1.0–2.4	Pat	F	This report; case 5
del(10)(q21.1)	1	RP11-430K23	2.5	Mat	M	Rosenberg et al., 2006; case 12
del(13)(q33.3q34)	2	fl RP11-141M24, RP11-40E6	NR	Mat	M	Shaw-Smith et al., 2004; case 10
del(15)(q13.1)	1	RP11-408F10	2.2	Mat	F	Rosenberg et al., 2006; case 11
del(15)(q15.3)	1[d]	RP11-263I19	0.9	Pat	F	Rosenberg et al., 2006; case 10
del(15)(q22.2)	1	RP11-231A23	0.2–3.2	Mat	F	Menten et al., 2006; case 17
del(X)(p11.23)	1[d]	RP1-54B20	1.8	Mat	M	Rosenberg et al., 2006; case 14
dup(2)(q21.2)	1	NR	<1	Pat	M	Vissers et al., 2003; case 4
dup(3)(p12.2)	3	RP11-425D6→RP11-359D24	0.5–2.1	Pat	M	Menten et al., 2006; case 5
dup(3)(p26.3p26.2)	2	fl RP11-95E11, RP11-10H6	NR	Pat	M	Shaw-Smith et al., 2004; case 8
dup(3)(q29qter)	2	GC-196F4, GC-56H22	0.4	Pat	F	Rosenberg et al., 2006; case 9
dup(6)(q13)	1	fl RP11-462G2	0.6	Mat	M	Shaw-Smith et al., 2004; case 9
dup(8)(p11.1)	1	CTD-2115H11	1.3	Mat	M	Rosenberg et al., 2006; case 16
dup(16)(p13.11p12.3)	3	RP11-489O1→RP11-288I13	1.5–7.0	Mat	F	This report; case 7
dup(18)(q23)	2	RP11-315M18, RP11-154H12	0.1–2	Mat	M	This report; case 8
dup(22)(q11.21)	1	XX-91c	0.1–4.2	Pat	F	Menten et al., 2006; case 27
dup(X)(p21.3)	2	RP11-37E19, RP6-27C10	0.3–1.2	Mat	M	Menten et al., 2006; case 28
dup(X)p22.3)	2	fl RP11-483M24, RP11-323F16	NR	Mat	F	Shaw-Smith et al., 2004; case 11
dup(X)(q11.2)	1	fl RP13-34C21	NR	Mat	M	Shaw-Smith et al., 2004; case 12
dup(X)(q28)	1	RP5-1087L19	1.3	Mat	M	Rosenberg et al., 2006; case 13

[a]   NR = Not reported; fl = flanking clones.
[b]   Mat = Maternal; Pat = paternal.
[c]   Homozygous deletion.
[d]   Partially deleted.

and vestibular dysgenesis were present. She has an atrial septal defect, a left renal agenesis and gonadotrophin deficiency. Mutation analysis of the *CHD7* gene was normal. The patient had a maternal duplication of three clones (1.5 to 7 Mb in size) of chromosome 16p13.11p12.3, karyotype 46,XX, arr cgh 16p13.11p12.3(RP11-489O1→RP11-288I13)×3.

Patient 8. As the only child to normal young parents, this adult man has short stature (167 cm), severe MR and behavioral problems. He has deep-set eyes, simple cupped ears and a pointed chin. He displays echolalia, is autistic and intransigent in his routine. The karyotype 46,XY, arr cgh 18q23(RP11-315M18, RP11-154H12)×3 indicates a 0.1–2-Mb duplication of chromosome 18q23.

Patient 9 (Menten et al., 2006; case 27). This 9-year-old girl with developmental delay/mental retardation had a short neck, long eyelashes, a wide nasal bridge, ptosis, preauricular pits on the left, and a unilateral cleft lip and palate. She had a truncus arteriosus, ureteronephrosis, dimples on the elbows, fetal finger pads, a hypotrophic left lower limb, a sandal gap of the toes and hypoplastic labia minora. The karyotype is 46,XX, arr cgh 22q11.21(XX-91c)×3.

Patient 10 (Menten et al., 2006; case 28). This 1-year-old boy with developmental delay, axial hypotonia, peripheral spasticity, microcephaly, upslanting palpebral fissures, wide

fingertips and fetal finger pads had a ventricular septal defect and an abdominal situs inversus. The karyotype was 46,XY, arr cgh Xp21.3(RP11-37E19, RP6-27C10)×3.

Review of the literature on imbalances inherited from normal parents

Table 1 summarizes the inherited chromosomal imbalances using array CGH at 1 Mb resolution as reported in the literature. Vissers et al. (2003) detected two of the five imbalances to be inherited in a total of 20 patients, Shaw-Smith et al. (2004) five of 12 cases with imbalances in 50 screened patients and Rosenberg et al. (2006) nine out of 20 imbalances detected in 81 patients. Overall, this amounts to a detection rate of 10% inherited imbalances, equivalent to 43% of the detected imbalances in this patient population. This is a low estimate since the origin of the imbalance could not be determined from four patients in the series of Rosenberg et al. (2006). De Vries et al. (2005) analyzed 100 patients with unexplained MR using an array with 100 kb resolution (32447 BACs). The ten de novo alterations were taken as pathologic whilst the reproducible DNA copy-number changes present in 97% of patients were considered as 'normal large-scale copy number variation'. Finally, Kriek et al. (2006) found six patients with chromosomal microduplications screening 105 patients with developmental delay and

MCA and another six with MCA without MR using a specialized array. Two had familial chromosome 7q11.23 duplications (1.4 to 1.7 Mb of paternal and 0.3 to 0.4 Mb of maternal origin), and one had a paternal 0.5–2.3-Mb chromosome 10q11.22 duplication.

From Table 1 it can be seen that by using the 1-Mb array 11 of the 12 familial deletions, and 12 of the 13 familial duplications spanned less than 4 Mb, mostly less than 2.0 Mb. The 6.9 to 11.8 Mb deleted in chromosome 5q34q35.1 and the 1.5 to 7.0 Mb duplicated chromosome 16p13.11p12.3 appear to be exceptions. The size of the imbalances is indeed larger in de novo than in inherited cases. The de novo deletions average 7.2 clones, de novo duplications 4.7 clones whilst inherited deletions average 1.75 clones and duplications 1.5 clones on the 1-Mb array (present study; Vissers et al., 2003; Shaw-Smith et al., 2004; Menten et al., 2006; Rosenberg et al., 2006). Interestingly, although in all series the patients found with microdeletions are at least twice as frequent as those with microduplications, the distribution is equal in inherited cases. The maternally inherited imbalances (62%) slightly outnumber the paternally inherited (38%) ones.

Discussion

The high frequency (around 40%) of imbalances in patients with MCA/MR inherited from a healthy parent and the identification of recurrent rare variants associated with a specific phenotype challenge the general view that familial variants are innocent and of no major phenotypic consequences. Some of these inherited imbalances will be truly *benign variants* and the finding of a developmental anomaly in the child will be purely coincidental, as is probably the situation in our cases 2, 5, 8 and 10. The 3p12.2 duplication of about 1 Mb in patient 2 is likely not causal for the phenotype as the only affected gene in this region codes for a glycogen-branching enzyme. It is unlikely that a gene dosage effect of this gene results in an MCA/MR phenotype (Menten et al., 2006). In patient 5 two chromosomal anomalies were detected. The 4.8–7.9-Mb de novo duplication of chromosome 17p11.2, the Smith-Magenis syndrome and adjacent regions, is most likely the dominant pathogenic component as it encompasses the 3.7-Mb duplication reported in a number of patients with a similar phenotype (Shaw et al., 2002). Hence, it is deemed unlikely that the small paternally inherited 9p21.3 deletion is causal for the phenotype. The maternally inherited duplication of chromosome 18q23 in patient 8 contains five protein coding genes, only one of which has been shown to be related to cataracts and a neuropathy. Since this is not the clinical presentation of this patient, we consider this duplication to be benign. Finally, the 0.3–1.3-Mb duplication of chromosome Xp21.3 in patient 10 is also found in his 26-year-old normal mother. This duplicated region overlaps with the *IL1RAPL1* gene, in which point mutations have been reported to cause non-specific mental retardation in males and learning disabilities in some female carriers, where this phenomenon is at-

tributed to different X-inactivation patterns. This duplication is, however, believed to be a polymorphism (our unpublished data).

Sharp et al. (2005) demonstrated that segmental duplications likely act as mediators of normal variation as well as genomic disease. It is thus not surprising that we find patients with normal or rare chromosomal imbalance variants, which are detected by screening of patients with MCA/MR but which may be true variants and not the cause of the problem.

On the other hand, it is imaginable that these rare or normal variants may cause pathology in a different genetic background, and it seems likely that a substantial number of these variants encompass disease *susceptibility loci* that through gene dosage imbalance can hamper normal human development. Cases with MCA/MR and similar imbalances to the ones reported here and being inherited from normal parents may support the potentially non-benign nature of these, examples of which are cases 1, 3, 4, 6, 7 and 9. The maternally inherited microdeletion in patient 1 involves similar clones to a de novo deletion previously reported (Menten et al., 2006; case 3) and a de novo 2.12-Mb duplication reported by de Vries et al. (2005; case 11) using a microarray containing 32,447 BACs. As all these cases presented with MCA/MR, the deletion in our patient is believed to be pathogenic, in spite of the fact that it is inherited from a phenotypically normal mother.

The region between the flanking markers of the paternally inherited 3p12.1 deletion in patient 2 contains one gene, *IGSF4D (SYNCAM2)*, coding for an immunoglobulin superfamily protein responsible for extracellular recognition and intercellular adhesion. The expression pattern and function of this gene is not yet elucidated, but the related *IGSF4 (SYNCAM1)* gene has 65% homology with those encoding the neural cell adhesion molecules 1 and 2 *(NCAM1* and *NCAM2)*. SYNCAM1 functions as a cell adhesion molecule at the synapse and immuno-reactivity against the protein is detected only in the brain. As patient 2 has brain anomalies, further analysis is required to elucidate the pathogenic role of this deletion. In patient 4, the deletion of chromosome 5q34q35.1 was inherited from a similarly affected mother and believed to be causal, as a number of similarly affected patients have been reported. The distal flanking clone RP11-20O22 in this patient is the one deleted de novo in another reported patient (Menten et al., 2006; case 8). The deleted clone in chromosome region 5q35.1 in this latter patient lies within the de novo 1.24-Mb duplicated region of a third patient (de Vries et al., 2005; case 4). It appears that there may be a common breakpoint in all three cases, in our case a proximal rearrangement, in the two others a distal one. Patient 6 has the same microdeletion as is found in her similarly affected sister, mildly affected mother and non-affected brother. Thus, this familial deletion is associated with phenotypic variation. It is of interest to note that one other patient has been reported with a breakpoint between clones RP11-231A23 and RP11-50C13 (Lalani et al., 2006). However, this patient had a deletion of at least 7.54 Mb proximal to clone RP11-231A23. Further cases are needed in order to assess whether this will be a relatively frequent breakpoint. Patient 7 with the maternally inherited duplication of 1.5–7.0 Mb in chromosome 16p (maximal region 16p13.11p12.3) (clones RP11-489O1, CTD-2504F3, RP11-288I13) exhibits one recurrent breakpoint. Kriek et al. (2006), using duplicon screening, reported one patient (case 5) with a de novo duplication of clones RP11-489O1 and CTD-2504F3 on chromosome 16p13.11 (size 0.8–2.4 Mb). A deletion of these same two clones has also been found in one patient in this series (parents not alive). She has severe mental retardation, short stature (height 143 cm), microcephaly (head circumference 51 cm), facial dysmorphism, suffers from epilepsy, has mood swings and has an ataxic gait. Therefore it seems that this deletion, at least in certain circumstances, results in a pathological phenotype. As this region contains many repeats, the precise breakpoints in these patients with a probable new microdeletion syndrome remain to be determined. That the mother of our patient did not manifest the syndrome as such is not unusual and is a phenomenon known to occur in other microdeletion/duplication syndromes as well. However, the size of the imbalance is exceptionally large. Alternatively, our findings may represent a polymorphism in this repeat-rich zone. The father of patient 9, with only mild learning disabilities, also has the 3-Mb duplication of chromosome 22q11.21. This duplication has previously been detected by array CGH screening (cases 19 and 20 – inheritance could not be determined; Rosenberg et al., 2006). The inheritance of this imbalance from a normal parent, and the variable expression, is well described in the literature (Portnoï et al., 2005; Yobb et al., 2005).

Recently, Barber (2005) described several potential mechanisms that could explain why a specific chromosomal imbalance only occasionally results in abnormal development: (1) phenotypic variation may extend into the normal range, (2) chromosomal non-penetrance, (3) unmasking of a recessive allele in the proband, (4) mosaicism in the parent, (5) imprinting at certain loci. At the molecular level different mechanisms may compensate for the abnormal dosages of expressed genes. (1) Allelic exclusion. At one locus, gene expression of dosage-sensitive genes may be variable. (2) Position effect variegation. Variability in expression near heterochromatic regions is well established in S. cerevisiae. Position effect variegation leads to silencing of genes in the euchromatic region. Thus far, it has only rarely been reported in humans (Schotta et al., 2003). (3) A hypothetical mechanism is transvection (Lupski and Stankiewicz, 2005). In transvection, interaction between similar alleles on homologous chromosomes would enable gene expression to be regulated *in trans*.

These models to explain phenotypic variability are mainly based on the assumption that the effect of an aneuploid phenotype is the sum of individual gene dosage effects. Wilson (1990) discussed an alternative hypothesis explaining aneuploid phenotypes. In the interactive hypothesis, aneuploid characteristics are viewed as network properties of genes within and outside the aneuploid segment. Networks of genes maintain homeostasis. Gene dosage imbalances may or may not, dependent on the dosage of all the players in the network, destabilize this homeostasis. It is clear from experimental evidence that both the additive and the interactive model may be at work and, dependent on the gene and phenotype under investigation, one or the other model may be more dominant. The genotype–phenotype collection efforts are mainly aimed at identifying these genes. However, if a gene is part of a larger homeostatic network, an imbalance may (1) not always have phenotypic consequences or (2) may not always result in a similar phenotype. Especially for the more complex congenital anomalies such as heart defects, facial malformations and many others, this latter process may be most important. To identify these genes, it thus will be important to collect not only data on de novo chromosomal imbalances but also the phenotypes and genotypes on affected patients with imbalances inherited from a normal parent.

These hypotheses also have an important clinical consequence. While, in general, the additive hypothesis will assume that a gene imbalance will recurrently result in a specific phenotype, the interactive hypothesis provides more room for variation. It is this latter hypothesis that variation may best explain why certain chromosomal imbalances are inherited from normal parents but may be causing developmental disorders in the offspring. Dependent on the genetic and environmental background, the homeostasis may be destabilized. The rare inherited imbalances from phenotypically 'normal' individuals may then sometimes result in disease. At the other end of the spectrum, imbalanced regions known to cause disorders can sometimes be tolerated. Examples are the scanty reports of subtelomeric imbalances in normal individuals (reviewed in Hochstenbach et al., 2006). The clinical consequence is that determining risk figures for rare chromosomal imbalances becomes difficult. Similarly, the detection of small imbalances during prenatal diagnosis will cause counseling dilemmas: whether a certain imbalance would result in a specific phenotype becomes subject to a higher degree of uncertainty.

In conclusion, a large number of rare small copy number variations, detected in patients with MCA/MR, are inherited from normal parents. While some of these imbalances may be benign variations, others are likely to represent susceptibility loci for disease. In order to obtain both more reliable clinical information and a better understanding of the potential role of the genes located within the imbalanced regions in the disease pathogenesis, it will be essential to compile both genotype and phenotype information on a large number of such patients. The clinical consequence is that providing recurrence risk figures for these rare imbalances is at present subject to speculation.

Acknowledgements

The authors wish to thank the MicroArray Facility, Flanders Interuniversity Institute for Biotechnology (VIB) for their help in the spotting of the arrays and the Mapping Core and Map Finishing groups of the Wellcome Trust Sanger Institute for the initial clone supply and verification.

References

Barber JC: Directly transmitted unbalanced chromosome abnormalities and euchromatic variants. J Med Genet 42:609–629 (2005).

Barber JCK, Maloney V, Hollox EJ, Stuke-Sontheimer A, du Bois G, et al: Duplications and copy number variants of 8p23.1 are cytogenetically indistinguishable but distinct at the molecular level. Eur J Hum Genet 13:1131–1136 (2005).

Bonaglia MC, Giorda R, Carrozzo R, Roncoroni ME, Grasso R, et al: 20-Mb duplication of chromosome 9p in a girl with minimal physical findings and normal IQ: narrowing of the 9p duplication critical area to 6 Mb. Am J Med Genet 112:154–159 (2002).

Conrad DF, Andrews TD, Carter NP, Hurles ME, Pritchard JK: A high-resolution survey of deletion polymorphism in the human genome. Nat Genet 38:75–81 (2006).

de Vries BBA, Pfundt R, Leisink M, Koolen DA, Vissers LELM, et al: Diagnostic genome profiling in mental retardation. Am J Hum Genet 77:606–616 (2005).

Feuk L, Carson AR, Scherer SW: Structural variation in the human genome. Nat Rev Genet 7:85–97 (2006).

Gardner RJM, Sutherland GR: Chromosome Abnormalities and Genetic Counselling. Third edition. (Oxford University Press, New York 2004).

Hinds DA, Kloek AP, Jen M, Chen X, Frazer KA: Common deletions and SNPs are in linkage disequilibrium in the human genome. Nat Genet 38:82–85 (2006).

Hochstenbach R, van Amstel HKP, Poot M: Microarray-based genome investigation: molecular karyotyping or segmental aneuploidy profiling? Eur J Hum Genet 14:262–265 (2006).

Iafrate AJ, Feuk L, Rivera MN, Listewnik ML, Donahoe PK, et al: Detection of large-scale variation in the human genome. Nat Genet 36:949–951 (2004).

Kriek M, White SJ, Szuhai K, Knijnenburg J, van Ommen G-JB, et al: Copy number variation in regions flanked (or unflanked) by duplicons among patients with developmental delay and/or congenital malformations; detection of reciprocal and partial Williams-Beuren duplications. Eur J Hum Genet 14:180–189 (2006).

Lalani SR, Sahoo T, Sanders ME, Peters SU, Bejjani BA: Coarctation of the aorta and mild to moderate developmental delay in a child with a de novo deletion of chromosome 15(q21.1q22.2). BMC Med Genet 7:8 (2006).

Lupski JR, Stankiewicz P: Genomic disorders: molecular mechanisms for rearrangements and conveyed phenotypes. PloS Genet 1:e49 (2005).

McCarroll SA, Hadnott TN, Perry GH, Sabeti PC, Zody MC, et al: Common deletion polymorphisms in the human genome. Nat Genet 38:86–92 (2006).

Menten B, Maas N, Thienpont B, Buysse K, Vandesompele J, et al: Emerging patterns of cryptic chromosomal imbalances in patients with idiopathic mental retardation and multiple congenital anomalies: a new series of 140 patients and review of the literature. J Med Genet 43:625–633 (2006).

Portnoï M-F, Lebas F, Gruchy N, Ardalan A, Biran-Mucignat V, et al: 22q11.2 duplication syndrome: two new familial cases with some overlapping features with DiGeorge/velocardiofacial syndromes. Am J Med Genet 137:47–51 (2005).

Rosenberg C, Knijnenburg J, Bakker E, Vianna-Morgante AM, Sloos W, et al: Array-CGH detection of micro rearrangements in mentally retarded individuals: clinical significance of imbalances present both in affected children and normal parents. J Med Genet 43:180–186 (2006).

Schotta G, Ebert A, Dorn R, Reuter G: Position-effect variegation and the genetic dissection of chromatin regulation in Drosophila. Semin Cell Dev Biol 14:67–75 (2003).

Schoumans J, Ruivenkamp C, Holmberg E, Kyllerman M, Anderlid B-M, Nordenskjöld M: Detection of chromosomal imbalances in children with idiopathic mental retardation by array based comparative genomic hybridisation (array-CGH). J Med Genet 42:699–705 (2005).

Sebat J, Lakshmi B, Troge J, Alexander J, Young J, et al: Large-scale copy number polymorphism in the human genome. Science 305:525–528 (2004).

Sharp AJ, Locke DP, McGrath SD, Cheng Z, Bailey JA, et al: Segmental duplications and copy-number variation in the human genome. Am J Hum Genet 77:78–88 (2005).

Shaw CJ, Bi W, Lupski JR: Genetic proof of unequal crossovers in reciprocal deletion and duplication of 17p11.2. Am J Hum Genet 71:1072–1081 (2002).

Shaw-Smith C, Redon R, Rickman L, Rio M, Willatt L, et al: Microarray based comparative genomic hybridisation (array-CGH) detects submicroscopic chromosomal deletions and duplications in patients with learning disability/mental retardation and dysmorphic features. J Med Genet 41:241–248 (2004).

Vissers LELM, de Vries BBA, Osoegawa K, Janssen IM, Feuth T, et al: Array-based comparative genomic hybridization for the genomewide detection of submicroscopic chromosomal abnormalities. Am J Hum Genet 73:1261–1270 (2003).

Wilson GN: Karyotype/phenotype controversy: Genetic and molecular implications of alternative hypotheses. Am J Hum Genet 36:500–505 (1990).

Yobb TM, Somerville MJ, Willatt L, Firth HV, Harrison K, et al: Microduplication and triplication of 22q11.2: A highly variable syndrome. Am J Hum Genet 76:865–876 (2005).

Cytogenet Genome Res 115:231–239 (2006)
DOI: 10.1159/000095919

Cytogenetic genotype-phenotype studies: Improving genotyping, phenotyping and data storage

I. Feenstra   H.G. Brunner   C.M.A. van Ravenswaaij

Radboud University Nijmegen Medical Centre, Department of Human Genetics, Nijmegen (The Netherlands)

Manuscript received 17 February 2006; accepted in revised form for publication by A. Geurts van Kessel, 2 May 2006.

Abstract. High-resolution molecular cytogenetic techniques such as genomic array CGH and MLPA detect submicroscopic chromosome aberrations in patients with unexplained mental retardation. These techniques rapidly change the practice of cytogenetic testing. Additionally, these techniques may improve genotype-phenotype studies of patients with microscopically visible chromosome aberrations, such as Wolf-Hirschhorn syndrome, 18q deletion syndrome and 1p36 deletion syndrome. In order to make the most of high-resolution karyotyping, a similar accuracy of phenotyping is needed to allow researchers and clinicians to make optimal use of the recent advances. International agreements on phenotype nomenclature and the use of computerized 3D face surface models are examples of such improvements in the practice of phenotyping patients with chromosomal anomalies. The combination of high-resolution cytogenetic techniques, a comprehensive, systematic system for phenotyping and optimal data storage will facilitate advances in genotype-phenotype studies and a further deconstruction of chromosomal syndromes. As a result, critical regions or single genes can be determined to be responsible for specific features and malformations.

Copyright © 2006 S. Karger AG, Basel

New molecular cytogenetic techniques like array-based comparative genomic hybridization (array CGH) (Pinkel et al., 1998; Speicher and Carter, 2005) and Multiplex Ligation-dependent Probe Amplification (MLPA) (Schouten et al., 2002) can be used to search for submicroscopic chromosome aberrations in patients with unexplained mental retardation (Koolen et al., 2004; de Vries et al., 2005). In addition, these techniques will improve genotype-phenotype studies of patients with microscopically visible chromosomal imbalances by precisely determining the genomic region affected. The exact determination of breakpoints needed for genotype-phenotype studies used to be very time-consuming and only feasible for rather common cytogenetic syndromes. Examples are the determination of the Wolf-Hirschhorn syndrome critical region on chromosome 4p and the cat-cry region on chromosome 5p in Cri du Chat syndrome (Niebuhr, 1978b; Wright et al., 1997). An overview of current cytogenetic and molecular techniques used in clinical cytogenetics is given in Table 1.

Nowadays, size and location of chromosome aneuploidies can be determined with very high accuracy by tiling path BAC arrays, oligonucleotide arrays or SNP arrays in one single test run (Barrett et al., 2004; Slater et al., 2005; Vissers et al., 2005).

As high-resolution genotyping is rapidly becoming routine, phenotyping with an equally high accuracy is needed to fully benefit from the advantages of these new techniques.

In this report the impact of new techniques on genotype-phenotype studies is reviewed on the basis of various chromosomal syndromes. Advantages and limitations of the new approaches will be discussed, as will the need for sophisticated phenotyping and data collection.

Request reprints from Ilse Feenstra
    Radboud University Nijmegen Medical Centre
    Department of Human Genetics 849, P.O. Box 9101
    NL–6500 HB Nijmegen (The Netherlands)
    telephone: +31 24 361 39 46; fax: +31 24 366 87 74
    e-mail: i.feenstra@antrg.umcn.nl

KARGER

Fax +41 61 306 12 34
E-Mail karger@karger.ch
www.karger.com

© 2006 S. Karger AG, Basel
1424–8581/06/1154–0231$23.50/0

Accessible online at:
www.karger.com/cgr

Deconstructing chromosomal syndromes

With the use of new molecular techniques, various chromosome syndromes have been analyzed in detail. Whereas in some a single gene appeared to be responsible for most of the phenotypic features, for other syndromes an increasing number of critical regions for specific clinical features can be determined. In this section we first describe the detection of critical regions and some candidate genes in a number of microscopically visible chromosome disorders. Subsequently, some examples are given of submicroscopic aberrations in which single genes appear to play a major role in the phenotypes of patients.

Cri du Chat syndrome (5p–)

Cri du Chat syndrome (CDC, OMIM 123450) was first described by Lejeune and co-workers in 1963 (Lejeune et al., 1963). The syndrome is caused by a partial deletion of the short arm of chromosome 5 and is characterized by a high-pitched cat-like cry, microcephaly, facial dysmorphology and mental retardation (Niebuhr, 1978a). Chromosome analysis showed different deletion sizes, but no clear association between deletion size and the clinical features could be demonstrated (Miller et al., 1969). In 1978, Niebuhr made an attempt to locate the genetic segment responsible for the clinical features of Cri du Chat syndrome by investigating 35 individuals with a 5p– karyotype (Niebuhr, 1978b). He concluded that the typical features of this syndrome were probably caused by a deletion of the midportion of the 5p15 segment, more specifically 5p15.2. This region is shown in the schematic overview in Fig. 1.

These findings have subsequently been confirmed (Overhauser et al., 1994; Church et al., 1995; Gersh et al., 1995; Mainardi et al., 2001).

Recently, Zhang and co-authors applied the new array CGH technique to analyze genomic DNA of 94 patients

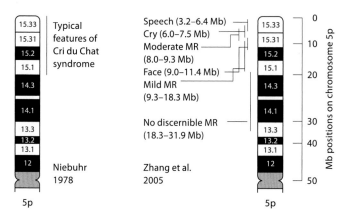

Fig. 1. Schematic overview of the clinical features of Cri du Chat syndrome and the associated critical regions on chromosome 5p. Array CGH was used in the study shown on the right, resulting in a significant refinement of the critical regions. MR = Mental retardation.

Table 1. Overview of techniques used in clinical cytogenetics

Technique	Resolution; deletion sizes to be detected	Detectable level of mosaicism	Detection of balanced aberrations	Turn-around time	Additional requirements	Relative estimated costs
Routine karyotyping	≥ 5–10 Mb	Depending on number of cells examined; ≥ 1%	Possible	3–10 days	– Experienced personnel for correct interpretation	Low
FISH	100 kb	≥ 20%	Possible	1–7 days	– Clinical indication of possible loci responsible – Labour intensive	High; depending on number of annual investigations
Multicolour FISH/SKY	2–3 Mb	10%	Possible	1–7 days	– Clinical indication of suspected loci responsible	High
Comparative genomic hybridisation	≥ 3–10 Mb	≥ 50%	Not possible	5–7 days	– Experienced personnel – Labour intensive	High
MLPA	~ 0.1 kb	≥ 40%	Not possible	1–4 days	– Clinical indication of possible loci responsible	Low; depending on number of annual investigations
BAC array (3–32 K)	Depending on number of clones; 100 kb–1 Mb	Depending on size of aberration and array coverage; ≥ 30%	Not possible	1–4 days	– Sophisticated equipment – Standardized storage system – Thorough statistical support	High
Oligonucleotide array	Depending on number of clones; 1–250 kb	Depending on size of aberration and array coverage; currently unknown	Not possible	1–4 days	– Sophisticated equipment – Standardized storage system – Thorough statistical support	Very high
SNP array (100–500 K)	Depending on number of clones; 10–250 kb	Depending on size of aberration and array coverage; currently unknown	Not possible	1–4 days	– Sophisticated equipment – Standardized storage system – Thorough statistical support	Very high

with known deletions of 5p (Zhang et al., 2005). A detailed clinical description was available for all patients. The authors were able to define three critical regions for the cry, speech delay, and facial dysmorphology on 5p15.31, 5p15.32→p15.33 and 5p15.2→p15.31, respectively. Moreover, they concluded that there were three adjacent regions on chromosome 5p that have differential effects on the level of mental retardation (MR) if deleted. A distal 1.2-Mb deletion in 5p15.31 produces moderate MR, whereas isolated deletions of more proximal located regions result in mild or no discernable MR. In Fig. 1 an overview of critical regions associated with the different clinical features is provided.

Wolf-Hirschhorn syndrome (4p–)

In 1965, groups led by Wolf and Hirschhorn each described a patient with a deletion of the short arm of chromosome 4 presenting with growth delay, mental retardation, and congenital anomalies suggestive of a midline fusion defect (Hirschhorn et al., 1965; Wolf et al., 1965). Numerous case-reports on similar patients followed.

One of the first studies in which the investigators tried to localize the segment of chromosome 4p associated with the clinical features of Wolf-Hirschhorn syndrome (WHS, OMIM 194190) was published in 1981 (Wilson et al., 1981). Giemsa-banding (GTG) was performed in 13 patients. The authors concluded that the critical region involved in WHS is within 4p16, the most distal band of the p-arm (Fig. 2).

However, a terminal deletion could not be detected in all patients displaying the clinical features of WHS by routine karyotyping. The contribution of new molecular cytogenetic techniques such as fluorescence in situ hybridisation (FISH), enabled the diagnosis of WHS in patients with submicroscopic interstitial or terminal deletions or subtle unbalanced translocations (Altherr et al., 1991; Johnson et al., 1994).

A preliminary phenotypic map of chromosome 4p16 was put forward in 1995. A systematic genotype-phenotype analysis was performed in 11 patients with chromosome 4p deletions and/or rearrangements (Estabrooks et al., 1995). It was suggested that specific regions within 4p16 correlated with different clinical features.

In 1997 the WHS critical region (WHSCR) was refined to 165 kb with FISH using a series of landmark cosmids from a collection of WHS patient-derived cell lines (Wright et al., 1997; see Fig. 2). The WHSCR is a gene-rich region and contains, among others, the *FGFR3* gene, which is mutant in achondroplasia and other skeletal dysplasias.

Another gene designated as Wolf-Hirschhorn Syndrome Candidate 1 *(WHSC1)* was described in 1998 (Stec et al., 1998). This 25 exon gene was found to be expressed ubiquitously in early development and to undergo complex alternative splicing and differential polyadenylation. It encodes a 136-kDa protein containing four domains also present in other developmental proteins. It is expressed preferentially in rapidly growing embryonic tissues, in a pattern corre-

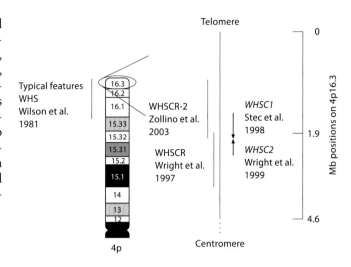

Fig. 2. Schematic overview of the deconstruction of the Wolf-Hirschhorn syndrome in critical regions and candidate genes. WHS = Wolf-Hirschhorn syndrome; WHSCR = WHS critical region; WHSCR-2 = WHS critical region 2; *WHSC1* = WHS candidate gene 1; *WHSC2* = WHS candidate gene 2.

sponding to the affected organs in WHS patients. The nature of the protein motifs, the expression pattern, and its mapping to the critical region led the authors to propose *WHSC1* as a good candidate gene for WHS. A second candidate gene *(WHSC2)* was identified one year later (Wright et al., 1999). The location of both candidate genes is depicted in Fig. 2.

In 2000 an Italian group reported the cytogenetic, molecular, and clinical findings in 16 WHS patients (Zollino et al., 2000). Submicroscopic deletions ranging from 2.8 to 4.4 Mb were detected in four patients. In one patient, no molecular deletion could be detected within the WHSCR. The precise definition of the cytogenetic defect permitted an analysis of genotype/phenotype correlations in WHS, leading to the proposal of a set of minimal diagnostic criteria. Deletions of less than 3.5 Mb resulted in a mild phenotype in which major malformations were absent. The authors proposed a 'minimal' WHS phenotype in which the clinical manifestations are restricted to the typical facial appearance, mild mental and growth retardation, and congenital hypotonia.

In 2003, the same group reported their findings in eight patients carrying a 4p16.3 microdeletion (Zollino et al., 2003). The WHSCR was fully preserved in one patient with a 1.9-Mb deletion, in spite of a typical WHS phenotype. Therefore, the authors proposed a new critical region, WHSCR2, a 300-kb interval located distally from the known WHSCR1 (Fig. 2). Furthermore, for the purpose of genetic counseling, they recommended dividing the WHS phenotype into two distinct clinical entities, i.e., a 'classical' and a 'mild' form, which are usually caused by cytogenetically visible and submicroscopic deletions, respectively. Another patient with a 1.9-Mb subtelomeric deletion was described in 2005, which supports the proposed WHSCR2 (Rodriguez et al., 2005).

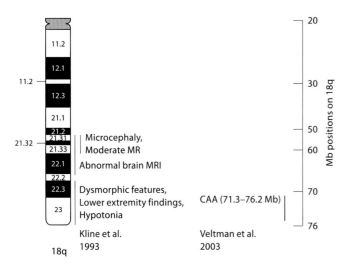

Fig. 3. Overview of the short arm of chromosome 18 and the critical regions defined for distinctive clinical features. MR = Mental retardation; CAA = congenital aural atresia.

A Belgian group reported six additional patients with an atypical 4p16.3 deletion, of whom five patients showed a (very) mild form of WHS and one patient had no clinical signs of WHS (Van Buggenhout et al., 2004). By means of a contiguous 4pter BAC array, the sizes and breakpoints were physically mapped and four terminal deletions (range 0.4–3.81 Mb) and two interstitial deletions (1.55 and 1.7 Mb) were revealed. This study enabled further refinement of the phenotypic map of this region, suggesting hemizygosity of *WHSC1* to cause the typical WHS facial appearance.

In summary, although molecular analysis allows a more detailed view of the WHS critical regions, the exact contribution of each of the proposed critical regions to the WHS phenotype still remains to be determined.

De Grouchy syndrome (18q–)

The 18q deletion syndrome (OMIM 601808) was described first in 1964 by de Grouchy et al. (1964). Most 18q cases are associated with terminal deletions and the phenotype of this syndrome is mainly characterized by mental retardation, hypotonia, short stature, ear anomalies and a flat midface. A first preliminary phenotypic map based on seven patients with deletions of 18q21.3 or 18q22.2 to 18qter was published in 1993 (Kline et al., 1993). In Fig. 3 an overview of clinical features and associated chromosome regions is provided.

Moreover, a substantial percentage of 18q– patients has congenital aural atresia (CAA), leading to hearing loss (Cody et al., 1999).

By applying array CGH, a critical region for CAA was mapped on 18q22.3→q23 (Veltman et al., 2003). The authors used a 670-kb resolution chromosome 18-specific BAC array to analyse genomic DNA of 20 patients with CAA. Of these, 18 patients had a microscopically visible 18q

deletion. In two patients, a submicroscopic 18q deletion was detected which allowed the mapping of CAA to a region of 5 Mb located in 18q22.3→q23 (Fig. 3).

2q deletions

Since 1988 a few patients with a deletion of 2q32→q33 have been described (Miyazaki et al., 1988; Palmer et al., 1990; Kreuz and Wittwer, 1993; Vogels et al., 1997).

BAC array and FISH analyses were used to delineate the deletion size to a critical region of 8.1 Mb in four patients (Van Buggenhout et al., 2005). Three patients displayed psychiatric and behavioural problems (hyperactivity, aggressiveness, anxiety) and shared a commonly deleted region of 0.5 Mb just proximal of the proximal deletion breakpoint of the fourth patient, who lacked behavioural problems. Within this region two genes are located that could cause the behavioural phenotype.

1p36 deletions

This relatively common chromosome aberration has been known for less than ten years as it was discovered only in 1997 (Shapira et al., 1997). With an estimated prevalence of one in 5,000 live births, monosomy of 1p36 (OMIM 607872) is the most common terminal deletion syndrome (Shaffer and Lupski, 2000). Because of the variability in deletion size, parental origin and clinical presentation, it has been proposed that monosomy 1p36 is a contiguous gene syndrome in which haploinsufficiency of functionally unrelated genes leads to the phenotypic features (Wu et al., 1999).

In 2003, a first physical map of 1p36 deletions was published (Heilstedt et al., 2003). First, DNA samples of 61 patients were screened with 25 microsatellite markers for the most distal part of 1p36. Then, a contig of 99 overlapping large-insert clones of this 10.5-Mb region was used to further refine the deletion size. Furthermore, clinical phenotypes of 30 patients were carefully defined. The authors proposed critical regions for hypotonia (2.2-Mb region from the telomere), a large fontanel (2.2 Mb), hearing loss (2.5 Mb), cardiomyopathy (3.1 Mb), hypothyroidism (4.1 Mb) and clefting (4.1 Mb). Because the terminal region of 1p36 is gene rich, no candidate genes could be determined.

In the same year, this group published their data using a dedicated 1p36 array CGH (Yu et al., 2003). This array was designed by using the previously assembled contig, consisting of 97 clones from 1p36, supplemented by clones for the subtelomeric regions of all chromosomes and clones for both sex-chromosomes. Genomic DNA of twenty-five patients with well-defined 1p36 deletions was studied and the array results agreed with the previously determined deletion sizes and breakpoint locations as detected by FISH and microsatellite analyses.

Recently, a tiling resolution BAC array covering 99.5% of the euchromatic parts of chromosome 1 has been applied to

Cytogenet Genome Res 115:231–239 (2006)

study six patients with a 1p36 deletion phenotype. In all patients a 1p36 deletion was confirmed, with sizes ranging from 2 to 10 Mb. Remarkably, in two clinically similar patients two non-overlapping deletions were detected. Therefore, the authors concluded that the 1p36 phenotype is a consequence of distinct and non-overlapping deletions having a positional effect rather than being a true contiguous gene deletion syndrome (Redon et al., 2005).

Cytogenetic microdeletion syndromes and the impact of single genes

In a number of (micro)deletion syndromes, the molecular determination of breakpoints together with a comparison of clinical features has resulted in such small critical regions that single genes appear to be responsible for the (majority of) phenotypic features.

An example is Smith-Magenis Syndrome (SMS, OMIM 182290), characterized by behavioural problems, speech delay, psychomotor and growth retardation and distinct craniofacial anomalies (Smith et al., 1998). About 75% of the SMS patients have a common deletion spanning 3.5 Mb in the 17p11.2 region, although deletion sizes vary from 1.5 to 9 Mb (Greenberg et al., 1991; Vlangos et al., 2003). Recently, a number of patients who fulfil the criteria for SMS but without the 17p11.2 deletion were analyzed for mutations of the *RAI1* gene, located within the central portion of the critical region for SMS, using PCR and sequencing strategies (Slager et al., 2003; Bi et al., 2004; Girirajan et al., 2005). This resulted in the identification of nine patients having *RAI1* mutations and to the conclusion that haploinsufficiency of this gene is associated with the craniofacial, behavioral and neurological symptoms of SMS.

The 22q13 deletion syndrome (OMIM 606232) is characterized by neonatal hypotonia, severe expressive language delay in combination with mild mental retardation (Prasad et al., 2000). Included in the critical region of this syndrome is the *SHANK3/ProSAP2* gene, which is preferentially expressed in the cerebral cortex and the cerebellum. DNA analysis of *SHANK3/ProSAP2* in a patient carrying a de novo balanced translocation between chromosomes 12 and 22, t(12;22)(q24.1;q13.3), revealed a disruption within exon 21 (Bonaglia et al., 2001). Since the patient displayed all 22q13.3 deletion features, the authors proposed that *SHANK3/ProSAP2* haploinsufficiency is the cause of the 22q13 deletion syndrome. This finding was supported by another group who tested 45 patients with variable sizes of 22q13 deletions, thereby confirming a deletion for the *SHANK3/ProSAP2* gene in all patients (Wilson et al., 2003). A recent study using array CGH for molecular characterization of nine patients with 22q13 aberrations identified deletion sizes ranging from 3.3 to 8.4 Mb (Koolen et al., 2005). The authors did not observe a relation between clinical features and deletion size, thereby supporting the idea that a gene in the 3.3-Mb minimal deleted region, notably *SHANK3/ProSAP2*, may be the major candidate gene in the 22q13 deletion syndrome. Another group using array CGH

Table 2. Examples of cytogenetic microdeletion syndromes in which single genes appear to be responsible for the (majority of) clinical features

Syndrome	Chromosome location	Gene responsible
Smith Magenis syndrome	17p11.2	*RAI1*
22q13 deletion syndrome	22q13.3	*SHANK3/ProSAP2*
9q34 deletion syndrome	9q34	*EHMT1*
Rubinstein-Taybi syndrome	16p13.3	*CREBBP, EP300*
Sotos syndrome	5q35	*NSD1*
DiGeorge/VCFS syndrome	22q11.2	*TBX1*

reported their findings in two unrelated 22q13.3 deletion patients (Bonaglia et al., 2006), which were consistent with the concept of *SHANK3/ProSAP2* being the best candidate gene for the neurological deficits in the 22q13.3 syndrome, although patients with the same kind of *SHANK3/ProSAP2* disruption can exhibit different degrees of severity in their phenotype.

Another terminal deletion syndrome is the 9q34 subtelomeric deletion syndrome. This syndrome is characterized by severe mental retardation, hypotonia, microcephaly and a typical face with midface depression, hypertelorism, everted lower lip, cupid bow configuration of the upper lip, and a prominent chin. The minimum critical region involved is ~1.2 Mb in size and encompasses at least 14 genes (Stewart et al., 2004). In a mentally retarded patient with a typical 9qter deletion phenotype, a balanced translocation t(X;9) (p11.23;q34.3) was detected (Kleefstra et al., 2005). Sequence analysis of the breakpoints revealed a disruption of *EHMT1*, indicating that haploinsufficiency of this gene may be responsible for the 9q subtelomeric deletion syndrome. In fact, we have since analysed the *EHMT1* gene in a series of patients with clinical phenotypes suggestive of a 9qter deletion whose telomere region was intact according to FISH and MLPA. We found a de novo nonsense mutation in one such patient and a frameshift in another (Kleefstra et al., 2006). This establishes that *EHMT1* haploinsufficiency is indeed the cause of the 9qter deletion phenotype.

Other examples of cytogenetic syndromes of which the (majority of) clinical features appear to be caused by mutations in single genes are Rubinstein-Taybi Syndrome (RSTS, OMIM 180849), Sotos syndrome (OMIM 117550) and DiGeorge/VCFS Syndrome (DGS, OMIM 188400) (Petrij et al., 1995; Jerome and Papaioannou, 2001; Kurotaki et al., 2002; Yagi et al., 2003; Roelfsema et al., 2005). Furthermore, it has been described that atypical deletions may be associated with variant phenotypes (Rauch et al., 2003, 2005).

These examples illustrate how the boundary between cytogenetic deletion syndromes and single gene conditions is becoming more and more indistinct. Ultimately, we should be able to assess the phenotype contribution of each gene within known microdeletion/microduplication syndromes.

An overview of the above-mentioned syndromes and the possible genes responsible for most phenotypic features is given in Table 2.

The phenotype; how and what to describe

The phenotype, defined as the appearance (physical, biochemical and physiological) of an individual which results from the interaction of the environment and the genotype, is usually presented in scientific articles by a clinical description, sometimes accompanied by clinical photographs. Any description of clinical features of a patient is inherently subjective. It varies between independent physicians and any emphasis on specific features may reflect the background speciality of the observer.

Description of phenotypes

To overcome the bias of subjectivity, proposals have been made to standardize the phenotype description by a systematic collection of clinical information (Freimer and Sabatti, 2003; Hall, 2003; Merks et al., 2003).

A detailed proposal for the organization and standardization of clinical descriptions of human malformations has recently been made (Biesecker, 2005). The author felt that, in contrast to the enormous improvements in molecular biology, the processes and approaches of the clinical component of molecular dysmorphology have not changed substantially. He argued that the current way of collecting phenotypic information holds several weaknesses. The quality and completeness of clinical descriptions published in the medical literature depend on the authors and editors involved. Another threat is confusion in understanding the terms used by the authors, due to the existence of synonyms, various definitions for one word, and sometimes overlapping of two different terms. The author pointed out a number of criteria for an ideal standardized clinical genetics nomenclature.

Standardization of phenotype descriptions will be crucial for a 'Human Phenome Project', in which comprehensive databases are created for such systematically collected phenotypic information (Freimer and Sabatti, 2003). The authors argued that phenotypic information should be collected on different levels: molecules, cells, tissues and whole organisms.

Visualization of phenotype

In a number of cytogenetic syndromes, such as WHS or 1p36 deletion syndrome, the clinical diagnosis is primarily based on characteristic facial features. Clinical geneticists are trained in recognizing specific patterns in different syndromes and can do this relatively well (Winter, 1996). Multiple efforts have been made to implement objective, quantitative criteria and analytical techniques for craniofacial assessments (Allanson, 1997; Shaner et al., 2001). In previous decades, anthropometry, photogrammetry and cephalometry have been applied as diagnostic methods (Garn et al., 1984, 1985; Richtsmeier, 1987; DiLiberti and Olson, 1991).

More recently, computer programs have been designed to analyze and identify faces of patients with certain syndromes on the basis of specific craniofacial features. In one study, standardized photographs of 55 patients with different syndromes were analyzed in a mathematical way by comparing feature vectors at 32 facial nodes (Loos et al., 2003). Over 75% of the patients were correctly classified by the computer, whereas clinicians who were shown the same pictures achieved a recognition rate of 62%.

More recently, a large study on computer-based three-dimensional (3D) imaging of the face of 696 individuals was published (Hammond et al., 2005). This study demonstrated the potential contributions of dense surface models (DSM) in clinical training, making clinical diagnoses and objective comparisons. Such mathematical pattern recognition might improve phenotype-genotype analyses, particularly in patients with rare or atypical chromosome aberrations.

A first application of 3D face surface models in genotype-phenotype studies was demonstrated in Williams-Beuren syndrome (WBS, OMIM 194050), involving a 7q11.23 deletion (Tassabehji et al., 2005). As the typical deletion size in WBS is 1.5 Mb and contains 28 genes, a clear genotype-phenotype correlation for craniofacial features could not be made so far. In this study, a patient with a small, atypical deletion was identified and 3D surface images of this patient's face were compared with those of WBS-individuals and controls. The patient was classified as borderline WBS with mildly dysmorphic features. Chromosome analysis revealed a heterozygous deletion at 7q11.23 of ~1 Mb, resulting in reduced expression of the *GTF2IRD1* gene. In mice, homozygous loss of *Gtf2ird1* results in craniofacial abnormalities reminiscent of those seen in WBS, together with growth retardation. These observations suggest that *GTF2IRD1* plays a role in mammalian craniofacial and cognitive development. The authors suggested that cumulative dosage of TFII-I family genes explains the main phenotypes of WBS. *Gtf2ird1*-null mice and classic WBS patients have two functional copies (*in trans* and *cis*, respectively), whereas the atypical patient had three functional genes of the *GTF2IRD1/GTF2I* cluster and showed a milder WBS phenotype.

Storage of genomic and clinical data

Cytogenetic and clinical information concerning specific chromosomal disorders are continuously published in the (inter)national medical literature. Thus, systematic collection and archiving are essential.

Many of these reports have been collected in the 'Catalogue of Unbalanced Chromosome Aberrations in Man', containing around 2,000 descriptions of patients with a rare chromosome aberration (Schinzel, 2001). This catalogue provides an unprecedented resource for genotype-phenotype studies in cytogenetically visible chromosome anomalies. In order to perform searches directed towards specific chromosome aberrations and/or clinical features, a computerized version is commercially available as the Zurich Cytogenetic Database, which contains cytogenetic and clinical information on more than 7,200 cases from the medical literature and references to the original papers (Schinzel, 1994).

In the past decennium, a number of internet databases have been created. These databases allow users online access to databases which are constantly being updated.

One of the databases collecting cytogenetic, molecular, and clinical information on patients with rare unbalanced chromosome aberrations is the ECARUCA database (http://www.ecaruca.net) (Feenstra et al., 2006). This database is based on information from the Zurich Cytogenetic Database, and is frequently supplemented by new data of patients with (sub)microscopic chromosomal aberrations by a European network of cytogenetic laboratories. In this password protected database, geneticists can search for information on more than 1,500 different chromosome aberrations of almost 4,100 cases. Frequent submission of new cases is performed by the account holders, thereby ensuring the up-to-date quality of the collection. In addition, data is centrally checked for usage of correct cytogenetic nomenclature and description of clinical features before inclusion in the database. ECARUCA is interactive, dynamic and has long-term possibilities to store molecular data. Also, parents of children whose data have been entered in the database can anonymously add follow-up information through the website.

A specialized database for submicroscopic chromosome aberrations is Decipher (http://www.sanger.ac.uk/PostGenomics/decipher/). This database currently contains information on 38 microdeletion/-duplication syndromes and, like ECARUCA, members are asked to actively participate in the submission of new cases.

Linking the above mentioned databases to genome browsers allows users to directly search for molecular information in their chromosome region of interest. By comparing the clinical features of different patients and their (non) overlapping aberrations at the molecular level, this can be a helpful tool in genotype-phenotype studies.

Analysing data stored in databases

Using a mathematical model, chromosome maps for specific malformation patterns based on the catalogue of unbalanced chromosome disorders and associated congenital malformations collected in the Zurich Cytogenetic Database were created (Brewer et al., 1998, 1999). The chromosomal deletion map was assembled through the analysis of 1,753 patients with a single, non-mosaic contiguous autosomal deletion and the presence of common major malformations. This resulted in 284 positive associations between specific malformations and deleted bands, distributed among 137 malformation-associated chromosome regions (MACRs).

In a second article, a chromosomal duplication map was described. Here, a total of 143 MACRs were identified, of which 21 were highly significant.

Obviously, such maps should always be interpreted with care. Although the number of cases available for analysis was high, the accuracy of breakpoints is not known since the cytogenetic analyses were mostly performed with standard karyotyping. Nonetheless, this type of analyses can point to those chromosome regions where the search for loci involved in congenital malformations is most likely to be successful. This has been abundantly proven in the case of holoprosencephaly, where at least four genes have been found based on chromosomal mapping of critical regions (Muenke et al., 1994; Brown et al., 1995, 1998; Overhauser et al., 1995; Schell et al., 1996; Wallis et al., 1999).

As more and more submicroscopic deletions and duplications are mapped, further candidate genes for specific malformations will be revealed. For instance, a recent study in 100 patients with mental retardation and malformations detected a small duplication in 5q35.1 in a patient with lobar holoprosencephaly (de Vries et al., 2005). This region contains seven known genes of which *FBXW11* is a likely candidate gene for holoprosencephaly (Koolen et al., 2006).

Conclusion and future prospects

There are many rapid advances in genotype-phenotype studies in chromosome disorders. Many improvements have been made in the field of genotyping, leading to the detection of smaller and smaller genomic deletions and duplications. Moreover, new cytogenetic molecular techniques allow for the exact determination of breakpoints in microscopically visible aberrations.

The capacity to investigate a high number of patients by undertaking automated genotyping projects is no longer the limiting step in elucidating the molecular basis of cytogenetic syndromes. Only an equally high accuracy of phenotyping will allow researchers and clinicians to make optimal use of the recent advances in genotyping. Objective, standardized descriptions and/or visualizations of the phenotype will be critical to determine the role of critical regions or candidate genes detected by new molecular techniques.

The combination of high-resolution cytogenetic techniques, a comprehensive, systematic approach for phenotyping and collection of this information in sophisticated databases will lead to advances in genotype-phenotype studies. Thereby, a further deconstruction of chromosomal syndromes in which critical regions or single genes appear to be responsible for specific features is to be expected.

Acknowledgements

The authors would like to thank Joris Veltman and Bert de Vries for critical reading of the manuscript.

References

Allanson JE: Objective techniques for craniofacial assessment: what are the choices? Am J Med Genet 70:1–5 (1997).

Altherr MR, Bengtsson U, et al: Molecular confirmation of Wolf-Hirschhorn syndrome with a subtle translocation of chromosome 4. Am J Hum Genet 49:1235–1242 (1991).

Barrett MT, Scheffer A, et al: Comparative genomic hybridization using oligonucleotide microarrays and total genomic DNA. Proc Natl Acad Sci USA 101:17765–17770 (2004).

Bi W, Saifi GM, et al: Mutations of RAI1, a PHD-containing protein, in nondeletion patients with Smith-Magenis syndrome. Hum Genet 115:515–524 (2004).

Biesecker LG: Mapping phenotypes to language: a proposal to organize and standardize the clinical descriptions of malformations. Clin Genet 68:320–326 (2005).

Bonaglia MC, Giorda R, et al: Disruption of the Pro-SAP2 gene in a t(12;22)(q24.1;q13.3) is associated with the 22q13.3 deletion syndrome. Am J Hum Genet 69:261–268 (2001).

Bonaglia MC, Giorda R, et al: Identification of a recurrent breakpoint within the SHANK3 gene in the 22q13.3 deletion syndrome. J Med Genet 43:822–828 (2006).

Brewer C, Holloway S, et al: A chromosomal deletion map of human malformations. Am J Hum Genet 63:1153–1159 (1998).

Brewer C, Holloway S, et al: A chromosomal duplication map of malformations: regions of suspected haplo- and triplolethality – and tolerance of segmental aneuploidy–in humans. Am J Hum Genet 64:1702–1708 (1999).

Brown J, Russo J, et al: The 13q- syndrome: the molecular definition of a critical deletion region in band 13q32. Am J Hum Genet 57:859–866 (1995).

Brown SA, Warburton D, et al: Holoprosencephaly due to mutations in ZIC2, a homologue of Drosophila odd-paired. Nat Genet 20:180–183 (1998).

Church DM, Bengtsson U, et al: Molecular definition of deletions of different segments of distal 5p that result in distinct phenotypic features. Am J Hum Genet 56:1162–1172 (1995).

Cody JD, Ghidoni PD, et al: Congenital anomalies and anthropometry of 42 individuals with deletions of chromosome 18q. Am J Med Genet 85:455–462 (1999).

De Grouchy J, Royer P, et al: Partial deletion of the long arms of the chromosome 18. Pathol Biol (Paris) 12:579–582 (1964).

de Vries BB, Pfundt R, et al: Diagnostic genome profiling in mental retardation. Am J Hum Genet 77:606–616 (2005).

DiLiberti JH, Olson DP: Photogrammetric evaluation in clinical genetics: theoretical considerations and experimental results. Am J Med Genet 39:161–166 (1991).

Estabrooks LL, Rao KW, et al: Preliminary phenotypic map of chromosome 4p16 based on 4p deletions. Am J Med Genet 57:581–586 (1995).

Feenstra I, Fang J, et al: European Cytogeneticists Association Register of Unbalanced Chromosome Aberrations (ECARUCA); An online database for rare chromosome abnormalities. Eur J Med Genet 49:279–291 (2006).

Freimer N, Sabatti C: The human phenome project. Nat Genet 34:15–21 (2003).

Garn SM, Smith BH, et al: Applications of pattern profile analysis to malformations of the head and face. Radiology 150:683–690 (1984).

Garn SM, Lavelle M, et al: Quantification of dysmorphogenesis: pattern variability index, sigma z. AJR Am J Roentgenol 144:365–369 (1985).

Gersh M, Goodart SA, et al: Evidence for a distinct region causing a cat-like cry in patients with 5p deletions. Am J Hum Genet 56:1404–1410 (1995).

Girirajan S, Elsas LJ 2nd, et al: RAI1 variations in Smith-Magenis syndrome patients without 17p11.2 deletions. J Med Genet 42:820–828 (2005).

Greenberg F, Guzzetta V, et al: Molecular analysis of the Smith-Magenis syndrome: a possible contiguous-gene syndrome associated with del(17)(p11.2). Am J Hum Genet 49:1207–1218 (1991).

Hall JG: A clinician's plea. Nat Genet 33:440–442 (2003).

Hammond P, Hutton TJ, et al: Discriminating power of localized three-dimensional facial morphology. Am J Hum Genet 77:999–1010 (2005).

Heilstedt HA, Ballif BC, et al: Physical map of 1p36, placement of breakpoints in monosomy 1p36, and clinical characterization of the syndrome. Am J Hum Genet 72:1200–1212 (2003).

Hirschhorn K, Cooper HL, et al: Deletion of short arms of chromosome 4–5 in a child with defects of midline fusion. Humangenetik 1:479–482 (1965).

Jerome LA, Papaioannou VE: DiGeorge syndrome phenotype in mice mutant for the T-box gene, Tbx1. Nat Genet 27:286–291 (2001).

Johnson VP, Altherr MR, et al: FISH detection of Wolf-Hirschhorn syndrome: exclusion of D4F26 as critical site. Am J Med Genet 52:70–74 (1994).

Kleefstra T, Smidt M, et al: Disruption of the gene Euchromatin Histone Methyl Transferase1 (EuHMTase1) is associated with the 9q34 subtelomeric deletion syndrome. J Med Genet 42:299–306 (2005).

Kleefstra T, Brunner HG, et al: Loss of function mutations in euchromatin histone methyl transferase 1 (EHMT1) cause the 9q34 subtelomeric deletion syndrome. Am J Hum Genet 79:370–377 (2006).

Kline AD, White ME, et al: Molecular analysis of the 18q- syndrome – and correlation with phenotype. Am J Hum Genet 52:895–906 (1993).

Koolen DA, Nillesen WM, et al: Screening for subtelomeric rearrangements in 210 patients with unexplained mental retardation using multiplex ligation dependent probe amplification (MLPA). J Med Genet 41:892–899 (2004).

Koolen DA, Reardon W, et al: Molecular characterisation of patients with subtelomeric 22q abnormalities using chromosome specific array-based comparative genomic hybridisation. Eur J Hum Genet 13:1019–1024 (2005).

Koolen DA, Herbergs J, et al: Holoprosencephaly and preaxial polydactyly associated with a 1.24 Mb duplication encompassing FBXW11 at 5q35.1. J Hum Genet 51:721–726 (2006).

Kreuz FR, Wittwer BH: Del(2q)–cause of the wrinkly skin syndrome? Clin Genet 43:132–138 (1993).

Kurotaki N, Imaizumi K, et al: Haploinsufficiency of NSD1 causes Sotos syndrome. Nat Genet 30:365–366 (2002).

Lejeune J, Lafourcade J, et al: 3 Cases of partial deletion of the short arm of chromosome 5. C R Hebd Seances Acad Sci 257:3098–3102 (1963).

Loos HS, Wieczorek D, et al: Computer-based recognition of dysmorphic faces. Eur J Hum Genet 11:555–560 (2003).

Mainardi PC, Perfumo C, et al: Clinical and molecular characterisation of 80 patients with 5p deletion: genotype-phenotype correlation. J Med Genet 38:151–158 (2001).

Merks JH, van Karnebeek CD, et al: Phenotypic abnormalities: terminology and classification. Am J Med Genet A 123:211–230 (2003).

Miller DA, Warburton D, et al: Clustering in deleted short-arm length among 25 cases with a Bp-chromosome. Cytogenetics 8:109–116 (1969).

Miyazaki K, Yamanaka T, et al: Interstitial deletion 2q32.1→q34 in a child with half normal activity of ribulose 5-phosphate 3-epimerase (RPE). J Med Genet 25:850–851 (1988).

Muenke M, Gurrieri F, et al: Linkage of a human brain malformation, familial holoprosencephaly, to chromosome 7 and evidence for genetic heterogeneity. Proc Natl Acad Sci USA 91:8102–8106 (1994).

Niebuhr E: The Cri du Chat syndrome: epidemiology, cytogenetics, and clinical features. Hum Genet 44:227–275 (1978a).

Niebuhr E: Cytologic observations in 35 individuals with a 5p- karyotype. Hum Genet 42:143–156 (1978b).

Overhauser J, Huang X, et al: Molecular and phenotypic mapping of the short arm of chromosome 5: sublocalization of the critical region for the cri-du-chat syndrome. Hum Mol Genet 3:247–252 (1994).

Overhauser J, Mitchell HF, et al: Physical mapping of the holoprosencephaly critical region in 18p11.3. Am J Hum Genet 57:1080–1085 (1995).

Palmer CG, Heerema N, et al: Deletions in chromosome 2 and fragile sites. Am J Med Genet 36:214–218 (1990).

Petrij F, Giles RH, et al: Rubinstein-Taybi syndrome caused by mutations in the transcriptional co-activator CBP. Nature 376:348–351 (1995).

Pinkel D, Segraves R, et al: High resolution analysis of DNA copy number variation using comparative genomic hybridization to microarrays. Nat Genet 20:207–211 (1998).

Prasad C, Prasad AN, et al: Genetic evaluation of pervasive developmental disorders: the terminal 22q13 deletion syndrome may represent a recognizable phenotype. Clin Genet 57:103–109 (2000).

Rauch A, Beese M, et al: A novel 5q35.3 subtelomeric deletion syndrome. Am J Med Genet A 121:1–8 (2003).

Rauch A, Zink S, et al: Systematic assessment of atypical deletions reveals genotype-phenotype correlation in 22q11.2. J Med Genet 42:871–876 (2005).

Redon R, Rio M, et al: Tiling path resolution mapping of constitutional 1p36 deletions by array-CGH: contiguous gene deletion or 'deletion with positional effect' syndrome? J Med Genet 42:166–171 (2005).

Richtsmeier JT: Comparative study of normal, Crouzon, and Apert craniofacial morphology using finite element scaling analysis. Am J Phys Anthropol 74:473–493 (1987).

Rodriguez L, Zollino M, et al: The new Wolf-Hirschhorn syndrome critical region (WHSCR-2): a description of a second case. Am J Med Genet A 136:175–178 (2005).

Roelfsema JH, White SJ, et al: Genetic heterogeneity in Rubinstein-Taybi syndrome: mutations in both the CBP and EP300 genes cause disease. Am J Hum Genet 76:572–580 (2005).

Schell U, Wienberg J, et al: Molecular characterization of breakpoints in patients with holoprosencephaly and definition of the HPE2 critical region 2p21. Hum Mol Genet 5:223–229 (1996).

Schinzel A: Zurich Cytogenetics Database (1994).

Schinzel A: Catalogue of Unbalanced Chromosome Aberrations in Man. (De Gruyter, Berlin 2001).

Schouten JP, McElgunn CJ, et al: Relative quantification of 40 nucleic acid sequences by multiplex ligation-dependent probe amplification. Nucleic Acids Res 30:e57 (2002).

Shaffer LG, Lupski JR: Molecular mechanisms for constitutional chromosomal rearrangements in humans. Annu Rev Genet 34:297–329 (2000).

Shaner DJ, Peterson AE, et al: Soft tissue facial resemblance in families and syndrome-affected individuals. Am J Med Genet 102:330–341 (2001).

Shapira SK, McCaskill C, et al: Chromosome 1p36 deletions: the clinical phenotype and molecular characterization of a common newly delineated syndrome. Am J Hum Genet 61:642–650 (1997).

Slager RE, Newton TL, et al: Mutations in *RAI1* associated with Smith-Magenis syndrome. Nat Genet 33:466–468 (2003).

Slater HR, Bailey DK, et al: High-resolution identification of chromosomal abnormalities using oligonucleotide arrays containing 116,204 SNPs. Am J Hum Genet 77:709–726 (2005).

Smith AC, Dykens E, et al: Behavioral phenotype of Smith-Magenis syndrome (del 17p11.2). Am J Med Genet 81:179–185 (1998).

Speicher MR, Carter NP: The new cytogenetics: blurring the boundaries with molecular biology. Nat Rev Genet 6:782–792 (2005).

Stec I, Wright TJ, et al: *WHSC1*, a 90 kb SET domain-containing gene, expressed in early development and homologous to a *Drosophila dysmorphy* gene maps in the Wolf-Hirschhorn syndrome critical region and is fused to *IgH* in t(4;14) multiple myeloma. Hum Mol Genet 7:1071–1082 (1998).

Stewart DR, Huang A, et al: Subtelomeric deletions of chromosome 9q: a novel microdeletion syndrome. Am J Med Genet A 128:340–351 (2004).

Tassabehji M, Hammond P, et al: *GTF2IRD1* in craniofacial development of humans and mice. Science 310:1184–1187 (2005).

Van Buggenhout G, Melotte C, et al: Mild Wolf-Hirschhorn syndrome: micro-array CGH analysis of atypical 4p16.3 deletions enables refinement of the genotype-phenotype map. J Med Genet 41:691–698 (2004).

Van Buggenhout G, Van Ravenswaaij-Arts C, et al: The del(2)(q32.2q33) deletion syndrome defined by clinical and molecular characterization of four patients. Eur J Med Genet 48:276–289 (2005).

Veltman JA, Jonkers Y, et al: Definition of a critical region on chromosome 18 for congenital aural atresia by array CGH. Am J Hum Genet 72:1578–1584 (2003).

Vissers LE, Veltman JA, et al: Identification of disease genes by whole genome CGH arrays. Hum Mol Genet 14 Spec No. 2:R215–223 (2005).

Vlangos CN, Yim DK, et al: Refinement of the Smith-Magenis syndrome critical region to approximately 950 kb and assessment of 17p11.2 deletions. Are all deletions created equally? Mol Genet Metab 79:134–141 (2003).

Vogels A, Haegeman J, et al: Pierre-Robin sequence and severe mental retardation with chaotic behaviour associated with a small interstitial deletion in the long arm of chromosome 2 (del(2)(q331q333)). Genet Couns 8:249–252 (1997).

Wallis DE, Roessler E, et al: Mutations in the homeodomain of the human *SIX3* gene cause holoprosencephaly. Nat Genet 22:196–198 (1999).

Wilson HL, Wong AC, et al: Molecular characterisation of the 22q13 deletion syndrome supports the role of haploinsufficiency of *SHANK3/PROSAP2* in the major neurological symptoms. J Med Genet 40:575–584 (2003).

Wilson MG, Towner JW, et al: Genetic and clinical studies in 13 patients with the Wolf-Hirschhorn syndrome [del(4p)]. Hum Genet 59:297–307 (1981).

Winter RM: What's in a face? Nat Genet 12:124–129 (1996).

Wolf U, Reinwein H, et al: Deficiency on the short arms of a chromosome No. 4. Humangenetik 1:397–413 (1965).

Wright TJ, Ricke DO, et al: A transcript map of the newly defined 165 kb Wolf-Hirschhorn syndrome critical region. Hum Mol Genet 6:317–324 (1997).

Wright TJ, Costa JL, et al: Comparative analysis of a novel gene from the Wolf-Hirschhorn/Pitt-Rogers-Danks syndrome critical region. Genomics 59:203–212 (1999).

Wu YQ, Heilstedt HA, et al: Molecular refinement of the 1p36 deletion syndrome reveals size diversity and a preponderance of maternally derived deletions. Hum Mol Genet 8:313–321 (1999).

Yagi H, Furutani Y, et al: Role of *TBX1* in human del22q11.2 syndrome. Lancet 362:1366–1373 (2003).

Yu W, Ballif BC, et al: Development of a comparative genomic hybridization microarray and demonstration of its utility with 25 well-characterized 1p36 deletions. Hum Mol Genet 12:2145–2152 (2003).

Zhang X, Snijders A, et al: High-resolution mapping of genotype-phenotype relationships in Cri du Chat syndrome using array comparative genomic hybridization. Am J Hum Genet 76:312–326 (2005).

Zollino M, Di Stefano C, et al: Genotype-phenotype correlations and clinical diagnostic criteria in Wolf-Hirschhorn syndrome. Am J Med Genet 94:254–261 (2000).

Zollino M, Lecce R, et al: Mapping the Wolf-Hirschhorn syndrome phenotype outside the currently accepted WHS critical region and defining a new critical region, WHSCR-2. Am J Hum Genet 72:590–597 (2003).

Cytogenet Genome Res 115:240–246 (2006)
DOI: 10.1159/000095920

Copy number variation in the genome; the human *DMD* gene as an example

S.J. White   J.T. den Dunnen

Human and Clinical Genetics, Leiden University Medical Center, Leiden (The Netherlands)

Manuscript received 2 March 2006; accepted in revised form for publication by A. Geurts van Kessel, 15 May 2006.

Abstract. Recent developments have yielded new technologies that have greatly simplified the detection of deletions and duplications, i.e., copy number variants (CNVs). These technologies can be used to screen for CNVs in and around specific genomic regions, as well as genome-wide. Several genome-wide studies have demonstrated that CNV in the human genome is widespread and may include millions of nucleotides. One of the questions that emerge is which sequences, structures and/or processes are involved in their generation. Using as an example the human *DMD* gene, mutations in which cause Duchenne and Becker muscular dystrophy, we review the current data, determine the deletion and duplication profile across the gene and summarize the information that has been collected regarding their origin. In addition we discuss the methods most frequently used for their detection, in particular MAPH and MLPA.

Copyright © 2006 S. Karger AG, Basel

There has been considerable recent interest in the analysis of copy number variation (CNV) in the human genome. Several studies have demonstrated that CNV is widespread throughout the genome, up to several Mb in size (Fredman et al., 2004; Iafrate et al., 2004; Sebat et al., 2004; Sharp et al., 2005). Other studies, using one or a few probes targeted at specific loci, have shown that CNV can involve wide ranges of copy numbers, from zero to >10 in apparently healthy individuals (Hollox et al., 2003; Aldred et al., 2005; Gonzalez et al., 2005; Stefansson et al., 2005). It is clear that considerable work is necessary with a range of different techniques to fully explore the true extent of CNV on a genome-wide level, as well as to determine its phenotypic consequences.

One of the questions that remain to be answered concerns the frequency and stability of de novo CNVs. Recently, it was proposed to use the *DMD* gene, involved in Duchenne and Becker Muscular Dystrophy (DMD), as a model for this subject (van Ommen, 2005). There are several features of this gene that make it attractive. It is the largest gene known (~2.3 Mb with 79 exons) (Den Dunnen et al., 1992) without any known repeat elements that lead to preferential rearrangement. In contrast to other regions of similar size that encompass whole genes, there is no selection bias in the detection of deletions versus duplications, as both lead to the same phenotype if they disturb the reading frame of the transcript (Monaco et al., 1988). Another significant advantage is that several thousand individuals have already been screened on an exon by exon basis (average probe density 30 kb), providing a thorough overview of the relative frequency and distribution of CNVs.

Here we will briefly discuss two methods currently used to detect CNV, in particular multiplex amplifiable probe hybridisation (MAPH; Armour et al., 2000) and multiplex ligation-dependent probe amplification (MLPA; Schouten et al., 2002), their application to study CNV, and the main differences with other methods. In addition, we will discuss work performed by others and ourselves to identify and characterize deletions and duplications in the *DMD* gene, and the lessons that can be learned from it.

Request reprints from Dr. J.T. den Dunnen
  Human and Clinical Genetics
  Leiden University Medical Center, Einthovenweg 20
  2333ZC NL–Leiden (The Netherlands)
  telephone: +31 71 526 9501/9400; fax: +31 71 526 8285
  e-mail: ddunnen@LUMC.nl

Methods for CNV detection

Many methods have been developed to study DNA copy number variations, i.e., deletions and duplications. In the past these methods were applied mainly to study local rearrangements in specific genomic regions, mostly in relation to genomic disease, e.g. Southern blotting, quantitative PCR, breakpoint PCR, and FISH. Recently, several new methods have been developed to study different regions in parallel or even genome wide, again in relation to genetic disease but, lately, also to explore the variation that is present in the human genome, e.g. MAPH, MLPA, array-CGH, SNP-chips, and ROMA. For diagnostic applications MAPH (Armour et al., 2000), and especially MLPA (Schouten et al., 2002), have become widely applied. Both techniques are simple and cost-effective and facilitate multiplex deletion/duplication screening of currently up to 50 loci simultaneously.

The high degree of multiplexing turns MAPH and MLPA into ideal techniques for targeted approaches, e.g. for confirming potential CNVs that have been identified using genome-wide approaches. Although both techniques are similar, the principle difference significantly affects the results obtained. MAPH is based on the hybridization of a single DNA fragment (Armour et al., 2000). As such, small changes within the target sequence are unlikely to have a significant effect on the result. In contrast, MLPA utilizes a ligation step to join two separate oligonucleotide half-probes after hybridization (Schouten et al., 2002). This means that sequence changes at or near the ligation site may disturb the ligase reaction such that the end result appears to be a deletion (Rooms et al., 2004; Janssen et al., 2005). This has obvious consequences for diagnostic testing, where a deletion detected with a single probe needs to be confirmed with another assay. The advantage of this extra sensitivity is that it allows the distinction of highly homologous sequences, by designing the half-probes such that a difference in sequence is located under the ligation site. This can be particularly important when analyzing duplicons, or for distinguishing a specific gene from a pseudogene.

It should be noted that nucleotide variants in the human genome can also significantly affect the results obtained by methods that use oligonucleotide arrays for genome-wide CNV screening. Both ROMA (Lucito et al., 2003) and Affymetrix SNP-chips (Bignell et al., 2004) use restriction enzyme digestion of genomic DNA, followed by the addition of linker sequences and PCR amplification to reduce sample complexity and to increase the signal obtained. Sequence changes (SNPs) will affect the digestion/amplification step; loss of an enzyme recognition site may make the expected fragment too large to amplify, whereas gain of a restriction site may interfere with probe hybridization. In addition, any variant in the genomic DNA complementary to the oligonucleotide probe on the array will cause a loss of signal.

Both MLPA and MAPH seem to be more sensitive than array-CGH in detecting small changes in copy number, and can be used as an initial screen for the presence or absence of CNV at duplicon sequences (Hollox et al., 2003; Fredman et al., 2004). More accurate determination of exact copy numbers can be performed with other, more precise approaches. Examples of the latter include quantitative PCR (Gonzalez et al., 2005), fiber-FISH (Florijn et al., 1995; Iafrate et al., 2004), and PFGE (Lemmers et al., 2001).

An important point that should not be neglected is that copy number is usually measured as the sum of two chromosomes. This is not only of importance with regard to expression levels (e.g. parent-of-origin effects), but it may also lead to incorrect assumptions regarding the de novo status of a given rearrangement. Based on copy number, a person having two copies of a gene on one chromosome and zero copies on the other chromosome might be normal and without a phenotype. However, when the other parent is normal, with one copy on each chromosome, children will inherit either three copies or one, both situations with potentially pathogenic consequences. When encountered in a family, the obvious but incorrect conclusion will be that there is a 'de novo CNV' with subsequent consequences for genetic counseling. Only when a second child is born, which again shows a 'de novo CNV', will detailed analysis reveal the true nature of the CNV. Situations like this have been encountered in several diseases, e.g. in SMA where CNV of the *SMN1* gene (a deletion on one chromosome combined with a duplication on the other chromosome) may disguise the presence of a deleterious deletion allele, until it is transmitted to the offspring.

Intrinsically, deletions must directly affect a gene. It should be noted, however, that this direct correlation does not apply to duplications. Theoretically, the second copy (the duplicated sequence) can be anywhere in the genome and it remains to be proven that it disrupts the original gene copy. In most cases this possibility is merely hypothetical because, as for example in DMD, patients have been selected based on a specific phenotype, making it unlikely that a mutation that has been found does not affect the gene of interest. Still, in some rare cases transpositional duplications have been identified. One recent example of this is the transpositional duplication of the *SRY* gene to chromosome 16 in an XX-male (Dauwerse et al., 2006).

A form of variation that most of the molecular methodologies discussed above fail to detect is a positional rearrangement, i.e., transposition, inversion or translocation. Because of the difficulty in detecting them by conventional means, inversions are easily missed. A famous example is hemophilia A where ~50% of the cases are caused by an intra-chromosomal inversion (Lakich et al., 1993). This defect was discovered several years after the original identification of the disease gene, when a detailed study included RNA analysis. Recent data has demonstrated that inversions on a genome-wide level may be more common than previously thought (Feuk et al., 2005). Indeed, the copy number variation seen for part of the *NSF* gene is also associated with an inversion (Stefansson et al., 2005). Intragenic inversions are obviously important, as they will change the coding sequence of the gene. Inversions of an entire gene or genes can, by altering their location relative to control sequences, be expected to have an effect on their expression and/or their predisposition to rearrangements (Osborne et al., 2001).

The detection of rearrangements in the *DMD* gene

The identification of the *DMD* gene was facilitated by translocations (Ray et al., 1985) and a large deletion (Kunkel et al., 1985), both visible under the microscope. The ultimate cloning of its cDNA allowed the detection of smaller deletions and duplications using Southern blotting (Koenig et al., 1987; Darras et al., 1988; Den Dunnen et al., 1989; Hu et al., 1990), sometimes combined with PFGE (Den Dunnen et al., 1987, 1989). By doing so, it became clear that the majority of mutations in DMD/BMD patients were rearrangements of this sort. Two deletion hotspots were identified (Koenig et al., 1987; Den Dunnen et al., 1989), and based on this information two multiplex PCR sets were developed, each amplifying nine exons (Chamberlain et al., 1988; Beggs et al., 1990). These primer sets were later expanded and modified using fluorescently-labeled primers and dosage analysis, allowing duplications to be detected as well (Abbs and Bobrow, 1992; Ioannou et al., 1992).

Currently, multiplex PCR kits allow the detection of ~98% of deletions. However, to allow a prediction regarding disease severity (DMD or BMD), the effect on the reading frame needs to be assessed. In order to do this, it is usually necessary to screen the entire gene for determination of the exact breakpoints of the rearrangement. Southern blot analysis using cDNA probes was for long the method of choice to establish the exact breakpoints. However, since seven hybridizations were required to screen all 79 exons of the gene this method was time-consuming and costly. In addition, the detection of duplications, especially in females, was challenging and only successful in the hands of experts. The development and implementation of two new methods as described above, i.e., MAPH (White et al., 2002) and MLPA (Schwartz and Duno, 2004; Dent et al., 2005; Janssen et al., 2005; Lalic et al., 2005; White et al., 2006), greatly simplified this analysis. The use of MLPA to screen for deletions and duplications in the *DMD* gene is now routine in many diagnostic laboratories around the world.

DMD gene deletion and duplication profiles

To obtain an overview of the deletion and duplication profiles of the *DMD* gene we analyzed all rearrangements reported to date as collected by the DMD deletion/duplication database at the Leiden Muscular Dystrophy pages (http://www.DMD.nl/, version March 2005). The data reported below are based exclusively on those approaches that analyzed the entire gene, i.e. Southern blotting, MAPH and MLPA. We excluded duplications detected using the Protein Truncation Test (PTT), since this approach is biased towards the detection of small duplications and fails to detect larger ones.

In total 2,609 deletions and 301 duplications meeting our criteria were detected. Further analysis of these anomalies revealed that both deletions (Fig. 1) and duplications (Fig. 2) are distributed non-randomly across the gene. Deletions clearly show the two hotspots reported previously (Koenig

et al., 1987; Den Dunnen et al., 1989) with a major deletion hotspot around exons 45–52 and a minor (25% frequency) hotspot around exons 3–19 (Fig. 1).

It is apparent that deletions in the major hotspot show a strong directional effect, i.e., most deletions have the 5′ end in introns 44 and 45 and the 3′ end in introns 50–55 (compare the graphs for 5′ and 3′ breakpoints, Fig. 1B). Overall, the gradual increase of deletion breakpoints to the center (exon 49) and the absence of local breakpoint hotspots give the impression that sequences from the central region have a propensity to get deleted, with the deletion end points fading out towards both sides. Why this region shows such a propensity for deletion remains to be determined.

Many interesting features of this region have been reported. At 248 kb intron 44 is the largest intron of the *DMD* gene. Studies have shown that deletion breakpoints within this intron do not cluster, but are distributed relatively evenly (Blonden et al., 1991). Sequencing a range of deletion breakpoints did not reveal the involvement of any specific motif (Sironi et al., 2003).

Intron 44 contains a hotspot for meiotic recombination, like intron 7, the minor deletion hotspot (Oudet et al., 1992), and it can be hypothesized that the double-stranded breaks (DSBs) that occur during recombination may be casually related to the increased deletion susceptibility observed. Matrix attachment regions (MARs) are sequences of DNA that are involved in DNA looping and attachment to the protein scaffold (Boulikas, 1995). A co-localization of MARs and replication origins within the *DMD* gene has been described (Iarovaia et al., 2004), with one MAR again falling within the major deletion hotspot. It has been proposed that a relative paucity of MAR sites might lead to greater torsional stress within these regions (McNaughton et al., 1998). This would lead to an increased chance of DNA breakage and subsequent rearrangement. In addition, correlations between Loop Anchorage Regions (LARs) and recombination have been described (Svetlova et al., 2001).

Replication origins have been associated with chromosomal fragility (Toledo et al., 2000). Interestingly, six origins of replication have been identified in the *DMD* gene (Verbovaia and Razin, 1997). One replication termination site was mapped to intron 44. Studies in prokaryotes have shown that such termination sites may also serve as deletion hotspots (Bierne et al., 1991). An attractive hypothesis is that the deletion sensitivity of this region is somehow related to DNA replication; a scarcity of replication origins in the region might lead to incomplete DNA replication when cell division is initiated, yielding a deletion of the non-replicated sequences. A consequence of this scarcity would be that duplications should further increase the replication problem. As a result, duplications of the region might be rare and when present, unstable. In fact, this is exactly what has been found for duplications in the *DMD* gene (see below).

An analysis of deletions in mosaic cases showed a highly significant difference in distribution when compared to the expected frequencies (Passos-Bueno et al., 1992). Whereas the ratio of proximal to distal deletions is 1:3 overall, this was reversed when only confirmed mosaic cases were ana-

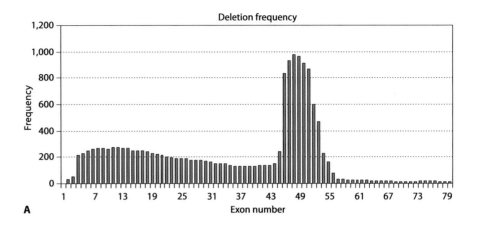

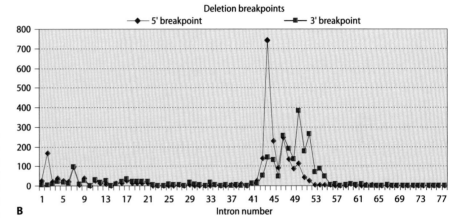

Fig. 1. Analysis of all deletions (2,609) reported in the Leiden Muscular Dystrophy database. Shown is the number of times each exon of the *DMD* gene is deleted (**A**) and how often a deletion breakpoint is located within an intron (**B**). Diamond = Start of deletion (5′ breakpoint); square = end of deletion (3′).

lyzed. Not only does this have consequences for genetic counseling when calculating risk estimates in apparently de novo cases (proximal rearrangements have a higher chance of recurring in a subsequent pregnancy), but it is also a clear illustration of the fact that 'hotspots' for rearrangement are dependent on various spatio-temporal factors, such as type of tissue, time of development (age), and type of cell division (meiotic or mitotic). This observation is not limited to the *DMD* gene, it was reported for *NF1* gene deletions that the extent of the rearrangement is dependent on whether it occurs during mitotic or meiotic cell division (Kehrer-Sawatzki et al., 2004).

Duplications

Because of a lack of sufficient data, the duplication profile of the *DMD* gene has not yet been reported. Our current analysis of the 301 duplications identified thus far shows that duplications in the *DMD* gene occur mostly near the 5′ end of the gene (Fig. 2), with exons 6 and 7 being duplicated most frequently (22% of cases). After this peak, the duplication frequency gradually decreases to 1% towards the 3′ end of the gene (exons 66–79) with small local increases at exons 18, 22, 38 and 51. Amongst these duplications there are 80 single-exon duplications, 26 of which are duplications of

exon 2 (9% overall frequency). The mean length of the duplications covers 7.1 exons (9.3 when single-exon duplications are excluded).

Figure 2B shows that most duplication breakpoints flank exon 2, 19% in total. A large fraction of these breakpoints seems to originate in intron 2 (67, or 11%), extending either towards exon 1 or, in a majority of the cases, towards exon 3 and further. The actual number of duplication breakpoints in intron 2 extending 5′ might be higher, as tandem duplications including the promoter region are not expected to disturb the reading frame, may not have a strong pathogenic effect and, therefore, would thus be missed.

Previous work studying duplications in the *DMD* gene has implicated cleavage sites for DNA topoisomerases (Hu et al., 1991). These proteins are known to play a role in DNA replication and transcription, breaking DNA molecules and altering chromatin conformation to allow these processes to take place (Wang et al., 1990; Gale and Osheroff, 1992). Whilst analyzing exon 2 duplications, we recently identified two ~6-kb hotspot regions within intron 2. Sequencing four breakpoints from this small region did not reveal any obvious homologous sequences at or near the breakpoints. At three of the duplication junctions multiple nucleotides were inserted (White et al., 2006), which is consistent with the process of non-homologous end joining (NHEJ) being involved in their generation.

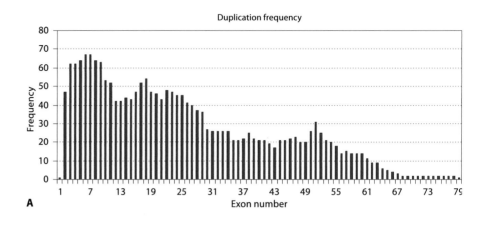

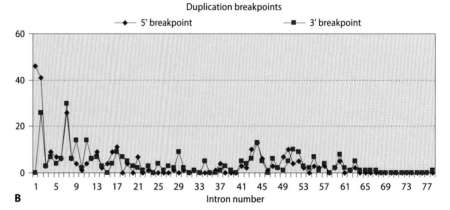

Fig. 2. Analysis of all duplications (301) reported in the Leiden Muscular Dystrophy database. Shown is the number of times each exon of the *DMD* gene is duplicated (**A**) and how often a duplication breakpoint is located within an intron (**B**). Diamond = Start of duplication (5′ breakpoint); square = end of duplication (3′).

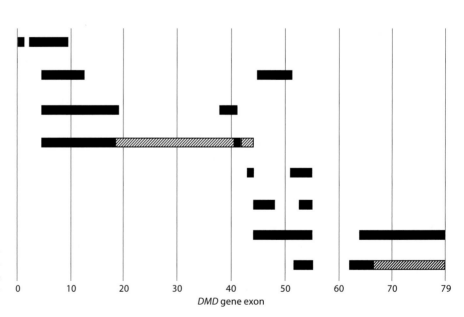

Fig. 3. The extent of all eight non-contiguous duplications described in the Leiden Muscular Dystrophy pages. Solid bars indicate duplicated exons; hatched bars indicate triplicated exons.

Interestingly, there are relatively few duplications in the deletion hotspot region, exons 45–55. If this deletion hotspot is related to a paucity of replication origins, then duplications can be expected to further increase the replication problem. As such one would expect, as is observed, a rather low duplication frequency for this region. Interestingly, the identification of non-contiguous duplications and triplications, nearly exclusively found in this region (Fig. 3), underscores the intrinsic instability of this region. Again this observation seems compatible with a local scarcity of replication origins, ultimately leading to a process reducing the size of the region to 'replicable length' (see above).

It should be noted that duplications can be more complex than expected. Using a combination of MLPA and RT-PCR we recently detected a multi-exon duplication (exons 52–62) that at the mRNA level leads, besides the duplication, to the unexpected deletion of a single exon, exon 63 (White et al., 2006). This result probably originates from a seemingly simple duplication, which in fact was a duplication/deletion event removing exon 63 from the original copy somewhere in the process of duplicating exons 52–63. This example, being one of few duplication cases analyzed at the mRNA level, shows that the reading frame rule (Monaco et al., 1988), often used to predict disease severity of *DMD* gene mutations, should be applied with great care and preferably only after analysis at the mRNA level. In case of non-contiguous duplications and triplications, one should not predict the effect on the transcript without further analysis. Analysis of duplications at other loci have also revealed complex rearrangements and transpositions, indicating that this phenomenon is not unique to the DMD locus (Gajecka et al., 2005; Woodward et al., 2005).

Conclusions

Locally duplicated sequences (duplicons) and low-copy repeats (LCRs) represent ~5% of the human genome. Several studies have shown that CNVs are overrepresented in regions overlapping with, or in close proximity of, duplicons and LCRs (Iafrate et al., 2004; Sebat et al., 2004; Sharp et al., 2005). Similarly, many genomic disorders are causally related to the local presence of such sequences (Inoue and Lupski, 2002). Although the *DMD* gene shows clear deletion and duplication hotspots, these rearrangements cannot be attributed to duplicons or LCRs. Clearly, other architectural features must lead to the increased rearrangement sus-

ceptibility at the DMD locus. It is anticipated that the human genome may harbor similar rearrangement hotspots.

Detailed analysis of the distribution and frequency of rearrangements within the *DMD* gene shows that regions prone to deletion may not necessarily have the same predisposition to duplications, and vice versa. A clear example of this is *DMD* exon 2. No deletions of only this exon have been reported, whereas its duplication is the most common rearrangement found. Several studies have recently identified a large number of loci that are commonly deleted (Conrad et al., 2006; Hinds et al., 2006; McCarroll et al., 2006). It seems attractive to use these loci to create a targeted 'rearrangement hotspot' array. Based on the observations made in the *DMD* gene, however, it seems clear that such an approach could easily miss those regions that may have a propensity to become duplicated.

Future prospects

Genome-wide studies have already identified a large number of potential loci showing non-pathogenic CNV, and these will only increase with further improvements in technologies (Iafrate et al., 2004; Sebat et al., 2004; Sharp et al., 2005; Conrad et al., 2006; Hinds et al., 2006; McCarroll et al., 2006). The next step is their confirmation, to identify their extent and frequency (including differences between populations) and to properly annotate and catalogue them. The latter will be very important to facilitate those studies that use the same tools to scan genome-wide for CNVs in relation to disease. Currently, the most problematic step in these studies is the follow-up of all CNVs detected, and determining which might be pathogenic. For this, an essential step will be to analyze a large series of normal control samples.

References

Abbs SJ, Bobrow M: Analysis of quantitative PCR for the diagnosis of deletion and duplication carriers in the dystrophin gene. J Med Genet 29: 191–196 (1992).

Aldred PM, Hollox EJ, Armour JA: Copy number polymorphism and expression level variation of the human alpha-defensin genes *DEFA1* and *DEFA3*. Hum Mol Genet 14:2045–2052 (2005).

Armour JA, Sismani C, Patsalis PC, Cross G: Measurement of locus copy number by hybridisation with amplifiable probes. Nucleic Acids Res 28:605–609 (2000).

Beggs AH, Koenig M, Boyce FM, Kunkel LM: Detection of 98 percent *DMD/BMD* gene deletions by polymerase chain reaction. Hum Genet 86: 45–48 (1990).

Bierne H, Ehrlich SD, Michel B: The replication termination signal terB of the *Escherichia coli* chromosome is a deletion hot spot. EMBO J 10: 2699–2705 (1991).

Bignell GR, Huang J, Greshock J, Watt S, Butler A, et al: High-resolution analysis of DNA copy number using oligonucleotide microarrays. Genome Res 14:287–295 (2004).

Blonden LAJ, Grootscholten PM, Den Dunnen JT, Bakker E, Abbs SJ, et al: 242 breakpoints in the 200-kb deletion-prone P20 region of the DMD-gene are widely spread. Genomics 10:631–639 (1991).

Boulikas T: Chromatin domains and prediction of MAR sequences. Int Rev Cytol 162A:279–388 (1995).

Chamberlain JS, Gibbs RA, Ranier JE, Nga Nguyen PN, Caskey CT: Deletion screening of the Duchenne muscular dystrophy locus via multiplex DNA amplification. Nucleic Acids Res 23: 11141–11156 (1988).

Conrad DF, Andrews TD, Carter NP, Hurles ME, Pritchard JK: A high-resolution survey of deletion polymorphism in the human genome. Nat Genet 38:75–81 (2006).

Darras BT, Blattner P, Harper JF, Spiro AJ, Alter S, Francke U: Intragenic deletions in 21 Duchenne muscular dystrophy (DMD)/Becker muscular dystrophy families studied with the dystrophin cDNA: location of breakpoints on *Hind*III and *Bgl*II exon-containing fragment maps, meiotic and mitotic origin of the mutations. Am J Hum Genet 43:620–629 (1988).

Dauwerse JG, Hansson KB, Brouwers AA, Peters DJ, Breuning MH: An XX male with the sex-determining region Y gene inserted in the long arm of chromosome 16. Fertil Steril 86:463.e1–e5 (2006).

Den Dunnen JT, Bakker E, Klein-Breteler EG, Pearson PL, Van Ommen GJB: Direct detection of more than 50% Duchenne muscular dystrophy mutations by field-inversion gels. Nature 329: 640–642 (1987).

Den Dunnen JT, Grootscholten PM, Bakker E, Blonden LAJ, Ginjaar HB, et al: Topography of the *DMD* gene: FIGE and cDNA analysis of 194 cases reveals 115 deletions and 13 duplications. Am J Hum Genet 45:835–847 (1989).

Den Dunnen JT, Grootscholten PM, Dauwerse JD, Monaco AP, Walker AP, et al: Reconstruction of the 2.4 Mb human DMD-gene by homologous YAC recombination. Hum Mol Genet 1: 19–28 (1992).

Dent KM, Dunn DM, von Niederhausern AC, Aoyagi AT, Kerr L, et al: Improved molecular diagnosis of dystrophinopathies in an unselected clinical cohort. Am J Med Genet A 134:295–298 (2005).

Feuk L, MacDonald JR, Tang T, Carson AR, Li M, et al: Discovery of human inversion polymorphisms by comparative analysis of human and chimpanzee DNA sequence assemblies. PLoS Genet 1:e56 (2005).

Florijn RJ, Blonden LAJ, Vrolijk H, Wiegant J, Vaandrager JW, et al: High-resolution FISH for genomic DNA mapping and colour bar-coding of large genes. Hum Mol Genet 4:831–836 (1995).

Fredman D, White SJ, Potter S, Eichler EE, Den Dunnen JT, Brookes AJ: Complex SNP-related sequence variation in segmental genome duplications. Nat Genet 36:861–866 (2004).

Gajecka M, Yu W, Ballif BC, Glotzbach CD, Bailey KA, et al: Delineation of mechanisms and regions of dosage imbalance in complex rearrangements of 1p36 leads to a putative gene for regulation of cranial suture closure. Eur J Hum Genet 13:139–149 (2005).

Gale KC, Osheroff N: Intrinsic intermolecular DNA ligation activity of eukaryotic topoisomerase II. Potential roles in recombination. J Biol Chem 267:12090–12097 (1992).

Gonzalez E, Kulkarni H, Bolivar H, Mangano A, Sanchez R, et al: The influence of CCL3L1 gene-containing segmental duplications on HIV-1/AIDS susceptibility. Science 307:1434–1440 (2005).

Hinds DA, Kloek AP, Jen M, Chen X, Frazer KA: Common deletions and SNPs are in linkage disequilibrium in the human genome. Nat Genet 38:82–85 (2006).

Hollox EJ, Armour JA, Barber JC: Extensive normal copy number variation of a beta-defensin antimicrobial-gene cluster. Am J Hum Genet 73:591–600 (2003).

Hu X, Ray PN, Murphy E, Thompson MW, Worton RG: Duplicational mutation at the Duchenne muscular dystrophy locus: its frequency, distribution, origin and phenotype/genotype correlation. Am J Hum Genet 46:682–695 (1990).

Hu X, Ray PN, Worton RG: Mechanisms of tandem duplication in the Duchenne muscular dystrophy gene include both homologous and nonhomologous intrachromosomal recombination. EMBO J 10:2471–2477 (1991).

Iafrate AJ, Feuk L, Rivera MN, Listewnik ML, Donahoe PK, et al: Detection of large-scale variation in the human genome. Nat Genet 36:949–951 (2004).

Iarovaia OV, Bystritskiy A, Ravcheev D, Hancock R, Razin SV: Visualization of individual DNA loops and a map of loop domains in the human dystrophin gene. Nucleic Acids Res 32:2079–2086 (2004).

Inoue K, Lupski JR: Molecular mechanisms for genomic disorders. Annu Rev Genomics Hum Genet 3:199–242 (2002).

Ioannou P, Christopoulos G, Panayides K, Kleanthous M, Middleton L: Detection of Duchenne and Becker muscular dystrophy carriers by quantitative multiplex polymerase chain reaction analysis. Neurol 42:1783–1790 (1992).

Janssen B, Hartmann C, Scholz V, Jauch A, Zschocke J: MLPA analysis for the detection of deletions, duplications and complex rearrangements in the dystrophin gene: potential and pitfalls. Neurogenetics 6:29–35 (2005).

Kehrer-Swatzki H, Kluwe L, Sandig C, Kohn M, Wimmer K, et al: High frequency of mosaicism among patients with neurofibromatosis type 1 (NF1) with microdeletions caused by somatic recombination of the JJAZ1 gene. Am J Hum Genet 75:410–423 (2004).

Koenig M, Hoffman EP, Bertelson CJ, Monaco AP, Feener CA, Kunkel LM: Complete cloning of the Duchenne muscular dystrophy (DMD) cDNA and preliminary genomic organization of the DMD gene in normal and affected individuals. Cell 50:509–517 (1987).

Kunkel LM, Monaco AP, Middlesworth W, Ochs HD, Latt SA: Specific cloning of DNA fragments absent from the DNA of a male patient with an X-chromosome deletion. Proc Natl Acad Sci USA 82:4778–4782 (1985).

Lakich D, Kazazian HHJ, Antonarakis SE, Gitschier J: Inversions disrupting the factor VIII gene are a common cause of severe haemophilia A. Nat Genet 5:236–241 (1993).

Lalic T, Vossen RH, Coffa J, Schouten JP, Guc-Scekic M, et al: Deletion and duplication screening in the DMD gene using MLPA. Eur J Hum Genet 13:1231–1234 (2005).

Lemmers RJL, de Kievit P, van Geel M, van der Wielen MJ, Bakker E, et al: Complete allele information in the diagnosis of facioscapulohumeral muscular dystrophy by triple DNA analysis. Ann Neurol 50:816–819 (2001).

Lucito R, Healy J, Alexander J, Reiner A, Esposito D, et al: Representational oligonucleotide microarray analysis: a high-resolution method to detect genome copy number variation. Genome Res 13:2291–2305 (2003).

McCarroll SA, Hadnott TN, Perry GH, Sabeti PC, Zody MC, et al: Common deletion polymorphisms in the human genome. Nat Genet 38:86–92 (2006).

McNaughton JC, Cockburn DJ, Hughes G, Jones WA, Laing NG, et al: Is gene deletion in eukaryotes sequence-dependent? A study of nine deletion junctions and nineteen other deletion breakpoints in intron 7 of the human dystrophin gene. Gene 222:41–51 (1998).

Monaco AP, Bertelson CJ, Liechti-Gallati S, Moser H, Kunkel LM: An explanation for the phenotypic differences between patients bearing partial deletions of the DMD locus. Genomics 2:90–95 (1988).

Osborne LR, Li M, Pober B, Chitayat D, Bodurtha J, et al: A 1.5 million-base pair inversion polymorphism in families with Williams-Beuren syndrome. Nat Genet 29:321–325 (2001).

Oudet C, Hanauer A, Clemens P, Caskey CT, Mandel JL: Two hot spots of recombination in the DMD-gene correlate with the deletion prone regions. Hum Mol Genet 1:599–603 (1992).

Passos-Bueno MR, Bakker E, Kneppers ALJ, Takata RI, Rapaport D, et al: Different mosaicism frequencies for proximal and distal Duchenne muscular dystrophy (DMD) mutations indicate difference in etiology and recurrence risk. Am J Hum Genet 51:1150–1155 (1992).

Ray PN, Belfall B, Duff C, Logan C, Kean V, et al: Cloning of the breakpoint of an X:21 translocation associated with Duchenne muscular dystrophy. Nature 318:672–675 (1985).

Rooms L, Reyniers E, van Luijk R, Scheers S, Wauters J, et al: Subtelomeric deletions detected in patients with idiopathic mental retardation using multiplex ligation-dependent probe amplification (MLPA). Hum Mutat 23:17–21 (2004).

Schouten JP, McElgunn CJ, Waaijer R, Zwijnenburg D, Diepvens F, Pals G: Relative quantification of 40 nucleic acid sequences by multiplex ligation-dependent probe amplification. Nucleic Acids Res 30:e57 (2002).

Schwartz M, Duno M: Improved molecular diagnosis of dystrophin gene mutations using the multiplex ligation-dependent probe amplification method. Genet Test 8:361–367 (2004).

Sebat J, Lakshmi B, Troge J, Alexander J, Young J, et al: Large-scale copy number polymorphism in the human genome. Science 305:525–528 (2004).

Sharp AJ, Locke DP, McGrath SD, Cheng Z, Bailey JA, et al: Segmental duplications and copy-number variation in the human genome. Am J Hum Genet 77:78–88 (2005).

Sironi M, Pozzoli U, Cagliani R, Giorda R, Comi GP, et al: Relevance of sequence and structure elements for deletion events in the dystrophin gene major hot-spot. Hum Genet 112:272–288 (2003).

Stefansson H, Helgason A, Thorleifsson G, Steinthorsdottir V, Masson G, et al: A common inversion under selection in Europeans. Nat Genet 37:129–137 (2005).

Svetlova EY, Razin SV, Debatisse M: Mammalian recombination hot spot in a DNA loop anchorage region: A model for the study of common fragile sites. J Cell Biochem 81:170–178 (2001).

Toledo F, Coquelle A, Svetlova E, Debatisse M: Enhanced flexibility and aphidicolin-induced DNA breaks near mammalian replication origins: implications for replicon mapping and chromosome fragility. Nucleic Acids Res 28:4805–4813 (2000).

van Ommen GJ: Frequency of new copy number variation in humans. Nat Genet 37:333–334 (2005).

Verbovaia LV, Razin SV: Mapping of replication origins and termination sites in the Duchenne muscular dystrophy gene. Genomics 45:24–30 (1997).

Wang JC, Caron PR, Kim RA: The role of DNA topoisomerases in recombination and genome stability: a double-edged sword? Cell 62:403–406 (1990).

White S, Kalf M, Liu Q, Villerius M, Engelsma D, et al: Comprehensive detection of genomic duplications and deletions in the DMD gene, by use of multiplex amplifiable probe hybridization. Am J Hum Genet 71:365–374 (2002).

White SJ, Aartsma-Rus A, Flanigan KM, Weiss RB, Kneppers ALJ, et al: Duplications in the DMD gene. Hum Mut 27:938–945 (2006).

Woodward KJ, Cundall M, Sperle K, Sistermans EA, Ross M, et al: Heterogeneous duplications in patients with Pelizaeus-Merzbacher disease suggest a mechanism of coupled homologous and nonhomologous recombination. Am J Hum Genet 77:966–987 (2005).

Cytogenet Genome Res 115:247–253 (2006)
DOI: 10.1159/000095921

Impact of low copy repeats on the generation of balanced and unbalanced chromosomal aberrations in mental retardation

F. Erdogan[a]   W. Chen[a]   M. Kirchhoff[b]   V.M. Kalscheuer[a]   C. Hultschig[a]
I. Müller[a]   R. Schulz[a]   C. Menzel[a]   T. Bryndorf[b]   H.-H. Ropers[a]   R. Ullmann[a]

[a]Max Planck Institute for Molecular Genetics, Department for Human Molecular Genetics, Berlin (Germany)
[b]Rigshospitalet, Department of Clinical Genetics, Copenhagen (Denmark)

Manuscript received 7 March 2006; accepted in revised form for publication by A. Geurts van Kessel, 19 May 2006.

Abstract. Low copy repeats (LCRs) are stretches of duplicated DNA that are more than 1 kb in size and share a sequence similarity that exceeds 90%. Non-allelic homologous recombination (NAHR) between highly similar LCRs has been implicated in numerous genomic disorders. This study aimed at defining the impact of LCRs on the generation of balanced and unbalanced chromosomal rearrangements in mentally retarded patients. A cohort of 22 patients, preselected for the presence of submicroscopic imbalances, was analysed using submegabase resolution tiling path array CGH and the results were compared with a set of 41 patients with balanced translocations and breakpoints that were mapped to the BAC level by FISH. Our data indicate an accumulation of LCRs at breakpoints of both balanced and unbalanced rearrangements. LCRs with high sequence similarity in both breakpoint regions, suggesting NAHR as the most likely cause of rearrangement, were observed in 6/22 patients with chromosomal imbalances, but not in any of the balanced translocation cases studied. In case of chromosomal imbalances, the likelihood of NAHR seems to be inversely related to the size of the aberration. Our data also suggest the presence of additional mechanisms coinciding with or dependent on the presence of LCRs that may induce an increased instability at these chromosomal sites.

Copyright © 2006 S. Karger AG, Basel

Low copy repeats (LCRs) are commonly defined as stretches of duplicated DNA that are larger than 1 kb in size and show sequence similarities exceeding 90%. LCRs are thought to constitute about 5% of the human genome and are clustered in the pericentromeric transition zones, the subtelomeres and several interspersed LCR hubs (Bailey et al., 2001, 2002; Cheung et al., 2001, 2003; Eichler, 2001; Horvath et al., 2001). A primate-specific burst of Alu retroposition activity about 35–40 million years ago has been implicated in their expansion (Bailey et al., 2003) and it has been speculated that this recent accumulation of LCRs may have driven primate speciation by generating new genes (Khaitovich et al., 2004; Stankiewicz et al., 2004 and references therein). In line with this notion, 33% of LCRs are found to be exclusively duplicated in humans, and not in chimpanzee (Cheng et al., 2005). Although LCRs may be important in an evolutionary sense, their existence poses a risk to the individual human genome, as non-allelic homologous recombination (NAHR) between these LCRs may lead to genomic instability, resulting in so-called genomic disorders (Lupski, 1998; Emanuel and Shaikh, 2001; Stankiewicz and Lupski, 2002). The probability of homologous recombination increases with sequence similarity (Elliott et al., 1998) and length of the duplicon. Nevertheless, the minimal efficiently processed segment necessary for recombination only requires a few hundred base pairs (Waldman and Liskay, 1988) and hot spots of recombination within duplicons have been encountered (Bi et al., 2003; Shaw et al., 2004; Visser et al., 2005). Double strand breaks (DSB) substantially increase the chance of homologous recombination, but there

Request reprints from Dr. Reinhard Ullmann
   Max Planck Institute for Molecular Genetics
   Department for Human Molecular Genetics
   Ihnestr. 73, DE–14195 Berlin (Germany)
   telephone: +49 30 8413 1251; fax: +49 30 8413 1383
   e-mail: ullmann@molgen.mpg.de
F.E. and W.C. contributed equally to this work.

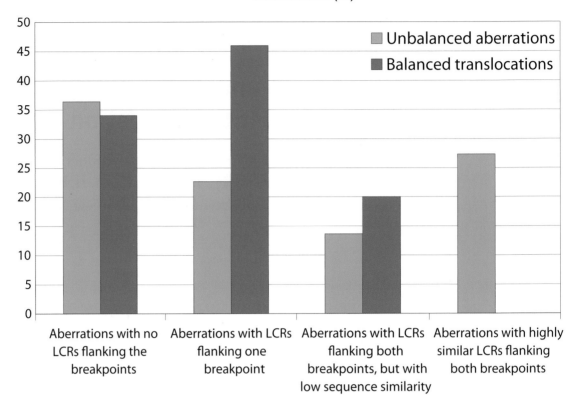

Fig. 1. Comparison of LCR frequency and sequence similarity at breakpoints of balanced and unbalanced aberrations. Data given in this chart are based on a 400-kb interval centered around the breakpoint (see Materials and methods section for details). LCR = Low copy repeat.

are mechanisms that suppress excessive NAHR in order to maintain genome stability (Elliott and Jasin, 2001). Although NAHR may represent a major pathway of DSB repair (Liang et al., 1998), non-homologous end joining (NHEJ) may therefore be the more common and less error-prone DSB repair mechanism in organisms with a large fraction of repetitive sequences (Lieber et al., 2003).

Less is known about the role of LCRs in constitutive balanced translocations. It appears that chromosomes 11, 17 and 22, mainly affecting regions with AT-rich palindromes embedded in LCRs, are more frequently involved and that they preferentially fuse with the telomeric regions of their translocation partner chromosomes (Kurahashi et al., 2000a, b, 2003, 2004; Edelmann et al., 2001; Kurahashi and Emanuel, 2001; Shaikh et al., 2001; Spiteri et al., 2003; Stankiewicz et al., 2003; Gotter et al., 2004). In this study we examined the impact of LCRs on the generation of balanced as well as unbalanced chromosomal rearrangements in mentally retarded patients. To this end, we have applied array CGH (Solinas-Toldo et al., 1997; Pinkel et al., 1998) to a set of 22 mentally retarded patients, pre-selected for the presence of unbalanced chromosomal aberrations, and compared these results with FISH mapping data from 41 mentally retarded patients with balanced translocations.

Materials and methods

Patient samples

For the present study, a cohort of 22 mentally retarded patients with unbalanced chromosomal anomalies was selected. In all but four cases, the imbalances were analysed and verified by HR-CGH (Kirchhoff et al., 1999, 2004). As controls we included three patients with known genomic disorders, i.e., Smith-Magenis syndrome (SMS) (case 16), Prader-Willi/Angelman syndrome (case 15) and 22q11 deletion/DiGeorge syndrome (case 7), respectively. The cohort used to estimate the role of LCRs in the generation of balanced translocations consisted of 41 mentally retarded patients, in whom the translocation breakpoints were fine mapped to the BAC level by FISH.

Array CGH

For array CGH a submegabase resolution tiling path BAC array was used, comprising the human 32k Re-Array set (http://bacpac.chori.org/pHumanMinSet.htm; clones and DNA kindly provided by Pieter de Jong) (Osoegawa et al., 2001; Ishkanian et al., 2004; Krzywinski et al., 2004), the 1 Mb Sanger set (clones kindly provided by Nigel Carter, Wellcome Trust Sanger Centre) (Fiegler et al., 2003), and a set of 390 subtelomeric clones (assembled by members of the COST B19 initiative: Molecular Cytogenetics of Solid Tumors). Cases 5, 7, 8 and 16 were hybridised on a 14 k array, with tiling path resolution only for chromosomes 4, 9, 10, 11, 16, 17, 21, 22, and X. All aberrations discussed in this paper were detected with a submegabase tiling path resolution. BAC DNA was amplified using linker-adapter ligation PCR. Amplified DNAs were ethanol precipitated, dissolved in 3× SSC, 1.5 M betaine

Table 1. Summary of LCR content of chromosomal breakpoint regions detected in 25 patients with mental retardation (400-kb interval). Cases are ordered according to aberration size. Three of these cases (7, 15 and 16 in bold) were known genomic disorders and were included as controls. Data given in this table are based on a 400-kb interval centered around the breakpoint (see Materials and methods section for details).

Case No.	LCR content[a] (upper breakpoint)	LCR content[a] (lower breakpoint)	Size of homologous sequence (bp)	Percentage of sequence identity	Size of aberration (bp)
1	3.088	2.898	146,337	0.996	651,903
2	5.162	4.37	310,722	0.957	1,620,202
3	1.218	1.615	44,532	0.995	1,620,803
4	0.0	0.0	0	0.0	1,742,093
5	2.299	3.041	200,031	0.987	2,042,922
6	1.454	1.769	48,352	0.987	2,347,885
7	**3.256**	**3.319**	**332,793**	**0.979**	**12,847,915**
8	1.835	0.0	0	0.0	3,354,593
9	0.0040	0.04	0	0.0	3,441,528
10	0.0	0.0	0	0.0	3,547,563
11	0.015	0.0	0	0.0	3,871,108
12	0.139	0.0080	0	0.0	4,335,684
13	0.0	0.0	0	0.0	4,353,899
14	0.0	0.0	0	0.0	4,391,984
15	**2.631**	**3.227**	**72,070**	**0.980**	**14,857,303**
16	**0.963**	**1.708**	**112,832**	**0.986**	**15,084,205**
17	0.0080	0.0	0	0.0	5,541,692
18	0.076	0.041	0	0.0	5,615,470
19	0.978	0.0	0	0.0	6,000,658
20	2.522	2.897	189,856	0.951	6,178,958
21	0.0	0.0	0	0.0	7,911,142
22	0.0080	0.0	0	0.0	9,136,740
23	0.0	0.0	0	0.0	9,353,455
24	0.0	0.0	0	0.0	12,902,226
25	0.0	0.0	0	0.0	14,231,923

[a] LCR = Low copy repeat; LCR content was calculated using the following formula ((Σ length of duplication · copy number)/length of flanking region).

(Diehl et al., 2001) and spotted on epoxy-coated slides (NUNC, Wiesbaden, Germany). In order to reach this high spotting density, advantage was taken of an in-house modified Qarray (originally from Genetix, now Milton, UK) and Pointech (Gibbon, MN) Tungston PTL 2,500 slit pins. Sonicated patient and reference DNAs were labelled by random priming (Bioprime Array CGH, Invitrogen, Carlsbad, Calif.) with Cy3 and Cy5 (Amersham Biosciences, Piscataway, N.J.), respectively. Subsequent hybridisations were performed overnight in a Slide-Booster (Advalytix, Munich, Germany) at 42°C. After high-stringency washes, slides were scanned using an Axon 4000B scanner and images were analysed using Genepix 5.0 (Axon Instruments, Union City, Calif.). Detailed step-by-step protocols can be obtained from our website (http://www.molgen.mpg.de/~abt_rop/ molecular_cytogenetics/).

Data analysis
The analysis and visualisation of array CGH data was performed using our software-package CGHPRO (Chen et al., 2005). No background subtraction was applied. Raw data were normalised by 'Subgrid LOWESS'. Copy number gains and losses were determined by conservative log2 ratio thresholds of 0.3 and –0.3, respectively. Aberrant ratios involving three or more neighbouring BAC clones were considered as genomic aberrations, unless they coincided with a known polymorphism as listed in the Database of Genomic Variants (http://projects. tcag.ca/variation/; version Dec 13, 2005). To estimate the LCR content of the breakpoint regions, a 400-kb interval centered around each breakpoint was screened in the Segmental Duplication Database (http://humanparalogy.gs.washington.edu/). Breakpoints of the chromosomal imbalances were defined as the midpoint between end and start of the two neighbouring clones with alternate states, i.e., the one with a normal and the other one with an aberrant ratio, respectively.

In balanced translocations, the position of breakpoints was defined as the midpoint of the respective breakpoint-flanking clones. All genomic coordinates and database annotations were based on the May 2004 NCBI assembly (build 35). In order to avoid any loss of information due to the method used for breakpoint definition, we repeated the whole procedure with different breakpoint intervals (200 kb and 1 Mb). When LCRs were found to occur in both breakpoint regions, the respective entries in the Segmental Duplication Database were checked for homology and degree of sequence similarity. A threshold of 90% was used to distinguish LCRs with low and high sequence similarity. Furthermore, we applied the same procedure to the imbalances detected in an independent cohort of mentally retarded patients described recently by de Vries et al. (2005).

Array CGH data discussed in this publication have been deposited in NCBIs Gene Expression Omnibus (GEO, Edgar et al., 2002; Barrett et al., 2005; http://www.ncbi.nlm.nih.gov/geo/) and are accessible through GEO Series accession number GSE4884.

Results and discussion

To shed more light on the mechanisms that give rise to chromosomal rearrangements in mentally retarded patients, we have assessed and compared the frequency of LCRs at the breakpoints of balanced and unbalanced chromosomal aberrations (Fig. 1, Tables 1 and 2; S1–S6, Supplementary Information, www.karger.com/doi/10.1159/

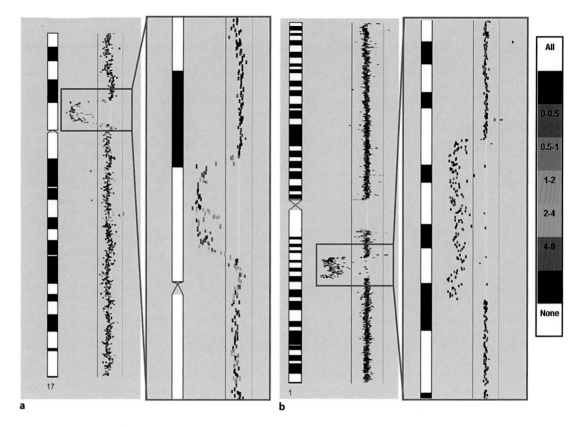

Fig. 2. Presence and absence of LCRs in chromosomal breakpoint regions. Deletions detected in cases 16 (**a**) and 25 (**b**) are shown. Cy3/Cy5 intensity ratios of each clone are plotted in a size-dependent manner along the chromosome ideograms. The red and green lines indicate the log2 ratio thresholds –0.3 (loss) and 0.3 (gain), respectively. For visualizing the content of low copy repeats in this figure, each BAC clone was classified into one out of seven categories and colour-coded as described previously (Chen et al., 2005). The color code is given by the color bar to the right (e.g. red = no low copy repeats).

000095921). Array CGH results including the size of the aberrations and locations of breakpoints are given in Table S7 (Supplementary Information, www.karger.com/doi/101159/000095921).

Unbalanced rearrangements can be grouped into four categories: (1) proximal and distal breakpoint regions are enriched for LCRs with high sequence similarity (6/22; 27.3%; Fig. 2), (2) proximal and distal breakpoint regions are enriched for LCRs, but with low sequence similarity (3/22; 13.6%), (3) only one breakpoint region harbours LCRs (5/22; 22.7%) and (4) no LCR lies in the vicinity of both breakpoints (8/22; 36.4%; Fig. 2). Results obtained with the independent dataset of de Vries et al. (2005) support these findings, although the distribution within these categories is slightly different (Tables S8–10; Supplementary Information, www.karger.com/doi/101159/000095921).

Thus we have shown that there is a conspicuous clustering of LCRs at or near the borders of sub-microscopic deletions and duplications that are associated with mental retardation. In 41% of these imbalances, both breakpoint regions carried LCRs, and in two thirds of these, their high degree of sequence similarity identified NAHR as the most likely cause of these rearrangements.

It is worthwhile to note that we have observed an inverse relationship between the size of the aberration and the likelihood of NAHR ($P = 0.018878$; Wilcoxon rank sum test). A higher sequence similarity of neighbouring LCRs could account for this size dependency. In addition, it has been reported that during meiosis equal crossovers could act as inter-chromosomal connections that prevent chromosomal slippage. Following this assumption, a small fragment with its lower probability of meiotic recombination would be more prone to NAHR (Inoue and Lupski, 2002).

The occurrence of LCRs at both breakpoints, yet with nearly no sequence similarity in 3/22 aberrations, however, already questions the necessity of NAHR to make those sites of LCR accumulation prone to rearrangements. LCRs at only one of the two breakpoints, as detected in 5/22 cases, are also unlikely to be involved in NAHR. Still, even in such situations, an involvement of NAHR cannot be ruled out, since many LCRs may not correctly be represented in the current version of the human genome sequence due to inherent problems with their sequencing and assembly (Cheung et al., 2003; She et al., 2004). In addition, the minimal homologous segment necessary for NAHR may be very small and, therefore, missed due to the resolution limits of this study. Although supportive for NAHR as a possible mechanism, it

Table 2. Summary of LCR content of chromosomal breakpoint regions detected in 41 mentally retarded patients with balanced translocation (400-kb interval). Data given in this table are based on a 400-kb interval centered around the breakpoint (see Materials and methods section for details).

Case No.	LCR content[a] (breakpoint 1)	LCR content[a] (breakpoint 2)	Size of homologous sequence (bp)	Percentage of sequence identity
1	0.009	0.0	0	0
2	0.0	0.0	0	0
3	0.000	0.0030	0	0
4	0.0	0.0	0	0
5	0.004	0.072	0	0
6	0.0	0.0	0	0
7	0.566	0.0	0	0
8	0.0	0.0	0	0
9	0.0	0.0	0	0
10	0.0	0.0	0	0
11	0.0	0.0	0	0
12	0.0	0.0	0	0
13	0.008	0.358	0	0
14	0.0	0.0	0	0
15	0.0	0.01	0	0
16	0.0	0.15	0	0
17	0.0	0.0	0	0
18	0.009	0.0	0	0
19	0.0	0.0	0	0
20	0.047	0.0	0	0
21	1.503	3.812	0	0
22	0.042	1.361	0	0
23	0.0	0.0	0	0
24	0.0	0.0070	0	0
25	0.0	0.0040	0	0
26	0.008	0.019	0	0
27	0.0	0.012	0	0
28	0.0	0.0	0	0
29	0.016	0.0070	0	0
30	0.0	0.087	0	0
31	6.382	0.0	0	0
32	0.0	0.0	0	0
33	1.987	0.0	0	0
34	0.0	0.032	0	0
35	0.007	0.0040	0	0
36	0.0	0.0030	0	0
37	0.0	0.0040	0	0
38	0.0	0.0030	0	0
39	0.0090	0.0	0	0
40	0.0080	0.358	0	0
41	0.133	0.0	0	0

[a] LCR = Low copy repeat; LCR content was calculated using the following formula ((Σ length of duplication $\cdot$ copy number)/length of flanking region).

would not explain the significance of accumulated LCRs at one breakpoint alone. In a recent report on Xq22.2 duplications analysed in Pelizaeus-Merzbacher syndrome (Woodward et al., 2005), the presence of LCRs at only one of the two chromosomal breakpoints has been explained by a mechanism described as coupled homologous and non-homologous recombination (Richardson and Jasin, 2000). But, since this process involves the generation of duplicated sequences, it does not provide any explanation for the deletions found in patients with only one breakpoint harbouring LCRs. In two other studies, one with a deletion associated with a Pelizaeus-Merzbacher-like phenotype (Inoue et al., 2002) and another one dealing with SMS (Shaw and Lupski, 2005), also a one-sided distribution of LCRs at the breakpoints was encountered. Subsequent detailed sequence analysis clearly suggested the occurrence of NHEJ in these cases.

In contrast to the findings in patients with small imbalances, supporting the involvement of NAHR in 6/22 cases examined, none of the 41 patients with constitutional balanced translocations studied exhibited highly similar LCRs in both breakpoint regions (Table 2, S5 und S6, Fig. 1). Although 8/41 (20%) balanced translocations displayed an increased LCR content at both breakpoint regions, the limited similarity between these LCRs strongly argues against a role of NAHR in the etiology of these rearrangements. In 19/41 (46%) balanced translocations only one breakpoint was enriched for LCRs, and 14/41 (34%) had no LCR in the vicinity of the two breakpoints at all.

Why NAHR is more common in small intra-chromosomal rearrangements than in translocations involving different chromosomes is as yet not clear, but there are at least two plausible explanations. First, LCRs on the same chromosome tend to be more similar than duplicated sequences elsewhere in the genome, because intra-chromosomal duplications occurred more recently during genome evolution (Zhang et al., 2005). Secondly, the physical distance between similar LCRs on heterologous chromosomes may drastically reduce the probability that such LCRs are recognized by the NAHR machinery.

In summary, we have found an accumulation of LCRs at breakpoint regions of balanced and unbalanced chromosomal aberrations. NAHR between LCRs seems to play no significant role in the etiology of balanced translocations. In cases with unbalanced chromosomal anomalies, we have observed an inverse relationship between the frequency of NAHRs and the sizes of the aberrations. Finally, our data suggest the presence of additional mechanisms coinciding with or dependent on the presence of LCRs that may cause increased instability at these chromosomal sites.

Acknowledgements

We would like to thank Pieter de Jong and the BACPAC Resources Centre (http://bacpac.chori.org) for providing DNA of the human 32 k BAC Re-Array Set, Nigel Carter and the Mapping Core and Map Finishing groups of the Wellcome Trust Sanger Institute for initial clone supply and verification of the 1-Mb array and the COST B19 Action 'Molecular Cytogenetics of Solid tumours' for the assembly of the subtelomere array.

References

Bailey JA, Yavor AM, Massa HF, Trask BJ, Eichler EE: Segmental duplications: organization and impact within the current human genome project assembly. Genome Res 11:1005–1017 (2001).

Bailey JA, Gu Z, Clark RA, Reinert K, Samonte RV, et al: Recent segmental duplications in the human genome. Science 297:1003–1007 (2002).

Bailey JA, Liu G, Eichler EE: An Alu transposition model for the origin and expansion of human segmental duplications. Am J Hum Genet 73:823–834 (2003).

Barrett T, Suzek TO, Troup DB, Wilhite SE, Ngau WC, et al: NCBI GEO: mining millions of expression profiles – database and tools. Nucleic Acids Res 1:33 Database Issue:D562–D566 (2005).

Bi W, Park SS, Shaw CJ, Withers MA, Patel PI, Lupski JR: Reciprocal crossovers and a positional preference for strand exchange in recombination events resulting in deletion or duplication of chromosome 17p11.2. Am J Hum Genet 73:1302–1315 (2003).

Chen W, Erdogan F, Ropers HH, Lenzner S, Ullmann R: CGHPRO – a comprehensive data analysis tool for array CGH. BMC Bioinformatics 6:85 (2005).

Cheng Z, Ventura M, She X, Khaitovich P, Graves T, et al: A genome-wide comparison of recent chimpanzee and human segmental duplications. Nature 437:88–93 (2005).

Cheung VG, Nowak N, Jang W, Kirsch IR, Zhao S, et al: Integration of cytogenetic landmarks into the draft sequence of the human genome. Nature 409:953–958 (2001).

Cheung J, Estivill X, Khaja R, MacDonald JR, Lau K, et al: Genome-wide detection of segmental duplications and potential assembly errors in the human genome sequence. Genome Biol 4:R25 (2003).

de Vries BB, Pfundt R, Leisink M, Koolen DA, Vissers LE, et al: Diagnostic genome profiling in mental retardation. Am J Hum Genet 77:606–616 (2005).

Diehl F, Grahlmann S, Beier M, Hoheisel JD: Manufacturing DNA microarrays of high spot homogeneity and reduced background signal. Nucleic Acids Res 29:E38 (2001).

Edelmann L, Spiteri E, Koren K, Pulijaal V, Bialer MG, et al: AT-rich palindromes mediate the constitutional t(11;22) translocation. Am J Hum Genet 68:1–13 (2001).

Edgar R, Domrachev M, Lash AE: Gene Expression Omnibus: NCBI gene expression and hybridization array data repository. Nucleic Acids Res 30:207–210 (2002).

Eichler EE: Recent duplication, domain accretion and the dynamic mutation of the human genome. Trends Genet 17:661–669 (2001).

Elliott B, Jasin M: Repair of double-strand breaks by homologous recombination in mismatch repair-defective mammalian cells. Mol Cell Biol 21:2671–2682 (2001).

Elliott B, Richardson C, Winderbaum J, Nickoloff JA, Jasin M: Gene conversion tracts from double-strand break repair in mammalian cells. Mol Cell Biol 18:93–101 (1998).

Emanuel BS, Shaikh TH: Segmental duplications: an 'expanding' role in genomic instability and disease. Nat Rev Genet 2:791–800 (2001).

Fiegler H, Carr P, Douglas EJ, Burford DC, Hunt S, et al: DNA microarrays for comparative genomic hybridization based on DOP-PCR amplification of BAC and PAC clones. Genes Chromosomes Cancer 36:361–374 (2003).

Gotter AL, Shaikh TH, Budarf ML, Rhodes CH, Emanuel BS: A palindrome-mediated mechanism distinguishes translocations involving LCR-B of chromosome 22q11.2. Hum Mol Genet 13:103–115 (2004).

Horvath JE, Bailey JA, Locke DP, Eichler EE: Lessons from the human genome: transitions between euchromatin and heterochromatin. Hum Mol Genet 10:2215–2223 (2001).

Inoue K, Lupski JR: Molecular mechanisms for genomic disorders. Annu Rev Genomics Hum Genet 3:199–242 (2002).

Inoue K, Osaka H, Thurston VC, Clarke JT, Yoneyama A, et al: Genomic rearrangements resulting in PLP1 deletion occur by nonhomologous end joining and cause different dysmyelinating phenotypes in males and females. Am J Hum Genet 71:838–853 (2002).

Ishkanian AS, Malloff CA, Watson SK, DeLeeuw RJ, Chi B, et al: A tiling resolution DNA microarray with complete coverage of the human genome. Nat Genet 36:299–303 (2004).

Khaitovich P, Muetzel B, She X, Lachmann M, Hellmann I, Dietzsch J, et al: Regional patterns of gene expression in human and chimpanzee brains. Genome Res 14:1462–1473 (2004).

Kirchhoff M, Gerdes T, Maahr J, Rose H, Bentz M, et al: Deletions below 10 megabasepairs are detected in comparative genomic hybridization by standard reference intervals. Genes Chromosomes Cancer 25:410–413 (1999).

Kirchhoff M, Pedersen S, Kjeldsen E, Rose H, Duno M, et al: Prospective study comparing HR-CGH and subtelomeric FISH for investigation of individuals with mental retardation and dysmorphic features and an update of a study using only HR-CGH. Am J Med Genet A 127:111–117 (2004).

Krzywinski M, Bosdet I, Smailus D, Chiu R, Mathewson C, et al: A set of BAC clones spanning the human genome. Nucleic Acids Res 32:3651–3660 (2004).

Kurahashi H, Emanuel BS: Long AT-rich palindromes and the constitutional t(11;22) breakpoint. Hum Mol Genet 10:2605–2617 (2001).

Kurahashi H, Shaikh TH, Hu P, Roe BA, Emanuel BS, Budarf ML: Regions of genomic instability on 22q11 and 11q23 as the etiology for the recurrent constitutional t(11;22). Hum Mol Genet 9:1665–1670 (2000a).

Kurahashi H, Shaikh TH, Zackai EH, Celle L, Driscoll DA, et al: Tightly clustered 11q23 and 22q11 breakpoints permit PCR-based detection of the recurrent constitutional t(11;22). Am J Hum Genet 67:763–768 (2000b).

Kurahashi H, Shaikh T, Takata M, Toda T, Emanuel BS: The constitutional t(17;22): another translocation mediated by palindromic AT-rich repeats. Am J Hum Genet 72:733–738 (2003).

Kurahashi H, Inagaki H, Yamada K, Ohye T, Taniguchi M, et al: Cruciform DNA structure underlies the etiology for palindrome-mediated human chromosomal translocations. J Biol Chem 279:35377–35383 (2004).

Liang F, Han M, Romanienko PJ, Jasin M: Homology-directed repair is a major double-strand break repair pathway in mammalian cells. Proc Natl Acad Sci USA 95:5172–5177 (1998).

Lieber MR, Ma Y, Pannicke U, Schwarz K: Mechanism and regulation of human non-homologous DNA end-joining. Nat Rev Mol Cell Biol 4:712–720 (2003).

Lupski JR: Genomic disorders: structural features of the genome can lead to DNA rearrangements and human disease traits. Trends Genet 14:417–422 (1998).

Osoegawa K, Mammoser AG, Wu C, Frengen E, Zeng C, et al: A bacterial artificial chromosome library for sequencing the complete human genome. Genome Res 11:483–496 (2001).

Pinkel D, Segraves R, Sudar D, Clark S, Poole I, et al: High resolution analysis of DNA copy number variation using comparative genomic hybridization to microarrays. Nat Genet 20:207–211 (1998).

Richardson C, Jasin M: Coupled homologous and nonhomologous repair of a double-strand break preserves genomic integrity in mammalian cells. Mol Cell Biol 20:9068–9075 (2000).

Shaikh TH, Kurahashi H, Emanuel BS: Evolutionarily conserved low copy repeats (LCRs) in 22q11 mediate deletions, duplications, translocations, and genomic instability: an update and literature review. Genet Med 3:6–13 (2001).

Shaw CJ, Lupski JR: Non-recurrent 17p11.2 deletions are generated by homologous and non-homologous mechanisms. Hum Genet 116:1–7 (2005).

Shaw CJ, Withers MA, Lupski JR: Uncommon deletions of the Smith-Magenis syndrome region can be recurrent when alternate low-copy repeats act as homologous recombination substrates. Am J Hum Genet 75:75–81 (2004).

She X, Jiang Z, Clark RA, Liu G, Cheng Z, et al: Shotgun sequence assembly and recent segmental duplications within the human genome. Nature 431:927–930 (2004).

Solinas-Toldo S, Lampel S, Stilgenbauer S, Nickolenko J, Benner A, et al: Matrix-based comparative genomic hybridization: biochips to screen for genomic imbalances. Genes Chromosomes Cancer 20:399–407 (1997).

Spiteri E, Babcock M, Kashork CD, Wakui K, Gogineni S, et al: Frequent translocations occur between low copy repeats on chromosome 22q11.2 (LCR22s) and telomeric bands of partner chromosomes. Hum Mol Genet 12:1823–1837 (2003).

Stankiewicz P, Lupski JR: Genome architecture, rearrangements and genomic disorders. Trends Genet 18:74–82. (2002).

Stankiewicz P, Shaw CJ, Dapper JD, Wakui K, Shaffer LG, et al: Genome architecture catalyzes nonrecurrent chromosomal rearrangements. Am J Hum Genet 72:1101–1116 (2003).

Stankiewicz P, Shaw CJ, Withers M, Inoue K, Lupski JR: Serial segmental duplications during primate evolution result in complex human genome architecture. Genome Res 14:2209–2220 (2004).

Visser R, Shimokawa O, Harada N, Kinoshita A, Ohta T, et al: Identification of a 3.0-kb major recombination hotspot in patients with Sotos syndrome who carry a common 1.9 Mb microdeletion. Am J Hum Genet 76:52–67 (2005).

Waldman AS, Liskay RM: Dependence of intrachromosomal recombination in mammalian cells on uninterrupted homology. Mol Cell Biol 8:5350–5357 (1988).

Woodward KJ, Cundall M, Sperle K, Sistermans EA, Ross M, et al: Heterogeneous duplications in patients with Pelizaeus-Merzbacher disease suggest a mechanism of coupled homologous and nonhomologous recombination. Am J Hum Genet 77:966–987 (2005).

Zhang L, Lu HH, Chung WY, Yang J, Li WH: Patterns of segmental duplication in the human genome. Mol Biol Evol 22:135–141 (2005).

Cytogenet Genome Res 115:254–261 (2006)
DOI: 10.1159/000095922

Whole-genome array-CGH screening in undiagnosed syndromic patients: old syndromes revisited and new alterations

A.C.V. Krepischi-Santos[a] A.M. Vianna-Morgante[a] F.S. Jehee[a]
M.R. Passos-Bueno[a] J. Knijnenburg[b] K. Szuhai[b] W. Sloos[b] J.F. Mazzeu[a, e]
F. Kok[a, c] C. Cheroki[a] P.A. Otto[a] R.C. Mingroni-Netto[a] M. Varela[a]
C. Koiffmann[a] C.A. Kim[d] D.R. Bertola[d] P.L. Pearson[a] ˙C. Rosenberg[a]

[a]Department of Genetics and Evolutionary Biology, University of São Paulo, São Paulo (Brazil)
[b]Department of Molecular Cell Biology, Leiden University Medical Center, Leiden (The Netherlands)
[c]Department of Neurology, Hospital das Clínicas, and [d]Genetics Unit, Department of Pediatrics, Instituto da
Criança, University of São Paulo, São Paulo (Brazil); [e]Robinow Syndrome Foundation, Anoka, MN (USA)

Manuscript received 15 May 2006; accepted in revised form for publication by A. Geurts van Kessel, 25 May 2006.

Abstract. We report array-CGH screening of 95 syndromic patients with normal G-banded karyotypes and at least one of the following features: mental retardation, heart defects, deafness, obesity, craniofacial dysmorphisms or urogenital tract malformations. Chromosome imbalances not previously detected in normal controls were found in 30 patients (31%) and at least 16 of them (17%) seem to be causally related to the abnormal phenotypes. Eight of the causative imbalances had not been described previously and pointed to new chromosome regions and candidate genes for specific phenotypes, including a connective tissue disease locus on 2p16.3, another for obesity on 7q22.1$\rightarrow$q22.3, and a candidate gene for the 3q29 deletion syndrome manifestations. The other causative alterations had already been associated with well-defined phenotypes including Sotos syndrome, and the 1p36 and 22q11.21 microdeletion syndromes. However, the clinical features of these latter patients were either not typical or specific enough to allow diagnosis before detection of chromosome imbalances. For instance, three patients with overlapping deletions in 22q11.21 were ascertained through entirely different clinical features, i.e., heart defect, utero-vaginal aplasia, and mental retardation associated with psychotic disease. Our results demonstrate that ascertainment through whole-genome screening of syndromic patients by array-CGH leads not only to the description of new syndromes, but also to the recognition of a broader spectrum of features for already described syndromes. Furthermore, on the technical side, we have significantly reduced the amount of reagents used and costs involved in the array-CGH protocol, without evident reduction in efficiency, bringing the method more within reach of centers with limited budgets.

Copyright © 2006 S. Karger AG, Basel

In the last couple of years, it has become evident by whole-genome array-CGH screening of patients with normal G-banded karyotypes and mental retardation as the cardinal phenotypic feature, that 13–16% present with de novo microdeletions or duplications apparently causing their phenotypes (Vissers et al., 2003; Shaw-Smith et al., 2004; Tyson et al., 2005; Menten et al., 2006; Rosenberg et al., 2006). A smaller proportion of patients (5–10%) carried alterations not previously described in normal individuals but which were also present in their phenotypically normal parents, and the significance of such imbalances is still unclear. Copy number variation of large genomic segments has recently been described in normal individuals (Iafrate et al.,

Request reprints from Carla Rosenberg, PhD
Departamento de Genética e Biologia Evolutiva
Instituto de Biociências – Universidade de São Paulo, C.P. 11461
05422-970 São Paulo, SP (Brazil)
telephone: +55 11 3091 7591; fax: +55 11 3091 7553
e-mail: carlarosenberg@uol.com.br

KARGER
Fax +41 61 306 12 34
E-Mail karger@karger.ch
www.karger.com

© 2006 S. Karger AG, Basel
1424–8581/06/1154–0254$23.50/0

Accessible online at:
www.karger.com/cgr

2004; Sebat et al., 2004), and information regarding these polymorphic segments has constantly been updated in the Genome Variation Database (http://projects.tcag.ca/variation). It remains to be determined which proportion of the inherited imbalances represent polymorphisms, and which proportion is causally related to the abnormal phenotypes through more complex mechanisms of manifestation (incomplete penetrance, variable expressivity, uncovering of recessive mutations or genomic imprinting).

Because of the limited number of patients initially described (~400) (Vissers et al., 2003; Shaw-Smith et al., 2004; Schoumans et al., 2005; Tyson et al., 2005; Menten et al., 2006; Rosenberg et al., 2006), copy number alterations detected by array-CGH appeared to be distributed randomly across the genome. More recently a pattern of recurrent alterations has begun to emerge, exemplified by the 3q29 (Willatt et al., 2005) and 9q22 (Redon et al., 2006) microdeletion syndromes, thus expanding the category of microimbalance syndromes, such as Charcot-Marie-Tooth (MIM 118220; OMIM, http://www3.ncbi.nlm.nih.gov/entrez/), Smith-Magenis (MIM 182290) and Miller-Dieker syndromes (MIM 247200). The introduction of whole-genome screening is now leading to recognition of patients with dissimilar congenital abnormalities associated with deletions or duplications of the same chromosome regions.

Here we report the results of whole-genome array-CGH screening of 95 Brazilian syndromic patients who had normal G-banded karyotypes. This study was enabled by collaboration with another academic institution that produced the arrays, namely, the Leiden University Medical Center, Netherlands. Some cost-effective changes to the standard protocol were successfully introduced without evident reduction in efficiency. Such modifications will certainly be of interest to other centers like ours with limited financial resources. Because our studies were performed mainly in collaboration with national reference centers for specific diseases, the range of congenital abnormalities represented in our sample is biased. Although most patients presented mental impairment, the primary ascertainment was most often made through other features, namely, heart defects, deafness, obesity, craniofacial dysmorphisms or urogenital tract malformations.

Materials and methods

Patient samples

All patients included in this study presented normal G-banded karyotypes but exhibited a syndromic phenotype, suggesting the presence of a chromosome alteration. These patients were part of samples of specific research/diagnostic groups at the University of São Paulo, and the need to reach a diagnosis due to their phenotype motivated the use of array-CGH to detect cryptic copy number alterations. Although not being the major or only selective criterion, almost all patients presented mental impairment. The 95 syndromic patients studied were selected and grouped according to the following criteria:

Group A (32 patients): Mental retardation and negative for fragile-X syndrome.

Group B (22 patients): Craniosynostosis, negative for mutations in the *TWIST, FGFR1, FGFR2* and *FGFR3* genes, and for deletions at *TWIST*, 9p24→p22 and 11q23 regions.

Group C (11 patients): Short stature, hypoplastic genitalia and hypertelorism (autosomal dominant Robinow syndrome features).

Group D (9 patients): Mental retardation and obesity. Five of the patients with clinical history compatible with Prader-Willy syndrome showed normal methylation pattern for the PWS region.

Group E (8 patients): Utero-vaginal aplasia with renal defects and negative for mutations in the *RARG, RXRA,* and *WNT4* genes.

Group F (7 patients): Heart defects, negative for 22q11.21 deletions by satellite marker analysis.

Group G (6 patients): Deafness, negative for mutations in *GJB2* (35delG and 167delT screening tests and SSCP), *GJB6* (delGJB6D13S1830 and delGJB6D13S1854) and the mitochondrial A1555G mutation.

Array-CGH

The array-CGH method used has been described previously (Knijnenburg et al., 2005; Rosenberg et al., 2006). Briefly, slides containing triplicates of ~3,500 large insert clones spaced at ~1.0 Mb density over the full genome were produced in the Leiden University Medical Center. The large insert clones set used to produce these arrays was provided by the Wellcome Trust Sanger Institute (UK), and information regarding the full set is available at the Wellcome Trust Sanger Institute mapping database site (Ensembl genome Browser: http://www.ensembl.org/). DNA amplification and spotting on the slides were based on published protocols (Fiegler et al., 2003). Hybridisation followed procedures of the same publication, with the following modifications: we used about half of the sample DNA (200 ng) and labelling reaction than originally described, reducing 2–3-fold the amount of labelling kit, fluorochrome-conjugated nucleotides and C_0t DNA. In addition, the use of columns after random priming labelling reaction to eliminate non-incorporated nucleotides seemed unnecessary since no qualitative differences in results following the use of separated or non-separated products were observed; therefore, this step was eliminated from our protocol. After hybridisation, the slides were scanned with a GenePix Personal 4100A scanner, and the spot intensities measured using GenePix Pro 4.1 software (Axon Instruments, Westburg BV, Leusden, Netherlands). Further analyses were carried out using Microsoft Excel 2000.

Target imbalances were determined based on log2 ratios of the average of the replicates, and sequences were considered as amplified or deleted when outside the ±0.33 range. We considered a patient to have a potentially causative chromosome imbalance when the amplification or deletion had not been previously documented in normal controls.

Array-CGH imbalances were validated either by fluorescence in situ hybridisation (FISH) or multiple ligation probe amplification (MLPA). FISH was also used to determine if an imbalance had been inherited. FISH was performed according to standard protocols. For MLPA, the kit P036B by MRC-Holland (Amsterdam, Netherlands) was used according to manufacturer's instructions.

Table 1. Frequency of copy number imbalances detected by array-CGH in 95 syndromic patients shown according to ascertainment group (see Materials and methods)

Ascertainment group	No. of patients investigated	No. of chromosome imbalances	No. of alterations probably causative of the phenotype
A	32	12	4
B	22	4	2
C	11	3	2
D	9	2	2
E	8	4	2
F	7	3	3
G	6	1	0
Total	95	29 (30%)	15 (16%)

Results

Through array-CGH analysis we detected 29 chromosome imbalances not previously described in normal individuals (Genome Variation Database) in our sample of 95 syndromic patients. A description of the imbalances and associated phenotypes was included in the database DECIPHER (http://www.sanger.ac.uk/PostGenomics/decipher).

Table 1 summarizes the frequency of alterations found in the array-CGH screening for each ascertainment group.

Tables 2 and 3 present the clinical features of the patients carrying chromosome imbalances, as well as the maximum size, position and mode of inheritance of the chromosome alterations.

Table 2 shows the chromosome imbalances considered as probably causative of the patients' abnormal phenotypes. We considered a chromosome imbalance as probably causative of the abnormal phenotype (patients 1–15) when it overlapped an already well-described deletion/duplication region for given phenotypes (patients 1–7), when it was de

Table 2. Description of probably causative chromosome imbalances: clinical features of the patients, ascertainment group, maximum size, position and mode of inheritance of the imbalances

Patient	Clinical description	Group	Type and maximum extent of genomic imbalance	Parental origin
1	12-year-old female with developmental delay, seizures, failure to thrive, dolichocephaly, hypertelorism, midface hypoplasia, coloboma of the right iris and coroid, depressed nasal bridge, macrostomia, micrognathia, 5th finger clinodactyly, hypoplasia of the labia minora, anteriorly displaced anus, patent ductus arteriosus and dextrocardia.	F	del 3.3 Mb at 1p36.32 (RP4-785P20)	de novo
2	13-year-old male with moderate mental retardation, low weight (<3rd centile) and short stature (3rd centile), microcephaly, low frontal hairline, long narrow face, myopia, large ears, narrow high-arched palate, simian palmar crease at left.	A	del 1.0 Mb at 3q29 (RP11-114F20)	de novo
3	3-year-old female with mental retardation, seizures, short stature, microcephaly, mesomelic shortening of limbs, radio-ulnar fusion, pectus excavatum, hypoplasic genitalia.	C	del 10.2 Mb at 4pter→p16.1 (GS-118-B13 – RP11-117J13) dup 8.0 Mb at 8pter→p23.1 (GS-77-L23 – CTD-2629I16)	de novo der(4)t(4;8) (p16.1;p23.1)
4	3-year-old female with developmental delay, frontal bossing and receding hair implantation, narrow palpebral fissures, hypertelorism, incompletely rotated large ears, kidney agenesis at left.	E	del 2.5 Mb at 5q35 (CTB-87L24 – RP11-564G9)	de novo
5	23-year-old female with mental retardation and schizophrenia, high-set malformed ears and full cheeks.	A	del 4.0 Mb at 22q11.21 (XX-91c)	de novo
6	4-year-old male with mild developmental delay, hypocalcaemia seizures, epicanthal folds and short neck, common truncus arteriosus, multicystic kidney at left and thymus agenesis.	F	del 4.0 Mb at 22q11.21 (XX-91c)	de novo
7	17-year-old female with learning disabilities, hypothyroidism, microcephaly, long face, prominent tubular blunt nose, short philtrum, high palate, slight dorso-lombar scoliosis, slight aortic arch ectasy, upper vaginal agenesis, very rudimentary uterus, kidney agenesis at right.	E	del 4.0 Mb at 22q11.21 (XX-91c)	de novo (Cheroki et al., 2006)
8	1-year-old male with developmental delay, short stature, hypotonia, hemiparesia at right, cleft palate, micropenis, hemivertebrae.	C	del 3.3 Mb at 1q41→q42.12 (RP11-308L13 – RP11-105I12)	de novo
9	7-year-old male with mental retardation, joint hyperextensibility with tendency to dislocation suggestive of connective tissue disease.	A	del 4.7 Mb at 2p16.3 (RP11-19A8 – RP11-335O22)	de novo
10	14-year-old female with developmental delay, mild mental retardation, abdominal obesity, hyperphagia, hypothyroidism.	D	del 2.7 Mb at 7q22.1→q22.3 (RP4-672O11 – RP11-148A10)	de novo
11	1-year-old female with developmental delay, hypotonia, weight and height <2.5 percentile, hypertelorism, atrial septal defect and pactent ductus arteriosus.	F	del 15.0 Mb at 8q21.11→q21.3 (RP11-48D4 – RP5-1089O20)	N.D.
12	4-year-old female with mental retardation, episode of seizures, brachycephaly, occipital groove, facial dysmorphisms, strabismus, hypopigmented skin, atrial septal and ventricular septal defects, and persistent ductus arteriosus.	A	del 1.0 Mb at 17q21.31 (RP5-843B9)	de novo (Varela et al., 2006)
13	2-year-old male severely hypotonic with mental retardation, microcephaly, trigonocephaly, facial dysmorphisms and hypospadias (FG syndrome). Deceased at the age of 4 years due to a generalized infection.	B	dup 5.8 Mb at Xq22.3 (RP11-230E14 – RP5-820B18)	inherited from normal mother (Jehee et al., 2005)
14	8-year-old male with developmental delay and bilateral coronal craniosynostosis.	B	del 1.1 Mb at Xq27.2 (RP11-518F7)	inherited from normal mother
15	14-year-old male with mental retardation, dolichocephaly, obesity, hypogenitalism.	D	dup ? Mb at Xq28 (RP11-402H20)	inherited from normal mother

N.D. = Not determined.

novo in non-familial cases (patients 8–12) or when a maternally inherited alteration was located on the X chromosome in a male (patients 13–15).

Table 3 lists the patients whose chromosome imbalances could not be clearly associated with the abnormal phenotypes. These were (a) de novo alterations that were not present in a similarly affected parent or sib (patients 16–19) and were considered as non-causative for the familial phenotype; (b) imbalances inherited from a normal parent (patients 20–29). Although several mechanisms can be invoked to explain the manifestation of aberrant phenotypes in unbalanced affected children but not in their phenotypically

normal carrier parents, we are not considering such alterations as being causative at this juncture. Equally we cannot exclude this possibility.

Discussion

We report 29 chromosome imbalances in a cohort of 95 syndromic patients not previously described as polymorphisms. We considered 15 of these copy number alterations as probably causative (patients 1–15; Table 2) while the significance of the imbalances in the remaining patients (Ta-

Table 3. Description of chromosome imbalances inherited from a normal parent or not present in similarly affected relatives: clinical features of the patients, ascertainment group, maximum size, position and mode of inheritance of the imbalances

Patient	Clinical description	Group	Type and maximum extent of genomic imbalance	Parental origin
16	4-year-old female with mental retardation, hydrocephaly, severe visual impairment. Deceased at the age of 4 years (unknown cause).	A	dup 0.8 Mb at 3p25.2 (RP11-163D23)	de novo; not present in brother with mental retardation, hydrocephaly and multiple malformations
17	Infant female with acrocephaly, skull asymmetry, syndactyly.	B	dup 0.4 Mb at 3q26.33 (RP11-534H15)	de novo; not present in similarly affected mother
18	6-year-old male with short stature, hypertelorism and shawl scrotum (Aarskog syndrome).	C	dup 0.5 Mb at 5q23.3 (CTB-104P14)	de novo; not present in similarly affected father
19	16-year-old male child with learning disabilities, cryptorchidism, perineo-scrotal hypospadias, macrorchidism at left, polycystic kidneys.	E	del 3.2 Mb at 22q11.22 (RP11-50L23)	de novo; not present in mother with urogenital abnormalities
20	3-year-old female with uterovaginal atresia, genital labia fusion, undetected ovaries at US examination, syndactyly of 2nd/3rd toes	E	dup 4.0 Mb at 1q21.1 (RP11-315I20 – RP11-301M17)	inherited from normal mother
21	2-year-old male with severe mental retardation, hypotonia, seizures, severe visual impairment, lissencephaly, genital hypoplasia (micropenis). Alterations in *ARX* (mutation analyses) and *MDCR* (FISH) genes excluded.	A	dup 0.8 Mb at 3p25.2 (RP11-163D23)	inherited from normal mother
22	17-year-old female with mental retardation, short stature, primary amenorrhea, brachydactyly.	A	dup 2.3 Mb at 5p15.2 (RP11-44C2)	inherited from normal father
23	2.5-year-old female with poor sucking, neonatal hypotonia, severe mental retardation, microcephaly, brachycephaly, mild to moderate hearing impairment, macrostomia, club feet.	A	del 1.3 Mb at 5q21.1 (RP11-560F8)	inherited from normal mother
24	3-year-old female with mild mental retardation, severe hearing impairment, ataxic gait, short stature (<3rd percentile), convergent strabismus, epicanthic folds, low-set ears, bifid nose, high-palate.	G	dup 1.5 Mb at 6q27 (RP3-470B24)	inherited from normal mother
25	7-year-old male with mental retardation, seizures, dysphagia, and marked motor and speech delay, thin long face, large ears with hypoplastic cartilage, high arched palate, bilateral cryptorchidism	A	dup 1.0 Mb at 9pter→p24.3 (RG-41-L13 – GS-43-N6)	inherited from normal mother
26	Infant female with developmental delay, hypoplasia of corpus callosum, hypertelorism, palpebral ptosis at left, cleft palate, inguinal herniae, duplicated left kidney, clubfeet, and hip joint dysplasia. Deceased at the age of 9 months (cardio-respiratory arrest).	A	dup 1.2 Mb at 11q22.3 (RP11-531F16)	inherited from normal father
27	5-year-old male with acrocephaly, trigonocephaly, skull asymmetry and syndactyly.	B	dup 0.5 Mb at 12q13.11 (RP3-432E18)	inherited from normal father
28	12-year-old male with developmental delay, narrow frontal bone, synophrys, frontal hirsutism, congenital cataract, severe visual impairment, nystagmus, small lop ears, high palate, joint hyperextensibility.	A	del 2.4 Mb at 16p13.11 (RP11-489O1 – CTD-2504F3)	inherited from normal mother
29	9-month-old male with developmental delay, lessening of white matter and enlargement of subarachnoidal space (MRI), square head with flat occipital and posterior asymmetry, prominent frontal bossing.	A	dup 3.8 Mb at Xp22.33 (RP11-457M7 – RP11-418N20)	inherited from normal father; FISH showed that the duplicated segment is translocated to Ypter both in father and child

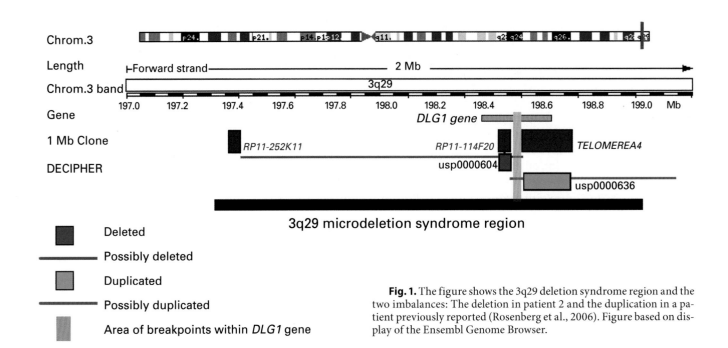

Fig. 1. The figure shows the 3q29 deletion syndrome region and the two imbalances: The deletion in patient 2 and the duplication in a patient previously reported (Rosenberg et al., 2006). Figure based on display of the Ensembl Genome Browser.

ble 3) is still unclear. None of the patients had abnormalities detected through karyotyping or routine screening for gene mutations related to their specific clinical phenotypes. Array-CGH has provided the basis for diagnosis and genetic counselling in the informative families. However, two of these cases should have been diagnosed in the previous routine investigations: Patient 6 would not have been included among the patients with idiopathic cardiological problems if the screening for 22q11 deletions had not missed it; in fact, the patient exhibited a typical DiGeorge phenotype. The second case involved a 15-Mb deletion of chromosome 8 (patient 11) which was well within the resolution of classical cytogenetics (400–600 bands resolution); however, sub-optimal metaphase preparations or imperfect cytogenetic analyses may lead to such errors, and large alterations (>10 Mb) first detected by microarray, and then retrospectively in G-banded preparations have been reported in most published array-CGH screens (Shaw-Smith et al., 2004; de Vries et al., 2005; Schoumans et al., 2005; Menten et al., 2006; Rosenberg et al., 2006). Table 1 suggests that the highest frequency of causative alterations in syndromic patients is found in individuals referred because of congenital heart abnormalities (group F). However, the two cases that were missed in the routine screening belonged to this group and resulted in overrepresentation of causative alterations associated with heart defects. Taking that into consideration, differences in frequencies of causative alterations observed among the clinical groups were not significant, given the small size of each sample.

The genomic alterations in individuals 1–7 have previously been associated with specific syndromes. However, the phenotypes of our patients were either not specific enough or were even atypical for these disorders, and there was insufficient reason to test them for alterations in the given chromosome regions purely on clinical grounds:

Patient 1 had an interstitial deletion fully contained in the 1p36 syndrome region (Shapira et al., 1997; Redon et al., 2005). Although she exhibited some features of this syndrome, she also showed some atypical signs such as coloboma of the right iris and coroid, dextrocardia, hypoplasia of labia minora and anteriorly displaced anus.

Patient 2 had the smallest deletion documented so far in the recently recognized 3q29 microdeletion syndrome region. Most of his clinical features (mental retardation, long face, microcephaly) are compatible with this disorder (Willatt et al., 2005), but are also common findings in many other genetic conditions. We have previously reported a duplication at 3q29 (Rosenberg et al., 2006), which is slightly distal to the 3q29 deletion in patient 2 (Fig. 1). A large gene, *DLG1* (synapse-associated protein 97), is certainly disrupted in both rearrangements. The duplication patient exhibited mental retardation, facial dysmorphisms and ataxia, the latter also present in some patients with 3q29 deletion. The *DLG1* gene encodes a scaffolding protein with multiple domains, probably involved in development, and appears as a strong candidate gene for the clinical manifestations of the 3q29 syndrome (MIM 601014).

The rearrangement carried by patient 3 has been described both in Pitt-Rogers-Danks (PRDS; MIM 262350) and Wolf-Hirschhorn (WHS; MIM 194190) syndromes. Although the size of the alterations (8–10 Mb) is within cytogenetics resolution, the presence of a duplicated segment of chromosome 8 on der(4) impairs the detection of the rearrangement. In addition to PRDS typical features, the patient exhibited some clinical signs less frequent or even never reported in PRDS syndrome, such as genital hypoplasia, radioulnar synostosis and mesomelic limb shortness.

Patient 4 was primarily investigated by array-CGH because the combination of mental retardation and renal agenesis was suggestive of chromosomal imbalance. Array-

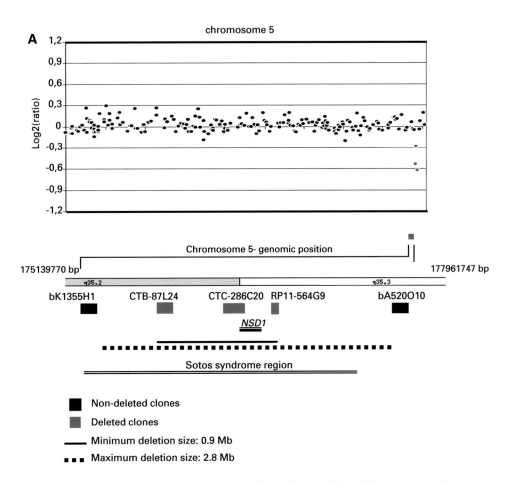

chromosome 5

Log2(ratio)

Chromosome 5- genomic position

175139770 bp   177961747 bp

q35.2   q35.3

bK1355H1   CTB-87L24   CTC-286C20 RP11-564G9   bA520O10

NSD1

Sotos syndrome region

■ Non-deleted clones

■ Deleted clones

— Minimum deletion size: 0.9 Mb

■■■ Maximum deletion size: 2.8 Mb

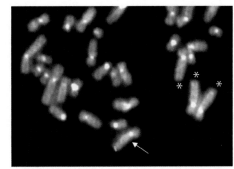

Fig. 2. De novo deletion at 5q35 from patient 4 demonstrated by array-CGH and confirmed by FISH. (**A**) Chromosome 5 array-CGH profile shows a deletion of three clones at 5q35. The figure also displays the relative position of the *NSD1* gene and the region commonly deleted in Sotos syndrome. (**B**) FISH using two of the deleted clones, CTC-286C20 (green) and RP11-564G9 (red), to metaphase chromosomes of patient 4. The signals from the two probes co-localize and are present in only one of the chromosomes 5 (arrow). The three unlabelled B-group chromosomes (chromosomes 4 and 5) are indicated by asterisks.

CGH disclosed a de novo 5q35 microdeletion (Fig. 2) encompassing the whole *NSD1* gene. Haploinsufficiency of *NSD1* is the cause of Sotos syndrome, a childhood disorder characterized by pre- and postnatal overgrowth, macrocephaly, developmental delay and typical craniofacial appearance (MIM 117550). Our patient did not present overgrowth or macrocephaly (at the age of 3 years, her weight was in the 25th centile, height in 50th centile and OFC between 25th and 50th centile). It is possible that the concomitant deletion of *NSD1* and *PROP1* (pituitary-specific homeodomain factor, associated with deficiency of growth hormone) genes balances the overgrowth effect in our and other patients with deletions in the 5q35 region. Retrospectively, after the deletion of *NSD1* gene had been detected in

our patient, her characteristic facial gestalt of Sotos syndrome could be recognized (Fig. 3). Although renal anomalies have sporadically been reported in Sotos syndrome patients (Nagai et al., 2003; Tatton-Brown et al., 2005), this is the first case with renal agenesis.

Patients 5–7 had deletions of clone XX-91c at 22q11.21, in the velocardiofacial/DiGeorge (VCFS/DGS) syndrome region. While patient 6 had clinical features typical of DiGeorge syndrome (DGS; MIM 188400), patients 5 and 7 were unlikely to be tested for deletion in the region based only on their phenotypes. Patient 5 was referred for mental retardation and psychotic disorder and, although schizophrenia is present in ~20% of 22q11 deletion syndrome patients, this adult woman had nothing else on her medical

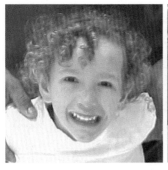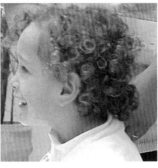

Fig. 3. Typical Sotos facial gestalt of patient 4 at the age of three years.

records suggestive of the syndrome. Patient 7, who was described in detail elsewhere (Cheroki et al., 2006), was referred because of primary amenorrhea and urogenital abnormalities that were not among the described signs of VCFS/DGS.

The detection of previously described imbalances in patients whose phenotypes are not strongly suggestive of associated syndromes is not too surprising when we consider that patients without the main features of a syndrome usually are not investigated for alterations in the candidate areas. Array-CGH provides an unbiased whole-genome screening of patients with congenital abnormalities, which will probably lead to a broadening of the phenotypic criteria associated with genetic changes at given loci.

The rearrangements of patients 8, 9, 10 and 12 were considered as probably causative because they were de novo. We still do not know, however, how often DNA segment copy number changes upon transmission from parents to children in normal individuals, and cannot exclude that this event in some cases is unrelated to the children's abnormal phenotypes. Assuming that these imbalances are in fact causative, the corresponding chromosome regions should indicate relevant genes for the specific phenotypes. Most of these rearrangements are too large to allow pinpointing major candidate genes. However, below we discuss some genes contained in the altered chromosome regions that seem to be interesting candidates for the patients' phenotypes:

In patient 9, in spite of the large size of the alteration (3.3–4.7 Mb at 2p16.3), the *NRX1B* gene (Neurexin 1) seems to be a suitable candidate for mental impairment in the patient: it codes for a neuronal cell surface protein and seems to play a role in the formation or maintenance of synaptic junctions. In addition, this gene is probably involved in the assembling of collagen, and its deletion might be connected to the abnormalities of conjunctive tissue observed in the patient (Fallahi et al., 2005).

Patient 10 had a small deletion at 7q22.1→q22.3 (1.1–2.7 Mb) encompassing the *RELN* gene, which, when mutated in mice, causes disruption of neuronal migration in several brain regions and gives rise to function deficits such as ataxic gate and trembling. It also seems to affect neuronal migration outside the brain (Yip et al., 2000). In addition, a mutation in the *RELN* gene has been described in three brothers with cerebral and cerebellar malformations and congenital lymphedema (Hourihane et al., 1993).

Patient 12 has a small deletion at 17q21.31, including the *MAPT* gene (microtubule-associated protein tau), for which variants are associated with late-onset neurodegenerative disorders, including Alzheimer and Parkinson-Dementia syndrome (MIM 260540). This patient is described in detail elsewhere (Varela et al., 2006).

Although the imbalances shown by patients 13–15 were inherited from their normal mothers, they were considered as possibly causative because they could behave as X-linked recessive, i.e., normal female carriers with affected male children. The large duplication at Xq22.3 in patient 13 is described elsewhere and contains a new locus for the FG syndrome (Jehee et al., 2005). The duplication carried by patient 15 is in accordance with the presence of genes associated with mental retardation, obesity and hypogenitalism at Xq28. However, there is still some uncertainty regarding the precise mapping of this BAC: our FISH studies confirmed the location at Xq28 of the duplicated probe RP11-402H20 (data not shown), but another clone from our array, RP11-296N8, co-localizes with this probe and showed normal copy number in our patient, indicating that there is a problem with mapping in this region. In fact, the information in the Ensembl Genome Browser (http://www.ensembl.org/) shows that sequencing of BAC-ends only confirmed the location of one side of RP11-402H20. According to the present mapping, this duplication is immediately distal to or may overlap the *MECP2* gene, which could be related to our patient's phenotype. However, other mental retardation genes have been described in the region, such as *GDI1*. Without a precise mapping of the alteration, the relationship of the patient's phenotype to chromosome alteration is highly speculative.

The alterations described in Table 3 were inherited from a normal carrier or were not present in other affected relatives. At this point, we have no evidence that these alterations are causative. Although other mechanisms of manifestation can be postulated to occur, such as incomplete penetrance, variable expressivity, uncovering of recessive mutations or genomic imprinting, these mechanisms combined with large segment copy number alterations detected by array-CGH so far have not been demonstrated. Genomic array is still a new tool, and the alterations with a dominant pattern of manifestation are likely to be described first. Patients 16 and 21 have duplications of the same BAC, RP11-163D23. In the first case, the alteration was not present in an affected brother; we suspect that the phenotypes of these affected sibs were not the same, and since the patient is now deceased we could not investigate the matter further. Patient 21 inherited the alteration from his normal mother. We did not uncover any additional alterations in the child that would explain his abnormal phenotype and the complete absence of any clinical phenotype in his mother. However, the presence of a never-previously described duplication in two affected individuals made us uncomfortable about whether genetic counselling should disregard the alteration or take it into account. We trust that public databases that compile information on 'polymorphic' and pathogenic copy number alterations, such as DECIPHER (http://www.sanger.ac.uk/PostGenomics/decipher) and ECARUCA (http://agserver01.azn.nl:8080/ecaruca/ecaruca.jsp) will allow clarification of the relevance of these inherited rearrangements and facilitate counselling in such complex cases.

Acknowledgements

The authors wish to thank the patients and their families for contributing to this study. We thank Ana Lucia Catelani, Fátima L.P.C. Baptista, Ligia S. Vieira, Maraisa de Castro Sebastião, Maria R.L.S. Pinheiro and Teresa Auricchio for technical assistance.

References

Cheroki C, Krepischi-Santos AC, Rosenberg C, Jehee FS, Mingroni-Netto RC, et al: Report of a del22q11 in a patient with Mayer-Rokitansky-Küster-Hauser (MRKH) anomaly and exclusion of *WNT-4*, *RAR-gamma*, and *RXR-alpha* as major genes determining MRKH anomaly in a study of 25 affected women. Am J Med Genet A 140:1339–1342 (2006).

de Vries BB, Pfundt R, Leisink MA, Koolen DA, Vissers LE, et al: Diagnostic genome profiling in mental retardation. Am J Hum Genet 77:606–616 (2005).

Fallahi A, Kroll B, Warner LR, Oxford RJ, Irwin KM, et al: Structural model of the amino propeptide of collagen XI alpha1 chain with similarity to the LNS domains. Protein Sci 14:1526–1537 (2005).

Fiegler H, Carr P, Douglas EJ, Burford DC, Hunt S, et al: DNA microarrays for comparative genomic hybridisation based on DOP-PCR amplification of BAC and PAC clones. Genes Chromosomes Cancer 36:361–374 (2003).

Hourihane JO, Bennett CP, Chaudhuri R, Robb SA, Martin ND: A sibship with a neuronal migration defect, cerebellar hypoplasia and congenital lymphedema. Neuropediatrics 24:43–46 (1993).

Iafrate AJ, Feuk L, Rivera MN, Listewnik ML, Donahoe PK, et al: Detection of large-scale variation in the human genome. Nat Genet 36:949–951 (2004).

Jehee FS, Rosenberg C, Krepischi-Santos AC, Kok F, Knijnenburg J, et al: An Xq22.3 duplication detected by comparative genomic hybridisation microarray (array-CGH) defines a new locus *(FGS5)* for FG syndrome. Am J Med Genet A 139:221–226 (2005).

Knijnenburg J, Szuhai K, Giltay J, Molenaar L, Sloos W, et al: Insights from genomic microarrays into structural chromosome rearrangements. Am J Med Genet A 132:36–40 (2005).

Menten B, Maas N, Thienpont B, Buysse K, Vandesompele J, et al: Emerging patterns of cryptic chromosomal imbalances in patients with idiopathic mental retardation and multiple congenital anomalies: a new series of 140 patients and review of published reports. J Med Genet 43:625–633 (2006).

Nagai T, Matsumoto N, Kurotaki N, Harada N, Niikawa N, et al: Sotos syndrome and haploinsufficiency of *NSD1*: clinical features of intragenic mutations and submicroscopic deletions. J Med Genet 40:285–289 (2003).

Redon R, Rio M, Gregory SG, Cooper RA, Fiegler H, et al: Tiling path resolution mapping of constitutional 1p36 deletions by array-CGH: contiguous gene deletion or 'deletion with positional effect' syndrome? J Med Genet 42:166–171 (2005).

Redon R, Baujat G, Sanlaville D, Le Merrer M, Vekemans M, et al: Interstitial 9q22.3 microdeletion: clinical and molecular characterisation of a newly recognised overgrowth syndrome. Eur J Hum Genet 14:759–767 (2006).

Rosenberg C, Knijnenburg J, Bakker E, Vianna-Morgante A, Sloos WC, et al: Array-CGH detection of micro rearrangements in mentally retarded individuals: Clinical significance of imbalances present both in affected children and normal parents. J Med Genet 43:180–186 (2006).

Schoumans J, Ruivenkamp C, Holmberg E, Kyllerman M, Anderlid BM, Nordenskjold M: Detection of chromosomal imbalances in children with idiopathic mental retardation by array based comparative genomic hybridisation (array-CGH). J Med Genet 42:699–705 (2005).

Sebat J, Lakshmi B, Troge J, Alexander J, Young J, et al: Large-scale copy number polymorphism in the human genome. Science 305:525–528 (2004).

Shapira SK, McCaskill C, Northrup H, Spikes AS, Elder FF, et al: Chromosome 1p36 deletions: the clinical phenotype and molecular characterization of a common newly delineated syndrome. Am J Hum Genet 61:642–650 (1997).

Shaw-Smith C, Redon R, Rickman L, Rio M, Willatt L, et al: Microarray based comparative genomic hybridisation (array-CGH) detects submicroscopic chromosomal deletions and duplications in patients with learning disability/mental retardation and dysmorphic features. J Med Genet 41:241–248 (2004).

Tatton-Brown K, Douglas J, Coleman K, Baujat G, Cole TR, et al: Genotype-phenotype associations in Sotos syndrome: an analysis of 266 individuals with *NSD1* aberrations. Am J Hum Genet 77:193–204 (2005).

Tyson C, Harvard C, Locker R, Friedman JM, Langlois S, et al: Submicroscopic deletions and duplications in individuals with intellectual disability detected by array-CGH. Am J Med Genet A 139:173–185 (2005).

Varela MC, Krepischi-Santos ACV, Paz JA, Knijnenburg J, Szuhai K, et al: A 17q21.31 microdeletion encompassing the *MAPT* gene in a mentally retarded patient. Cytogenet Genome Res 114:89–92 (2006).

Vissers LE, de Vries BB, Osoegawa K, Janssen IM, Feuth T, et al: Array-based comparative genomic hybridisation for the genomewide detection of submicroscopic chromosomal abnormalities. Am J Hum Genet 73:1261–1270 (2003).

Willatt L, Cox J, Barber J, Cabanas ED, Collins A, et al: 3q29 microdeletion syndrome: clinical and molecular characterization of a new syndrome. Am J Hum Genet 77:154–160 (2005).

Yip JW, Yip YP, Nakajima K, Capriotti C: Reelin controls position of autonomic neurons in the spinal cord. Proc Natl Acad Sci USA 97:8612–8616 (2000).

Cytogenet Genome Res 115:262–272 (2006)
DOI: 10.1159/000095923

Array-based comparative genomic hybridization and copy number variation in cancer research

E.K. Cho[a]   J. Tchinda[a]   J.L. Freeman[a]   Y.-J. Chung[b]   W.W. Cai[c]   C. Lee[a]

[a]Department of Pathology, Brigham and Women's Hospital and Harvard Medical School, Boston, MA (USA)
[b]Department of Microbiology, The Catholic University of Korea, Seoul (South Korea)
[c]Department of Molecular and Human Genetics, Baylor College of Medicine, Houston, TX (USA)

Manuscript received 14 July 2006; accepted in revised form for publication by A. Geurts van Kessel, 16 July 2006.

Abstract. Array-based comparative genomic hybridization (aCGH) is a molecular cytogenetic technique used in detecting and mapping DNA copy number alterations. aCGH is able to interrogate the entire genome at a previously unattainable, high resolution and has directly led to the recent appreciation of a novel class of genomic variation: copy number variation (CNV) in mammalian genomes. All forms of DNA variation/polymorphism are important for studying the basis of phenotypic diversity among individuals. CNV research is still at its infancy, requiring careful collation and annotation of accumulating CNV data that will undoubtedly be useful for accurate interpretation of genomic imbalances identified during cancer research.

Copyright © 2006 S. Karger AG, Basel

Chromosomal comparative genomic hybridization (CGH) was designed for the identification of relatively large chromosomal regions (i.e. chromosomal regions greater than several megabases in size) that are recurrently lost or gained in tumors (Kallioniemi et al., 1992). However, chromosomal CGH had major practical problems that limited its widespread use. It required template chromosome spreads of maximum length with minimal chromosomal overlaps. Optimal chromosome denaturation and hybridization conditions also varied considerably between chromosomal preparations. Most of all, single copy gains or losses involving regions smaller than 5–10 Mb were not reliably detected using chromosomal CGH (Forozan et al., 1997; Lee et al., 2000). For the detection of such smaller genomic imbalances, a higher-resolution technique was required. Array-based CGH (aCGH) combined genome-wide screening for genomic imbalances with an increased resolution made possible by densely spotted DNA clones or oligonucleotides on solid glass supports.

Array-based comparative genomic hybridization

aCGH was first used to identify segmental alterations in specific chromosomal regions associated with disease. Segmental genomic alterations of 75–130 kb in size were identified using an array which contained large-insert clones spanning the 13q14 and other specific chromosomal regions (Solinas-Toldo et al., 1997). Such arrays (often referred to as 'targeted' arrays) are naturally biased toward selected regions of the genome and require a priori knowledge of specific regions of interest.

Genome-wide arrays provided a more comprehensive analysis of the entire genome and were employed to overcome regional genomic biases inherent with targeted aCGH platforms. One of the first genome-wide aCGH approaches used cDNA microarrays constructed for gene expression

J.T. is supported in part by a German Research Foundation Fellowship Award.

Request reprints from Charles Lee
    Department of Pathology, Brigham and Women's Hospital
    20 Shattuck Street, Thorn 612A
    Boston, MA 02115 (USA)
    telephone: +1 617 278 0031; fax: +1 617 264 6861
    e-mail: cle@rics.bwh.harvard.edu

KARGER   Fax +41 61 306 12 34
            E-Mail karger@karger.ch
            www.karger.com

© 2006 S. Karger AG, Basel
1424–8581/06/1154–0262$23.50/0

Accessible online at:
www.karger.com/cgr

profiling experiments (Pollack et al., 1999). The advantage of using these arrays was that the same assays used to detect amplification and certain deletions could also be used to directly assess and correlate gene expression levels (e.g. Pollack et al., 1999, 2002). However, the low signal-to-noise ratios and the variable signal intensities obtained were major concerns that often arose with the use of cDNA clones as targets for detecting genomic copy-number alterations (Davies et al., 2005). Hence, when genome-wide, bacterial artificial chromosomes (BAC)-based arrays were subsequently constructed and utilized for genomic imbalance profiling, they became favored because larger insert clones provided superior signal-to-noise ratios compared to smaller insert clones or cDNAs. One of the initial large-insert, genome-wide arrays to be constructed for CGH assays contained 2,460 PAC and P1 clones and provided an average marker interval of ~1.4 Mb (Snijders et al., 2001).

With the ongoing demand for increased resolution, a variety of oligonucleotide arrays are now being constructed and used in aCGH experiments. For example, genotyping arrays containing 25-mer oligonucleotides (originally designed to detect human single-nucleotide polymorphisms (SNPs)) are being used to gather signal intensity data to infer copy number changes at specific genomic regions (e.g. Bignell et al., 2004; Zhao et al., 2004; Komura et al., in press). The use of such arrays provides the added advantage that the same platform can identify both loss of heterozygosity regions as well as relative copy number information (e.g. Garraway et al., 2005; Slater et al., 2005). It should be noted that aCGH experiments with oligo-based arrays either use a representational genomic sample that has been reduced in complexity (e.g. Kennedy et al., 2003; Lucito et al., 2003) or can utilize total genomic DNA if the spotted oligonucleotides are long (i.e. >50mer) and isothermic (i.e. all oligonucleotides on the array platform may not be exactly the same length but have similar melting temperatures (Tm); e.g. Barrett et al., 2004; Selzer et al., 2005).

aCGH provides a powerful entry point for cancer studies, due to its ability to efficiently detect genomic imbalances from a wide variety of specimens in an unbiased fashion. High-resolution and comprehensive genome-wide analyses of tumors are needed for the discovery of genes involved in the initiation and progression of a disease. For tumor specimens with appropriate clinical information, aCGH has the potential of rapidly identifying candidate oncogenes (genes that are usually gained or amplified in the tumor) and candidate tumor suppressor genes (genes usually seen as DNA losses) that are associated with a particular tumor type and stage of disease.

Genomic imbalances that are recurrently seen in multiple, unrelated individuals with similar disease should be differentiable from imbalances that arise randomly due to genomic instability. If a recurrent genomic imbalance is correlated in a statistically significant fashion with a particular tumor type or disease stage, it becomes an important candidate biomarker for use in clinical testing. Indeed, association of specific DNA copy number aberrations with disease prognosis has already been appreciated for a variety of tumors, including prostate cancer (e.g. Paris et al., 2004), breast cancer (e.g. Callagy et al., 2005), lung cancer (e.g. Kim et al., 2005), gastric cancer (e.g. Weiss et al., 2004), chronic lymphocytic leukemia (e.g. Schwaenen et al., 2004) and lymphomas (e.g. Martinez-Climent et al., 2003; Rubio-Moscardo et al., 2005).

One of the main limitations of aCGH is its inability to detect genomic aberrations that do not result in copy number changes (i.e. balanced chromosomal translocations and inversions). Moreover, aCGH has difficulties in reliably detecting low levels of mosaicism. The level of mosaicism that can be detected is primarily dependent on two factors: (1) the size and probe coverage within the region of mosaic genomic imbalance and (2) the extent of the copy number change within the region of imbalance (e.g. a 1-copy deletion vs. a 20-fold amplification). Shaw et al. (2004) suggested that a one-copy change of a single DNA clone on an array can be detected when the aberration is present in at least 50% of the cells. Our experiences have been that a one-copy change of a single DNA clone with a 100-kb or larger insert can be detected in a dye-swap assay when at least 30% of the cells have gained or lost the entire clone. One-copy changes of whole chromosomes, found in at least 10% of the cells being analyzed, are also detectable by dye-swap aCGH assays. This limitation is particularly important in cancer research where DNA samples being interrogated can be genetically heterogeneous and may often include surrounding, non-tumor cells that render genomic imbalances (even if present in 100% of the tumor cells), equivalent to a mosaic state in a given aCGH assay.

Wide-spread copy number variation in the human genome

Some of the earliest evidence for human genetic variation began with the identification of microscopically visible chromosomal alterations corresponding to large genomic regions that varied in size, morphology and staining properties among different individuals but had no apparent effect on phenotype (e.g. de la Chapelle, 1974; Lee, 2005). However, there were only a dozen or so, such well known chromosomal polymorphisms.

Since the completion of the human genome project, there have been substantial strides in describing and cataloguing different forms of human genetic variation. The most prevalent form of genetic variation was believed to be single nucleotide polymorphisms (SNPs), which accounted for 0.1% or 3 million nucleotides of genetic variability in a given individual. Currently, the total number of documented SNPs in the human genome exceeds 10 million (Altshuler et al., 2000).

In 2004, two groups used different aCGH platforms to independently identify the widespread presence of a newly appreciated class of genetic variation in the human genome: copy number variation (Iafrate et al., 2004; Sebat et al., 2004). Copy number variants (CNVs) can be defined as DNA segments of 1 kb or larger that vary in copy number

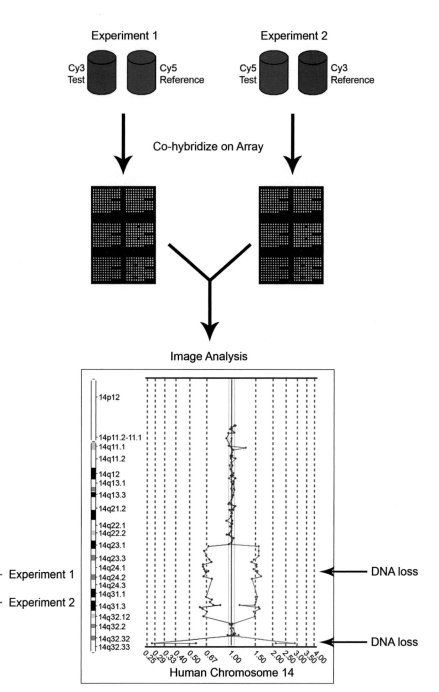

Fig. 1. Test and reference DNAs are differentially labeled with fluorescent dyes (typically cyanine-3 and cyanine-5) and cohybridized to DNA fragments which are spotted on a glass slide. The test and reference DNAs competitively bind to the spotted DNA fragments and the resulting fluorescence intensity ratios of both DNAs reflect their relative concentrations in the original DNA samples. To reduce the false-positive error rate, the two profiles of a dye-swap experiment are compared. Data are normalized so that the ratio is set to a standard value, typically 1.0 on a linear scale or 0.0 on a logarithmic scale. Each dot on the graph represents a particular DNA fragment on the array. A blue tracing to the left and a red tracing to the right of the '1.0' vertical line indicates a loss of a genomic region. Conversely, a blue tracing to the right and a red tracing to the left indicates a genomic gain. Blue and red tracings at the '1.0' vertical line indicate no copy number change.

among individuals (Feuk et al., 2006; Freeman et al., 2006) with current estimates suggesting that as much as 12% or more (>360 million bases of DNA) of the human genome is copy number variable (Redon et al., unpublished data). CNVs can be simple in structure (i.e. a deletion or a localized tandem duplication) or complex (involving multiple chromosomal loci). And more than one quarter of known CNVs appear to be flanked or associated with segmental duplications (Iafrate et al., 2004; Redon et al., unpublished data). CNVs that are associated with segmental duplications are thought to arise and be maintained via non-allelic homologous recombination-mediated events (reviewed in

Stankiewicz and Lupski, 2002), while the mechanisms for generating and maintaining CNVs not associated with segmental duplications remain ill defined.

Some CNVs could influence gene expression levels either by directly altering the copy number of the gene itself, or by altering the copy number of gene regulatory elements, or via altered position effects. Expression levels of genes within CNV regions could correlate positively (e.g. duplication of the gene leads to increased gene expression) or negatively (e.g. deletion of a negative regulator for a gene could lead to increased gene expression). Interestingly, CNV regions appear to be enriched for 'environmental sensor genes' (Sebat

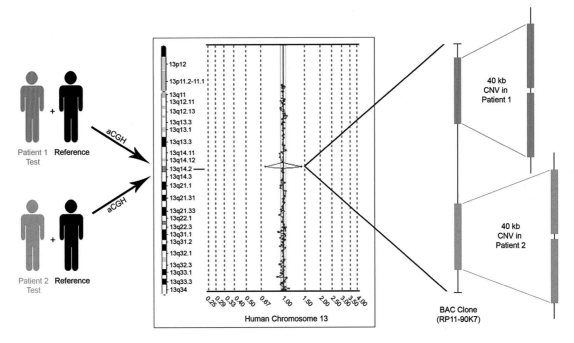

Fig. 2. Two patients who each have different single-copy duplications within the BAC clone (RP11-90K7) would have indistinguishable aCGH results.

et al., 2004; Tuzun et al., 2005) that include genes involved in cell adhesion, sensory perception, cell surface antigens and integrity, drug detoxification, immune response, and inflammation (Feuk et al., 2006; Freeman et al., 2006). While some CNVs (particularly larger CNVs that harbor multiple, developmentally important genes) may be shown to directly cause rare, early-onset and highly penetrant genomic disorders (Stankiewicz and Lupski, 2002), it is believed that other CNVs will actually turn out to be susceptibility factors for common human diseases. For example, the *Ccl3l1* gene and the *Fcgr3* gene have recently been associated with differential susceptibility to acquired immune deficiency syndrome (AIDS) and immunologically-related glomerulonephritis, respectively (Gonzales et al., 2005; Aitman et al., 2006).

Knowing that CNVs are a ubiquitous feature of the human genome, researchers should now be more cautious when interpreting aCGH data from human tumor specimens. When available, aCGH experiments designed to explore somatic changes occurring during tumorigenesis, should use the tumor sample as the test DNA source and a matching, non-tumor sample from the same individual as the reference DNA source (Fig. 1). Such an aCGH strategy should eliminate the identification of the patient's CNVs, allowing researchers to appreciate the specific somatic genomic changes that are more likely to be involved in disease initiation and progression. If non-tumor DNA from the patient is unavailable, aCGH can be performed using a reference DNA that is a mixture of DNAs from multiple healthy individuals. This strategy leads to reduced observation of common CNVs, but may still allow rare CNVs to be ob-

served in the aCGH assays. Subsequently, researchers could turn to a number of publically available databases that are collating known CNVs (e.g. the Database of Genomic Variants: http://projects.tcag.ca/variation; the Human Structural Variation Database: http://paralogy.gs.washington. edu/structuralvariation) to determine which of their observed imbalances are more likely to be CNVs. The caveat to this strategy is that many of the CNVs collated in these databases have ill-defined breakpoints and are based on large insert clones (e.g. BAC/PAC/P1 clones of ~120–150 kb in size). Thus, imbalances observed with a given BAC clone may actually be the result of different non-overlapping CNVs within a representative BAC clone (Fig. 2). This becomes less of an issue as the boundaries of the CNVs in these databases are better defined and researchers employ well-validated, higher-resolution array platforms for their experiments.

Recent studies have shown that over 500 CNVs can commonly exist as heterozygous (1 copy) or homozygous (2 copy) deletions among healthy individuals (e.g. Conrad et al., 2006; Hinds et al., 2006; McCarroll et al., 2006). Consistent with Knudson's two-hit theory of cancer causation, CNVs that are heterozygously deleted in multiple healthy individuals may still harbor a candidate tumor suppressor gene that becomes 'unmasked' when a functional mutation (or other small alteration) in the other allele results in tumorigenesis (Fig. 3). Conversely, CNVs that are homozygously deleted in multiple, unrelated healthy individuals are less likely to be directly involved in the genesis or proliferation of a given tumor.

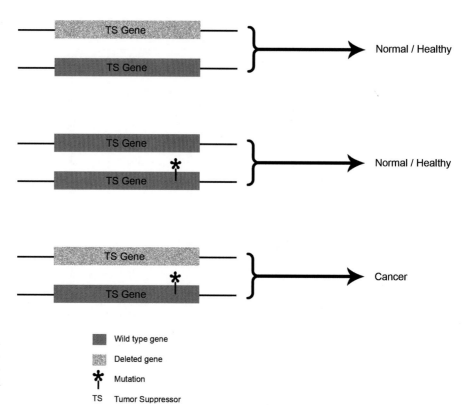

Fig. 3. An individual who has a heterozygous deletion or mutation of tumor suppressor gene alone can be a healthy carrier. However, an individual who has both the deletion and a mutation could develop cancer.

Wild type gene

Deleted gene

* Mutation

TS Tumor Suppressor

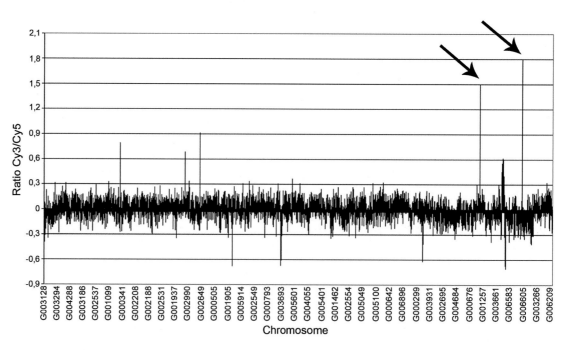

Fig. 4. aCGH profile of an individual with chronic myelogenous leukemia (CML). Arrows show two single BAC clone gains on chromosomes 18 and 22 that have an increased frequency (as much as 80%) in CML samples with an additional deletion at chromosome region 9q34.

While specific CNVs may not directly lead to the genesis of a tumor, it remains to be determined if certain CNVs are associated with susceptibility for certain types of tumors. Indirect evidence for such a phenomenon would include observing an increased frequency of certain CNVs in specific tumors (e.g. Fig. 4). For example, Braude et al. (2006) identified a CNV (CNV 14q12) that was present as a genomic gain or loss in 10% of control DNA derived from cytogenetically normal individuals, but the incidence of this CNV increased to 72% in a cohort of chronic myelogenous leukemia samples that had a microdeletion on one of their derivative chromosomes 9 and is associated with poor prognosis. Susceptibility to tumorigenesis should not be limited to individual CNVs but may also be extended to specific combinations of CNVs. For example, a homozygous deletion of any of three CNVs may be benign in nature, but homozygous deletions of all three CNVs in an individual may be associated with increased occurrence of a certain type of lymphoma. To properly assess whether acquired or inherited CNVs may be associated with the onset or progression of neoplasia, larger genome-wide studies need to be performed in conjunction with architectural definition of known human CNVs.

Copy number variation also occurs in mice and may be associated with certain QTLs

The mouse is the most commonly used model system for genetic research of human disease processes, including cancer. Many biological attributes, such as development, pathology, and physiology are shared among mammalian species. Hence, genetic manipulation and studies in mice rapidly lead to critical insights on the function of corresponding genes in humans.

Similar to that observed among humans, mice were also found to harbor many CNVs that differentiate inbred mouse strains (Li et al., 2004; Adams et al., 2005). In an initial study by Li et al. (2004), a minimal tiling-path mouse genomic array containing 19,200 BAC clones from the RP23 library (Gregory et al., 2002; Fig. 5) was used to compare the genomes of 13 commonly used mouse strains. In total, 216 BAC clones consistently showed a relative loss compared to genomic DNA from the C57BL/6J strain and 130 BAC clones consistently showed a relative gain compared to this same mouse strain. Many of these BACs were overlapping clones and showed abnormalities in more than one mouse strain, and some of these regions spanned more than one megabase and were detected by multiple BAC clones. Between any two inbred strains, CNVs totaling a few megabases could be detected.

Although the biological function of these CNVs in mice remains to be established, we suspect that some of these

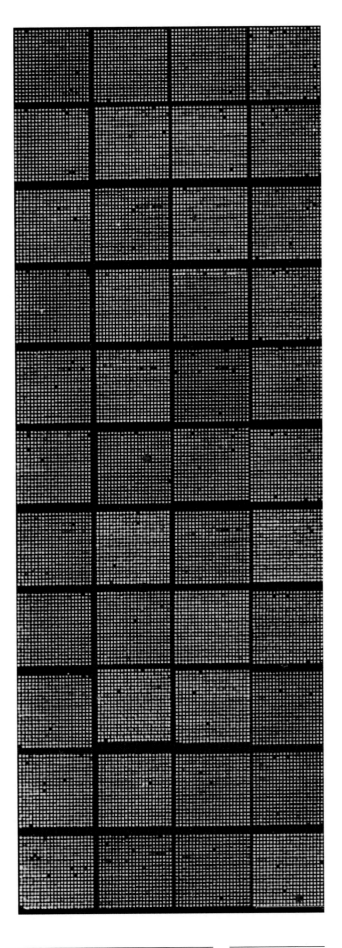

Fig. 5. A first-generation, minimal tiling path mouse array containing 19,200 mouse BAC clones chosen from the RP23 library.

Table 1. List of mouse QTLs overlapping with known CNVs

Trait	QTL marker	QTL peak position (Mb)	Overlapping CNV position (Mb)	Reference
Immunity	D13Mit63	42	40.7–40.9	Azuara and Pereira (2000)
Immunity	D17Mit41	82.9	90.5–90.7	Azuara and Pereira (2000)
Infectious disease	D1Mit396	153		Mitsos et al. (2000)
Infectious disease	D3Mit241	66.8		Mitsos et al. (2000)
Infectious disease	D7Mit117	18.9	11.5–23.5	Mitsos et al. (2000)
Obesity/diabetes	D2Mit413	162		Drake et al. (2001)
Obesity/diabetes	D3Mit14	118.8	144–146	Drake et al. (2001)
Obesity/diabetes	D6Mit198	120	130–131	Drake et al. (2001)
Obesity/diabetes	D7Mit80	27.6	11.5–23.5	Drake et al. (2001)
Obesity/diabetes	D15Mit13	83.4		Drake et al. (2001)
Arthritis	D6Mit124	71.5		Yang et al. (1999)
Arthritis	D10Mit64	74.7		Yang et al. (1999)
Arthritis	D7Mit34	91.4	92.6–102	Yang et al. (1999)
Angiogenesis	chr4	32	41.4–47.4	Rogers et al. (2004)
Angiogenesis	chr13	21.4	40.7–40.9	Rogers et al. (2004)
Angiogenesis	chr15	53.6	51.6–51.8	Rogers et al. (2004)
Angiogenesis	chr18	79.2		Rogers et al. (2004)
Glaucoma	D6Mit355	63.4		Chang et al. (1999)
Glaucoma	D4Mit178	65.5	41.4–47.5	Chang et al. (1999)
Cancer	D4Mit31	105.4	107–120	Lee et al. (1995)
Cancer	D10Mit15	66.7		Lee et al. (1995)

polymorphisms may play a role in conferring subtle phenotypic differences inherent in the diverse mouse strains and could even ultimately affect the outcome of certain genetic manipulation experiments. If this were the case, it may provide some explanation as to why the same gene knockout experiment results in inconsistent phenotypes among different mouse genetic backgrounds.

Since quantitative trait loci (QTLs) are subtle phenotypic differences that have a spectrum of values among individual organisms, it is possible that certain CNVs contribute in some manner to certain mouse QTLs. Past efforts in finding QTL genes have focused exclusively on identifying SNPs in candidate genes. However, with the discovery of CNVs as a common phenomenon in mouse genomes, researchers are now encouraged to explore the contribution of CNVs to specific QTLs. Indeed, at the molecular level, a gene's activity is thought to be controlled by the gene's specificity and its expression level. The gene's specificity is stipulated by the gene sequence and therefore specific nucleotide changes within a gene can have a dramatic effect on the individual's phenotype. On the other hand, change of gene copy number, particularly with duplications, may only minimally alter the equilibrium of associated biochemical processes. This subtle genetic effect of gene dosage differences has been extensively exemplified in some studies of tumor susceptibility of various mouse knockout models (e.g. Dumon-Jones et al., 2003; Avanzo et al., 2004; Li et al., 2004; Drusco et al., 2005; Guo et al., 2005).

To support the hypothesis that mouse CNVs harbor genes for quantitative traits, we searched the literature for mapped QTLs in mice of DBA/2J and C57BL/6J background to determine if statistically significant overlaps exist between QTLs and CNVs. DBA/2J and C57BL/6J are the most commonly used mouse strains for QTL studies because of the availability of publicly-available recombinant inbred and congenic strains developed from these two genetic backgrounds. As most of the QTL mapping only reaches a resolution of 10 cM (approximately 20 Mb) around the peak markers, the entire mouse genome has ~150 QTL loci with an apparent correlation between CNVs and traits with a high number of QTLs. We then focused our search on traits with a relatively small number of QTLs and pooled the number of QTLs overlapping with CNVs to calculate statistical significance. Between strain DBA/2J and C57BL/6J, we discovered 24 CNVs (Li et al., 2004). When comparing the peak QTL positions of the seven traits with nearby CNVs, we found that for every trait, there was at least one overlap between a QTL and known CNVs. In total, we have identified 12 out of 21 QTLs overlapping with CNVs for the seven traits analyzed (Table 1). The association between CNVs and QTLs is highly significant ($\chi^2 = 22.2$, $P < 10^{-5}$). Among the seven traits examined, three have QTLs significantly overlapping with CNVs (immunity, $\chi^2 = 8.8$, $P < 0.006$; obesity/diabetes, $\chi^2 = 6.0$, $P < 0.03$; angiogenesis, $\chi^2 = 8.7$, $P < 0.007$). These data support the idea that some QTLs are significantly associated with CNVs.

Zebrafish aCGH in cancer research

The zebrafish is well established as a genetic system for studying vertebrate development due to its small size, short generation time, high fecundity, and transparent embryos. More recently, investigators have begun applying zebrafish to the study of cancer genetics (Amatruda et al., 2002). One of the major advantages for using the zebrafish system is the amount of information that can be obtained in a short period of time because large numbers of zebrafish can be easily sectioned at specific time points after carcinogen treatment, on a scale that would be difficult to achieve with other organisms such as mice. A variety of tumors, including carcinomas, germ cell tumors, small blue round cell tumors and sarcomas, have already been seen in cancer toxicology experiments of zebrafish (Spitsbergen et al., 2000a, b). These neoplasms histologically resemble human cancers, including the capacity to invade neighboring tissues. For example, hepatocellular carcinoma is one of the more common tumors seen in carcinogen-treated zebrafish. Histologically, these tumors exhibit a wide spectrum of severity – from small foci of uncertain malignant potential to aggressive neoplasms with significant nuclear pleomorphism. It is likely that this morphologic spectrum reflects differences in underlying genetic changes. Hence, understanding the genetics of tumor progression in this system may be a foundation for the identification of prognostic indicators and targets for early therapeutic intervention in humans.

Although the production and phenotypic analysis of zebrafish mutations has progressed at an amazing pace over the past few years (Driever et al., 1996; Haffter et al., 1996), zebrafish genomics has not advanced as far as that for human and mouse. Currently, meiotic microsatellite maps, expressed sequence tagged (EST) sequencing projects, radiation hybrid (RH) panels, and the anticipated sequencing of the entire zebrafish genome in approximately 1–2 years facilitate the identification of genes important for cellular regulation (Thisse and Zon, 2002). However, to enhance the use of the zebrafish as a cancer model, additional genomic resources are required.

Recently, an array CGH platform has been developed for the zebrafish to assess genomic imbalances in tumor specimens. BAC clones containing zebrafish orthologs to known human oncogenes and tumor suppressor genes were chosen for inclusion on this platform. These BAC clones were first hybridized onto metaphase chromosome spreads from wildtype zebrafish, along with a known chromosome marker (Lee and Smith, 2004) to chromosomally localize the BAC clone and determine whether it uniquely mapped to a single chromosome region (e.g. Fig. 6a). BAC clones hybridizing to multiple chromosomal loci (e.g. Fig. 6b) were subsequently excluded from the array. Ultimately, an array containing 200 validated zebrafish BAC clones including 45

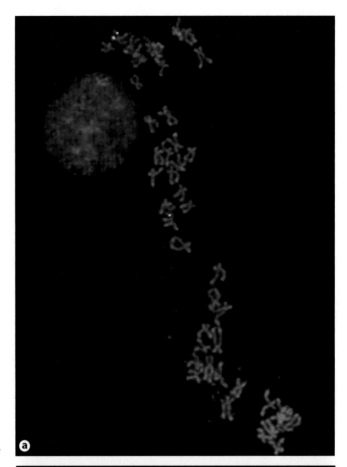

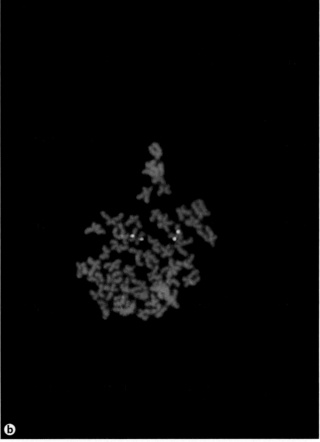

Fig. 6. FISH mapping of zebrafish BAC clones upon metaphase spreads from wild type zebrafish. (**a**) A BAC clone observed to have a unique signal (in green) cohybridized with the near-telomeric BAC clone (in red) for linkage group chromosome 1 (LG 1). (**b**) A BAC clone giving multiple signals throughout the genome (in red) cohybridized with a near-centromeric BAC clone (in green) for LG 21. BAC clones yielding multiple signals would not be ideal for array CGH.

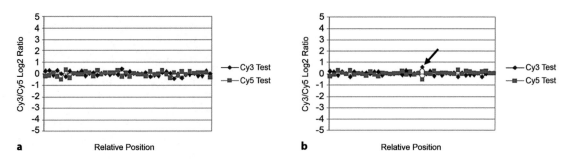

Fig. 7. Tumor analysis on the zebrafish cancer array CGH platform. (**a**) Analysis with matched tumor DNA and non-tumor DNA from the same fish. (**b**) Analysis with the same tumor DNA with wild type (i.e., non-tumor) DNA from a different fish. A gain in one BAC clone (denoted by the arrow in **b**) is observed in the analysis of the DNA from the two different fish. This imbalance was not detected in the matched DNA analysis (**a**), suggesting that this gain is a copy number variant and not related specifically to the tumor.

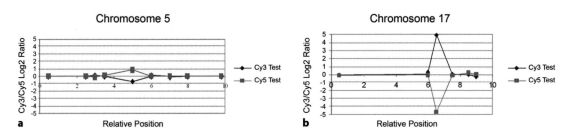

Fig. 8. Examples of genomic imbalances being observed on the validated zebrafish cancer array. (**a**) A loss on chromosome 5. (**b**) A gain on chromosome 17.

clones containing known oncogenes and 45 clones containing known tumor suppressor genes as well as 110 clones from chromosome-specific landmarks was constructed. This zebrafish array is now being used to assess genomic imbalances in zebrafish melanomas, rhabdomyosarcomas, T-cell acute lymphatic leukemias, and other tumors. All aCGH experiments are being conducted with tumor DNA matched to non-tumor DNA from the same fish. Clearly, if tumor DNA and non-tumor DNA from the same fish were not used in such experiments, there is a risk of identifying genomic imbalances that are not necessarily related to the tumors, but instead are copy number variants among the fish specimens (e.g. Fig. 7). This zebrafish cancer array is proving to be a valuable tool in the identification of previously unknown DNA copy number gains and losses in the tumor specimens being studied (e.g. Fig. 8).

Conclusion

aCGH is a molecular cytogenetic technique particularly useful in detecting and mapping DNA copy number alterations. In the past decade, aCGH has been successfully used in detecting genomic amplification and deletions of many types of tumors. Now, it is very important to distinguish 'benign' copy number variants and generalized genomic instability from genomic imbalances that are more likely to be involved in the initiation and specific etiology of a given tumor. Continued research into CNVs will clearly impact the success of future cancer genetic studies.

Acknowledgements

The authors would like to thank Ms. Shona Hislop for her assistance with Figs. 1–3.

References

Adams DJ, Dermitzakis ET, Cox T, Smith J, Davies R, et al: Complex haplotypes, copy number polymorphisms and coding variation in two recently divergent mouse strains. Nat Genet 37: 532–536 (2005).

Aitman, TJ, Dong R, Vyse TJ, Norsworthy PJ, Johnson MD, et al: Copy number polymorphism in *Fcgr3* predisposes to glomerulonephritis in rats and humans. Nature 16:851–855 (2006).

Altshuler D, Pollara VJ, Cowles CR, Van Etten WJ, Baldwin J, et al: An SNP map of the human genome generated by reduced representation shotgun sequencing. Nature 407:513–516 (2000).

Amatruda JF, Shepard JL, Stern HM, Zon LI: Zebrafish as a cancer model system. Cancer Cell 1:229–231 (2002).

Avanzo JL, Mesnil M, Hernandez-Blazquez FJ, Mackowiak II, Mori CM, et al: Increased susceptibility to urethane-induced lung tumors in mice with decreased expression of connexin43. Carcinogenesis 25:1973–1982 (2004).

Azuara V, Pereira P: Genetic mapping of two murine loci that influence the development of IL-4 producing Thy-1dull gamma delta thymnocytes. J Immunol 165:42–48 (2000).

Barrett MT, Scheffer A, Ben-Dor A, Sampas N, Lipson D, et al: Comparative genomic hybridization using oligonucleotide microarrays and total genomic DNA. Proc Natl Acad Sci USA 101: 17765–17770 (2004).

Bignell GR, Huang J, Greshock J, Watt S, Butler A, et al: High-resolution analysis of DNA copy number using oligonucleotide microarrays. Genome Res 14:287–295 (2004).

Braude I, Vukovic B, Prasad M, Marrano P, Turley S, et al: Large scale copy number variation (CNV) at 14q12 is associated with the presence of genomic abnormalities in neoplasia. BMC Genomics 7:138 (2006).

Callagy G, Pharoah P, Chin SF, Sangan T, Daigo Y, et al: Identification and validation of prognostic markers in breast cancer with the complementary use of array-CGH and tissue microarrays. J Pathol 205:388–396 (2005).

Chang B, Smith RS, Hawes NL, Anderson MG, Zabaleta A, et al: Interacting loci cause severe iris atrophy and glaucoma in DBA/2J mice. Nat Genet 21:405–409 (1999).

Conrad DF, Andrews TD, Carter NP, Hurles ME, Pritchard JK: A high-resolution survey of deletion polymorphism in the human genome. Nat Genet 38:75–81 (2006).

Davies JJ, Wilson IM, Lam WL: Array CGH technologies and their applications to cancer genomes. Chromosome Res 13:237–248 (2005).

de la Chapelle A, Schroder J, Stenstrand K, Fellman J, Herva R, et al: Pericentric inversions of human chromosomes 9 and 10. Am J Hum Genet 26:746–766 (1974).

Drake TA, Schadt E, Hannani K, Kabo JM, Krass K, et al: Genetic loci determining bone density in mice with diet-induced atherosclerosis. Physiol Genomics 5:205–215 (2001).

Driever W, Solnica-Krezel L, Schier AF, Neuhauss SC, Malicki J, et al: A genetic screen for mutations affecting embryogenesis in zebrafish. Development 123:37–46 (1996).

Drusco A, Zanesi N, Roldo C, Trapasso F, Farber JL, et al: Knockout mice reveal a tumor suppressor function for Testin. Proc Natl Acad Sci USA 102:10947–10951 (2005).

Dumon-Jones V, Frappart PO, Tong WM, Sajithlal G, Hulla W, et al: *Nbn* heterozygosity renders mice susceptible to tumor formation and ionizing radiation-induced tumorigenesis. Cancer Res 63:7263–7269 (2003).

Feuk L, Carson AR, Scherer SW: Structural variation in the human genome. Nat Rev Genet 7: 85–97 (2006).

Forozan F, Karhu R, Kononen J, Kallioniemi A, Kallioniemi OP: Genome screening by comparative genomic hybridization. Trends Genet 13: 405–409 (1997).

Freeman JL, Perry GH, Feuk L, Redon R, McCarroll SA, et al: Copy number variation: New insights in genome diversity. Genome Res 16:949–961 (2006).

Garraway LA, Widlund HR, Rubin MA, Getz G, Berger AJ, et al: Integrative genomic analyses identify *MITF* as a lineage survival oncogene amplified in malignant melanoma. Nature 436: 117–122 (2005).

Gonzalez, E, Kulkarni H, Bolivar H, Mangano A, Sanchez R, et al: The influence of *CCL3L1* gene-containing segmental duplications on HIV-1/AIDS susceptibility. Science 307:1434–1440 (2005).

Gregory SG, Sekhon M, Schein J, Zhao S, Osoegawa K, et al: A physical map of the mouse genome. Nature 418:743–750 (2002).

Guo Y, Cleveland JL, O'Brien TG: Haploinsufficiency for *Odc* modifies mouse skin tumor susceptibility. Cancer Res 65:1146–1149 (2005).

Haffter P, Granato M, Brand M, Mullins MC, Hammerschmidt M, et al: The identification of genes with unique and essential functions in the development of the zebrafish, *Danio rerio*. Development 123:1–36 (1996).

Hinds DA, Kloek AP, Jen M, Chen X, Frazer KA: Common deletions and SNPs are in linkage disequilibrium in the human genome. Nat Genet 38:82–85 (2006).

Iafrate AJ, Feuk L, Rivera MN, Listewnik ML, Donahoe PK, et al: Detection of large-scale variation in the human genome. Nat Genet 36:949–951 (2004).

Kallioniemi A, Kallioniemi OP, Sudar D, Rutovitz D, Gray JW, et al: Comparative genomic hybridization for molecular cytogenetic analysis of solid tumors. Science 258:818–821 (1992).

Kennedy GC, Matsuzaki H, Dong S, Liu WM, Huang J, et al: Large-scale genotyping of complex DNA. Nat Biotechnol 21:1233–1237 (2003).

Kim TM, Yim SH, Lee JS, Kwon MS, Ryu JW, et al: Genome-wide screening of genomic alterations and their clinicopathologic implications in non-small cell lung cancers. Clin Cancer Res 11:8235–8242 (2005).

Komura D, Shen F, Ishikawa S, Fitch KR, Chen W, et al: Genome-wide detection of human copy number variations using high density DNA oligonucleotide arrays. Genome Res (in press).

Lee C: Vive la difference! Nat Genet 37:660–661 (2005).

Lee C, Smith A: Molecular cytogenetic methodologies and a bacterial artificial chromosome (BAC) probe panel resource for genomic analyses in zebrafish. Methods Cell Biol 77:241–254 (2004).

Lee GH, Bennett LM, Carabeo RA, Drinkwater NR: Identification of hepatocarcinogen-resistance genes in DBA/2 mice. Genetics 139:387–395 (1995).

Lee C, Rens W, Yang F: Multicolor fluorescence in situ hybridization (FISH) approaches for simultaneous analysis of the entire human genome; in Dracopoli NC, Haines JL, Korf BR, Morton CC, Seidman CE, et al (eds): Current Protocols in Human Genetics, pp 4.9.1–11 (John Wiley and Sons, New York 2000).

Li AG, Lu SL, Zhang MX, Deng C, Wang XJ: *Smad3* knockout mice exhibit a resistance to skin chemical carcinogenesis. Cancer Res 64:7836–7845 (2004).

Lucito R, Healy J, Alexander J, Reiner A, Esposito D, et al: Representational oligonucleotide microarray analysis: a high-resolution method to detect genome copy number variation. Genome Res 13:2291–2305 (2003).

Martinez-Climent JA, Alizadeh AA, Segraves R, Blesa D, Rubio-Moscardo F, et al: Transformation of follicular lymphoma to diffuse large cell lymphoma is associated with a heterogeneous set of DNA copy number and gene expression alterations. Blood 101:3109–3117 (2003).

McCarroll SA, Hadnott TN, Perry GH, Sabeti PC, Zody MC, et al: International HapMap Consortium. Common deletion polymorphisms in the human genome. Nat Genet 38:86–92 (2006).

Mitsos LM, Cardon LR, Fortin A, Ryan L, LaCourse R, et al: Genetic control of susceptibility to infection with *Mycobacterium tuberculosis* in mice. Genes Immun 1:467–477 (2000).

Paris PL, Andaya A, Fridlyand J, Jain AN, Weinberg V, et al: Whole genome scanning identifies genotypes associated with recurrence and metastasis in prostate tumors. Hum Mol Genet 13: 1303–1313 (2004).

Pollack JR, Perou CM, Alizadeh AA, Eisen MB, Pergamenschikov A, et al: Genome-wide analysis of DNA copy-number changes using cDNA microarrays. Nat Genet 23:41–46 (1999).

Pollack JR, Sorlie T, Perou CM, Rees CA, Jeffrey SS, et al: Microarray analysis reveals a major direct role of DNA copy number alteration in the transcriptional program of human breast tumors. Proc Natl Acad Sci USA 99:12963–12968 (2002).

Rogers MS, Rohan RM, Birsner AE, D'Amato RJ: Genetic loci that control the angiogenic response to basic fibroblast growth factor. FASEB J 18:1050–1059 (2004).

Rubio-Moscardo F, Climent J, Siebert R, Piris MA, Martin-Subero JI, et al: Mantle-cell lymphoma genotypes identified with CGH to BAC microarrays define a leukemic subgroup of disease and predict patient outcome. Blood 105:4445–4454 (2005).

Schwaenen C, Nessling M, Wessendorf S, Salvi T, Wrobel G, et al: Automated array-based genomic profiling in chronic lymphocytic leukemia: development of a clinical tool and discovery of recurrent genomic alterations. Proc Natl Acad Sci USA 101:1039–1044 (2004).

Sebat J, Lakshmi B, Troge J, Alexander J, Young J, et al: Large-scale copy number polymorphism in the human genome. Science 305:525–528 (2004).

Selzer RR, Richmond TA, Pofahl NJ, Green RD, Eis PS, et al: Analysis of chromosome breakpoints in neuroblastoma at sub-kilobase resolution using fine-tiling oligonucleotide array CGH. Genes Chromosomes Cancer 44:305–319 (2005).

Shaw CJ, Stankiewicz P, Bien-Willner G, Bello SC, Shaw CA, et al: Small marker chromosomes in two patients with segmental aneusomy for proximal 17p. Hum Genet 115:1–7 (2004).

Slater HR, Bailey DK, Ren H, Cao M, Bell K, et al: High-resolution identification of chromosomal abnormalities using oligonucleotide arrays containing 116,204 SNPs. Am J Hum Genet 77: 709–726 (2005).

Snijders AM, Nowak N, Segraves R, Blackwood S, Brown N, et al: Assembly of microarrays for genome-wide measurement of DNA copy number. Nat Genet 29:263–264 (2001).

Solinas-Toldo S, Lampel S, Stilgenbauer S, Nickolenko J, Benner A, et al: Matrix-based comparative genomic hybridization: biochips to screen for genomic imbalances. Genes Chromosomes Cancer 20:399–407 (1997).

Spitsbergen JM, Tsai HW, Reddy A, Miller T, Arbogast D, et al: Neoplasia in zebrafish (*Danio rerio*) treated with N-methyl-N′-nitro-N-nitrosoguanidine by three exposure routes at different developmental stages. Toxicol Pathol 28:716–725 (2000a).

Spitsbergen JM, Tsai HW, Reddy A, Miller T, Arbogast D, et al: Neoplasia in zebrafish (*Danio rerio*) treated with 7,12-dimethylbenz[a]anthracene by two exposure routes at different developmental stages. Toxicol Pathol 28:705–715 (2000b).

Stankiewicz P, Lupski JR: Genome architecture, rearrangements and genomic disorders. Trends Genet 18:74–82 (2002).

Thisse C, Zon LI: Organogenesis – heart and blood formation from the zebrafish point of view. Science 295:457–462 (2002).

Tuzun E, Sharp AJ, Bailey JA, Kaul R, Morrison VA, et al: Fine-scale structural variation of the human genome. Nat Genet 37:727–732 (2005).

Weiss MM, Kuipers EJ, Postma C, Snijders AM, Pinkel D, et al: Genomic alterations in primary gastric adenocarcinomas correlate with clinicopathological characteristics and survival. Cell Oncol 26:307–317 (2004).

Yang HT, Jirholt J, Svensson L, Sundvall M, Jansson L, et al: Identification of genes controlling collagen-induced arthritis in mice: striking homology with susceptibility loci previously identified in the rat. J Immunol 163:2916–2921 (1999).

Zhao X, Li C, Paez JG, Chin K, Janne PA, et al: An integrated view of copy number and allelic alterations in the cancer genome using single nucleotide polymorphism arrays. Cancer Res 64:3060–3071 (2004).

Cytogenet Genome Res 115:273–282 (2006)
DOI: 10.1159/000095924

Genome wide measurement of DNA copy number changes in neuroblastoma: dissecting amplicons and mapping losses, gains and breakpoints

E. Michels[a]   J. Vandesompele[a]   J. Hoebeeck[a]   B. Menten[a]   K. De Preter[a]
G. Laureys[b]   N. Van Roy[a]   F. Speleman[a]

[a]Center for Medical Genetics and
[b]Department of Pediatric Hematology and Oncology, Ghent University Hospital, Ghent (Belgium)

Manuscript received 16 February 2006; accepted in revised form for publication by A. Geurts van Kessel, 3 May 2006.

Abstract. In the past few years high throughput methods for assessment of DNA copy number alterations have witnessed rapid progress. Both 'in house' developed BAC, cDNA, oligonucleotide and commercial arrays are now available and widely applied in the study of the human genome, particularly in the context of disease. Cancer cells are known to exhibit DNA losses, gains and amplifications affecting tumor suppressor genes and proto-oncogenes. Moreover, these patterns of genomic imbalances may be associated with particular tumor types or subtypes and may have prognostic value. Here we summarize recent array CGH findings in neuroblastoma, a pediatric tumor of the sympathetic nervous system. A total of 176 primary tumors and 53 cell lines have been analyzed on different platforms. Through these studies the genomic content and boundaries of deletions, gains and amplifications were characterized with unprecedented accuracy. Furthermore, in conjunction with cytogenetic findings, array CGH allows the mapping of breakpoints of unbalanced translocations at a very high resolution.

Copyright © 2006 S. Karger AG, Basel

Neuroblastoma (NB) is a pediatric tumor arising from primitive sympathetic nervous cells. The median age of diagnosis is two years and almost 90% of patients are diagnosed before the age of five years. Neuroblastomas have a remarkably variable clinical behavior ranging from spontaneous regression to widespread metastasis and fatal outcome (Brodeur, 2003). As a step towards more efficient treatment and better survival for children with aggressive NB, improved risk assessment and prognostic staging is needed. Also, insights into the genetic defects and altered molecular pathways governing NB oncogenesis are urgently required in order to design new, more efficient and less toxic therapeutic strategies.

DNA copy number alterations in the pre-FISH era

NB is one of the first tumors in which proto-oncogene amplification was discovered and used in therapy stratification (Alitalo et al., 1983; Schwab et al., 1983; Brodeur et al., 1984; Seeger et al., 1985; Schwab, 1999). Cytogenetically, aggressive NB tumors and cell lines derived from high-stage NB were shown to contain double minute chromatin bodies or homogeneously staining chromosome regions. Molecular analyses revealed that these unusual chromosomal alterations represented high-level amplification of a new pro-

Request reprints from Frank Speleman
    Center for Medical Genetics
    Ghent University Hospital, De Pintelaan 185
    BE–9000 Ghent (Belgium)
    telephone: +32 9 240 2451; fax: +32 9 240 6549
    e-mail: Franki.Speleman@UGent.be

KARGER   Fax +41 61 306 12 34
              E-Mail karger@karger.ch
              www.karger.com

© 2006 S. Karger AG, Basel
1424–8581/06/1154–0273$23.50/0

Accessible online at:
www.karger.com/cgr

to-oncogene with high homology to the previously discovered *MYC* gene. Hence, the amplified gene in NB was coined *MYCN* (Alitalo et al., 1983; Schwab et al., 1983). In addition to the high level amplification, these neuroblastoma cells often showed 1p-deletions or unbalanced translocations leading to distal 1p-loss (Brodeur et al., 1977; Maris et al., 2000). Further contribution of classical cytogenetics to the study of NB was restricted, especially by the difficulty of obtaining good metaphases, in particular in NB without *MYCN* amplification which roughly represents two thirds of all cases. Independent DNA content measurements and study of rare karyotypes indicated that a subset of these NB, in particular those with low stage, show near triploidy (Look et al., 1984; Kaneko et al., 1987). Further analyses of DNA copy number changes in NB were based on loss of heterozygosity studies, focussing on delineation of the critical region for 1p-deletions (Maris and Matthay, 1999; Bown, 2001; White et al., 2005) but also leading to the discovery of other important recurrent regions of loss at chromosome 3p, 11q and 14q (Takita et al., 1995; Hallstensson et al., 1997; Ejeskar et al., 1998; Guo et al., 1999; Theobald et al., 1999; Hoshi et al., 2000a, b; Plantaz et al., 2001; Thompson et al., 2001). Although these studies contributed to our insights in NB genetics, LOH analyses typically focused on one or a few specific regions and, at best, analyzed the entire genome at low resolution. Consequently, a genome-wide view of the detailed patterns of genomic imbalances associated with the different NB subtypes could not be described until the advent of chromosomal comparative genomic hybridisation (CGH).

From FISH, M-FISH and metaphase CGH to array CGH

The introduction of fluorescent in situ hybridisation (FISH) and chromosomal CGH analyses led to a number of remarkable findings in the analysis of genetic alterations in NB. The power of FISH was best illustrated by the finding of whole chromosome 17 and partial 17q gain as the most frequent recurrent chromosomal change in NB (Savelyeva et al., 1994; Van Roy et al., 1994; Vandesompele et al., 1998, 2001; Speleman and Bown, 2000). Only one cytogenetic study referred to chromosome 17 involvement in NB, all other previously conducted cytogenetic analysis overlooked the non-random involvement of chromosome 17 in NB (Gilbert et al., 1984; Brodeur and Fong, 1989). FISH studies including 24-colour M-FISH (Speicher et al., 1996) revealed gain of 17q in the majority of cell lines and high-stage tumors, most often as the result of unbalanced translocations (Van Roy et al., 2001; Schleiermacher et al., 2003). Although many partner chromosomes can be involved in these translocations, chromosome 1p and 11q seemed to be preferentially involved, leading to combined 17q gain and loss of putative tumor suppressor loci as a result of one single genetic event. It has been hypothesized that 17q gain contributes to NB oncogenesis due to copy number gain of one or more critical dosage sensitive genes (Speleman and Bown, 2000; De Preter et al., in preparation).

The introduction of chromosomal CGH in the study of NB opened up new possibilities (Kallioniemi et al., 1992; du Manoir et al., 1993). CGH was rapidly recognized as a powerful method for detection of DNA copy number imbalances in tumors, in particular for those that were difficult to karyotype or for retrospective studies on frozen or formalin fixed samples. CGH indeed yielded a number of fundamental new insights in NB (Altura et al., 1997; Brinkschmidt et al., 1997, 1998; Lastowska et al., 1997; Plantaz et al., 1997, 2001; Van Gele et al., 1997; Van Roy et al., 1997; Vandesompele et al., 1998, 2001; Hirai et al., 1999; Breen et al., 2000; Cunsolo et al., 2000; Vettenranta et al., 2001; Iehara et al., 2002). Most importantly, this method provided a genome-wide overview of genomic imbalances occurring in these tumors and, for the first time, the association of all these alterations within tumors and subgroups could be analyzed. This series of investigations allowed us and others to categorize NB into three major subgroups: favorable near triploid NB with a recognizable pattern of predominantly numerical gains and losses (losses of chromosome 3, 4, 9, 11, 14 and gains of chromosomes 6, 7, 17 and 18) (subtype 1) and two subtypes of unfavorable NB with either 11q-loss without *MYCN* amplification (subtype 2A) or those with *MYCN* amplification and 1p-deletions (subtype 2B). The latter two subtypes both typically present with 17q gain. Multi-center studies revealed 17q gain as the strongest independent genetic prognostic marker in NB (Bown et al., 1999; Vandesompele et al., 2005).

Although CGH has been an important tool in the investigation of large genomic changes in NB, the technique also suffers from a number of limitations. Most importantly, this method is rather time consuming and, due to the use of chromosome preparations in the analysis, the resolution remains restricted at about ~10 Mb for single copy changes in most studies. Array CGH has overcome these two limitations and is now providing fast assays with a resolution at the kilobase level. Although the principle of array CGH had been reported as early as 1997 by Solinas-Toldo and colleagues (Solinas-Toldo et al., 1997), it has taken several years before this methodology became more widely used. Below, we review the results obtained with various array CGH platforms in the genetic study of NB.

Platforms for array CGH

In total, 11 array CGH studies on neuroblastoma have been performed using a variety of platforms including BAC, custom made cDNA and commercial oligonucleotide arrays (Beheshti et al., 2003; Mosse et al., 2003, 2005; Chen et al., 2004; De Preter et al., 2004, 2005; Scaruffi et al., 2004; Selzer et al., 2005; Stallings et al., 2006; Hoebeeck et al., in press; Michels et al., in preparation). A representative overview of the three types of neuroblastomas analysed by array CGH is shown in Fig. 1. Typically, the resolution of the arrays depends on the number and size of reporters that are tested. BAC arrays were initially developed in house by a number of pioneering groups (Solinas-Toldo et al., 1997; Snijders et al.,

Type 1

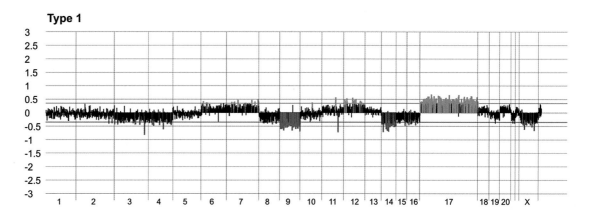

Type 2A

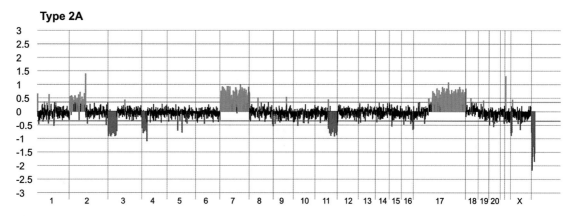

Type 2B

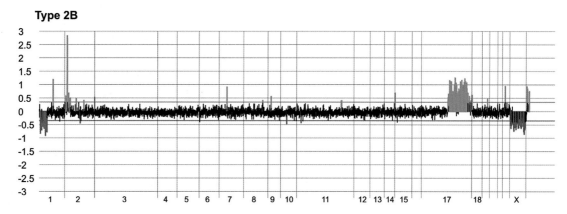

Fig. 1. ArrayCGH visualisation of representative neuroblastoma tumors, each belonging to a specific subtype (**1**, **2A**, **2B**). The X-axis represents the chromosomes, the Y-axis the ratio tumor versus control material.

2001; Cai et al., 2002; Wessendorf et al., 2002; Fiegler et al., 2003; Greshock et al., 2004). At the same time, oligonucleotide arrays were explored for DNA copy number change measurements (Lucito et al., 2003; Bignell et al., 2004).

The availability of a set of BAC clones with an average spacing of 1 Mb across the genome and further improvements in the protocols (Fiegler et al., 2003) as well as the production of reliable commercial platforms (Agilent, NimbleGen, Spectral Genomics, Affymetrix) have given a major boost to wide implementation of array CGH in the field of cancer genetics. The great interest in the potential of array

CGH has led to further increase in resolution, e.g. by producing tiling path arrays for given chromosomal regions (Fix et al., 2004; Hoebeeck et al., in press; Michels et al., in preparation) as well as whole genome tiling path BAC arrays (Garnis et al., 2003; Ishkanian et al., 2004; van Duin et al., 2005).

Similarly, oligonucleotide arrays have been produced with up to 40,000 oligos or more (Agilent), SNP chips probing about 500,000 SNPs (Affymetrix) or NimbleGen chips with up to 385,000 features. The SNP chips offer the additional advantage of allele status determination, as illustrat-

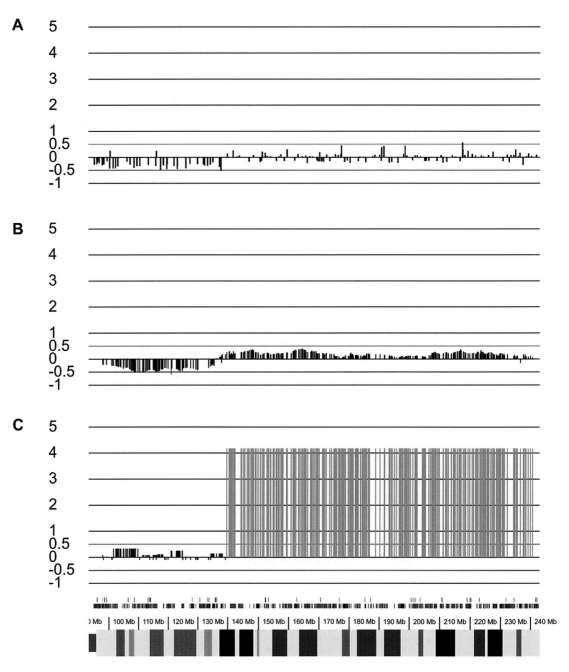

Fig. 2. Comparison of arrayCGH platforms focused on chromosome 2q in NB cell line SJNB-12. Part **A** depicts arrayCGH with a 1-Mb BAC set. Parts **B** and **C** represent Affymetrix SNP data, assessed for DNA copy number changes (**B**) or allele status determination (loss of heterozygosity) (**C**) (LOH-value out of Affymetrix GeneChip Chromosome Copy Number Analysis Tool was divided by 20 for rescaling reasons).

ed for chromosome 2 in NB cell line SJNB-12 (Fig. 2). This allows simultaneous copy number measurement, and detection of extended regions of homozygosity, even without copy number change (Bignell et al., 2004; Zhao et al., 2004). As a disadvantage, oligonucleotide and cDNA arrays typically produce more noise than BAC arrays (presumably due to the limited size of the reporter). Interpretation of copy number status for a given locus therefore requires combination of several adjacent reporters. Using the approach of a sliding window, good results can be produced, but at the cost of resolution. However, thanks to the recent production of (ultra) high-density oligonucleotide arrays, sensitivity remains very high even when 10–50 reporters have to be combined for copy number analysis at a given region. This is probably best illustrated by the current Affymetrix Gene Chip Mapping 500K Array set (3–5 kb) and NimbleGen chips that offer a standard 6 kilobase resolution but can even go up to an amazing resolution of 10 basepairs.

276

84

Cytogenet Genome Res 115:273–282 (2006)

Dissection of amplicons

In total 53 NB cell lines and 176 tumors have been investigated by several groups (Beheshti et al., 2003; Chen et al., 2004; De Preter et al., 2004, 2005; Scaruffi et al., 2004; Mosse et al., 2005; Selzer et al., 2005; Stallings et al., 2006; Hoebeeck et al., in press; Michels et al., in preparation). See also the Wellcome Trust Sanger Institute Cancer Genome Project web site (http://www.sanger.ac.uk/genetics/CGP). With respect to amplicon dissection, the *MYCN* locus, amplified in most of these cell lines, has been investigated in great detail in previous studies (Manohar et al., 1995; Kuroda et al., 1996; Reiter and Brodeur, 1996, 1998). Recent array CGH investigations focused on detailed dissection of complex *MYCN* amplicons as well as rare but putatively important amplicons involving other loci than those on the short arm of chromosome 2 (De Preter et al., 2004).

NB cell line IMR-32 contains a known complex non-contiguous amplicon including *MYCN* (Shiloh et al., 1985; Van Roy et al., 1997; Jones et al., 2000; Spieker et al., 2001) and was included in several array CGH studies (Beheshti et al., 2003; Chen et al., 2004; Mosse et al., 2005; Michels et al., in preparation). These revealed, in addition to *MYCN* and adjacent genes, also involvement of non-contiguous segments from the chromosome 2 short arm. In addition to our standard BAC array analysis we also studied this cell line with 10K SNP chips and Agilent Human Genome CGH Micro-Array 44A oligonucleotide chips. Furthermore, IMR-32 was included in a PCR based subtractive cloning procedure in our laboratory (De Preter et al., 2004). Deposition of the subtracted cDNA clones on a custom microarray and hybridization with IMR-32 DNA, resulted in the identification of clones that were overexpressed due to gene amplification. Using this approach, amplification of all previously reported amplified genes in this cell line was detected. Furthermore, four additional clones were found to be amplified, including the *ANTXR1* gene on 2p13.1, two anonymous transcripts, and a fusion transcript resulting from 2p13.3 and 2p24.3 juxtaposed sequences. Table 1 and Fig. 3 summarize the results of all studies on the 2p amplicon in IMR-32 (Beheshti et al., 2003; Chen et al., 2004; De Preter et al., 2004; Mosse et al., 2005; Michels et al., in preparation). Clearly, array CGH is well suited for amplicon dissection but it is of interest that the combined subtractive cloning and array CGH yielded complementary data. Involvement of other regions of 2p in *MYCN* amplicon formation was also detected in a few other cell lines and primary tumors (Beheshti et al., 2003; Chen et al., 2004; Mosse et al., 2005).

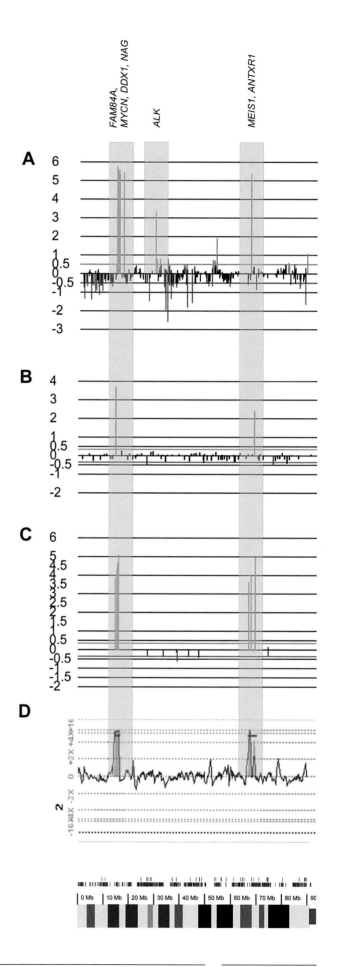

Fig. 3. Dissection of the 2p amplicons on IMR32 by the use of different platforms. (**A**) = Affymetrix 10K SNP chip, (**B**) = BAC array CGH, (**C**) = combined subtractive cDNA cloning and BAC array CGH and (**D**) = Agilent Human Genome CGH MicroArray 44A oligonucleotide chips.

Table 1. Summary of all studies on the 2p amplicon in NB cell line IMR-32

Methodology	Publication	MEIS1 2p14–p13	ANTXR1 2p13.1	FAM84A 2p24.3	NAG 2p24	DDX1 2p24	MYCN 2p24.1	ALK 2p23
CGH on cDNA microarrays	Beheshti et al. (2003)	×		×	×		×	
Combined subtractive cDNA cloning and BAC array CGH	De Preter et al. (2004)	×	×	×	×	×	×	
CGH on cDNA microarrays	Chen et al. (2004)	×	×	×	×	×	×	
BAC arrayCGH	Michels et al. (in prep.)	×	×	×	×	×	×	
Agilent	Michels et al. (in prep.)	×	×	×	×	×	×	
Affymetrix SNP chip	Michels et al. (in prep.)	×		×	×	×	×	×

Table 2. Dissection of amplicons in NB cell line NGP

Methodology	Publication	TSPAN31 12q13.3	CDK4 12q14	AVIL 12q14.1	CTDSP2 12q13–q15	MDM2 12q14.3–q15	CNOT2 12q15	FOXN4 12q24.11	ANAPC5 12q24.31	RSN 12q24.3	KNTC1 12q24.31
Hybridization of total genomic DNA to cDNA microarrays	Heiskanen et al. (2000)	×	×		×	×					
Array CGH	Michels et al. (in prep.)					×	×			×	×
Affymetrix SNP chip	Michels et al. (in prep.)	×	×	×		×	×	×	×	×	×

NB cell line NGP contains, in addition to the *MYCN* amplicon, also a second non-contiguous complex amplicon consisting of 12q14 and 12q24 sequences (Corvi et al., 1995; Van Roy et al., 1995). This cell line and its amplified sequences were investigated in several array CGH studies (Heiskanen et al., 2000; Chen et al., 2004; Mosse et al., 2005), including a BAC and SNP array analysis in our series of investigations (De Preter et al., 2004; Michels et al., in preparation). These analyses revealed a number of previously not recognized genes implicated in the amplicon formation on 12q in NB cell line NGP; i.e. *CNOT2* at 12q15, *FOXN4* at 12q24.11 and *KNTC1* at 12q24.31. The amplification status of all above-mentioned genes was validated and confirmed by FISH analysis (Table 2). Interestingly, positional expression mapping yielded evidence for a subset of primary NB with 12q amplification (Su et al., 2004).

Yet another nice illustration of the resolving power of array CGH but also of the importance of including metaphase FISH data, which allow interpretation of array CGH data in the context of the genomic position of the aberrant clones, was obtained through the study of the SJNB-12 NB cell line. This cell line is unusual as it is the only NB cell line with amplified sequences in the absence of *MYCN* amplification. Initial CGH and FISH studies showed amplification of sequences derived from 16q22.2 → q22.3 including the *ATBF1* transcription factor (Van Roy et al., 2001). Literature data (Boon et al., 2001) demonstrating *MYC* amplification in this cell line prompted us to perform dual-colour FISH with a *MYC* and *ATBF1* clone. This showed amplification of *MYC* and *ATBF1* on double minutes. The detection of a reciprocal t(8;16) with breakpoints in the chromosomal regions containing *ATBF1* and *MYC* suggested that this translocation might have triggered or accompanied amplicon formation in these tumor cells. A combination of FISH, SNP chip and BAC array CGH allowed us to map the amplified sequences, amplicon borders and a total of nine breakpoints that were implicated in a complex process of translocation-excision-deletion-amplification mechanism leading to nonsyntenic co-amplification of *MYC* and *ATBF1* (Van Roy et al., 2006).

Our array CGH screening of 75 primary NB tumors and 29 NB cell lines also revealed amplicons on 11q in five samples, which were confirmed with q-PCR at the genomic level (Michels et al., in preparation). All 11q amplicons were located at chromosomal band 11q13 containing the *CCND1* gene in keeping with previous findings of Molenaar et al. (2003).

Fix et al. (2004) analysed 1p-amplicons located at 1p34.2 and 1p36.3, respectively, found in two neuroblastomas by chromosomal CGH. Array CGH on a medium-resolution genomic array containing 178 PACs/BACs from 1p and subsequent high-resolution arrays containing contigs of overlapping PACs/BACs from the amplified regions, enabled precise mapping and delineation of both amplicons. The 1p34.2 amplicon appeared as a homogeneous amplification unit, whereas the 1p36.3 amplicon exhibited a more complex structure, with two non-contiguous, highly amplified regions and several moderately amplified units.

Genome-wide assessment of chromosomal gains and losses

In total 176 primary tumors and 53 cell lines have been tested by array CGH for chromosomal gains and losses. This approach has several advantages as compared to previous loss of heterozygosity studies using polymorphic markers. First, a genome wide appraisal for gains and losses is obtained in one single experiment by array CGH whereas LOH analysis requires a rather labour-intensive series of PCRs, even when multiplexing is performed. Second, the resolution that is obtained for mapping deletion borders is superior to LOH, in particular when high density oligonucleotide arrays or BAC tiling path arrays are used. Finally, although LOH studies have the advantage of detecting uniparental disomies, interpretation of allelic imbalance in hyperdiploid tumors or losses in tumors with substantial infiltrating normal cells can be problematic. Recent studies, as well as our analyses on a number of cell lines have shown that SNP arrays could be instrumental in the detection of losses and in particular regions of uniparental disomy. In leukemia, a screening of 64 AML cases with normal karyotypes indicated as much as 20% of samples with disomy for particular chromosomal segments (Raghavan et al., 2005). Subsequent analysis for selected genes in these regions showed the presence of mutations e.g. in *RUNX1*, indicating that loss of the normal homologue and reduplication of the chromosome containing the mutated allele contributed to tumor formation (Fitzgibbon et al., 2005). Such an extensive analysis has not been performed in NB and it remains to be determined whether this mechanism of oncogenesis is also implicated in neuroblastoma. For chromosome 2 in SJNB-12, uniparental disomy has been observed (Fig. 2).

In view of the frequent occurrence of 1p and 11q deletions, previous studies using conventional techniques on a large series of tumors have allowed a detailed delineation of the critical regions of loss. The recent array CGH studies have also contributed to the detection and delineation of losses at other chromosomal regions. We have focused specifically on 3p deletions in NB using a chromosome 3p BAC tiling path array. This allowed us to detect small interstitial deletions in NB cell lines as well as a number of critically important distal deletions in tumors which defined in total three putative SROs. Interestingly, the two most convincing SROs were located within regions that are frequently affected in common tumors such as lung and breast cancers (Hoebeeck et al., in press). Array CGH analysis was also used in an effort to fine map the region for 11q deletion in NB. In a previous study, functional evidence for a neuroblastoma suppressor gene on chromosome 11 was obtained through microcell mediated chromosome transfer, indicated by differentiation of neuroblastoma cells with loss of distal 11q upon introduction of chromosome 11 (Bader et al., 1991). Interestingly, some of these microcell hybrid clones were shown to harbor deletions in the transferred chromosome 11. This model system was further exploited as a means to identify candidate tumor suppressor or differentiation genes located on chromosome 11. To this purpose, array CGH was performed to evaluate the chromosome 11 status in the hybrids and allowed the delineation of three putative regions that could harbor the responsible differentiation gene on chromosome 11: 11q25, 11p15.1→p13 and 11p15.3 (De Preter et al., 2005).

Chromosome breakpoint analysis

Apart from the delineation of breakpoints of deleted regions and amplicons, array CGH analysis also allowed us to pinpoint the breakpoints of unbalanced translocations that result in partial gains and losses. In the absence of karyotypes, the nature of the chromosomal rearrangement leading to these gains and/or losses is difficult to determine. For cell lines however, karyotypes and (M)-FISH data are available, thus facilitating the interpretation of the array CGH findings. As mentioned above, gain of 17q represents the most frequent alteration in high-stage NB and typically results from unbalanced rearrangements with involvement of various partner chromosomes. Given the frequency and prognostic importance of 17q gain in NB, we performed array CGH with a chromosome 17 tiling path with an average resolution of 130 kb on a total of 28 NB cell lines and 69 primary tumors (Vandesompele et al., in preparation). One of the primary aims was to define a small critical region of gain in order to facilitate the identification of the genes contributing to NB pathogenesis. In total, twenty-one different chromosome 17 breakpoint regions were identified at the BAC level. The most proximal and distal breakpoints mapped at position 28.58 Mb (17q11.2) and 44.3 Mb (17q21.32), respectively and no small interstitial gains were found (Ensembl version 36). Given the fact that we did not find more distal 17q breakpoints in this series, we hypothesize that one or more critical genes sensitive to a gene dosage effect contributing to neuroblastoma oncogenesis could be located just telomeric to the region harboring the most distally located breakpoint at 17q21.32. Data-mining of gene expression profiles from primary NB tumors for genes located within this presumed critical 1–2 Mb segment allowed the identification of a number of interesting candidate genes (De Preter et al., in preparation; Vandesompele et al., in preparation). Also, we performed an innovative data-mining approach using the L2L (list-to-lists) concept of microarray data analysis which allowed us to compare our expression data of fetal neuroblasts and primary NB with published microarray gene lists (http://medgen.UGent.be/NBGS/) (Pattyn et al., in preparation). This provided additional genes of possible interest in NB development.

Breakpoints can be analyzed at an even higher resolution up to 50 bp to 10 kb. This was illustrated by recent papers by Selzer et al. (2005) and Stallings et al. (2006) who used fine-tiling oligonucleotide array CGH in the study of, amongst others, 17q breakpoints in NB cell lines and primary NB tumors.

Future challenges for array CGH in NB

The results summarized in this review clearly illustrate the analytical power of array CGH methods in the study of genomic imbalances in NB. Array CGH offers a rapid and detailed genome-wide picture of amplifications, deletions and gains and, in conjunction with cytogenetic data, allows high-resolution mapping of unbalanced translocation breakpoints. An increasing number of studies are now focusing on the combined analysis of gene expression and DNA copy number alteration profiling data, as also illustrated in this review. This approach will add more power to the data-mining efforts of the large expression data sets, e.g. for matching genomic subclasses of tumors with particular sets of differentially expressed genes and for focusing on altered gene expression in regions affected by genomic alterations in order to facilitate identification of candidate tumor suppressor genes in the deleted regions or proto-oncogenes in the gained or amplified chromosomal segments.

At the individual patient level, particular patterns of genomic imbalances may have important prognostic predictive value and, therefore, array CGH profiling might become an important aspect of the genetic diagnostic workup of certain tumors. Currently, the widespread use of this methodology is prevented by the high costs of the procedure but it is anticipated that due to further developments and the huge potential market for these products, array CGH will become a standard procedure for genome-wide detection of chromosomal imbalances.

Acknowledgements

We would like to thank The Wellcome Trust Sanger Institute (Hinxton, Cambridge, UK) for providing us with the 1 Mb BAC probes, as well as N. Carter, H. Fiegler, J. Knijnenburg and K. Szuhai for technical assistance. Jo Vandesompele and Nadine Van Roy are postdoctoral researchers with the Foundation for Scientific Research, Flanders (FWO). This text presents research results of the Belgian program of Interuniversity Poles of attraction initiated by the Belgian State, Prime Minister's Office, Science Policy Programming (IUAP).

References

Alitalo K, Schwab M, Lin CC, Varmus HE, Bishop JM: Homogeneously staining chromosomal regions contain amplified copies of an abundantly expressed cellular oncogene (c-myc) in malignant neuroendocrine cells from a human colon carcinoma. Proc Natl Acad Sci USA 80: 1707–1711 (1983).

Altura RA, Maris JM, Li H, Boyett JM, Brodeur GM, Look AT: Novel regions of chromosomal loss in familial neuroblastoma by comparative genomic hybridization. Genes Chromosomes Cancer 19:176–184 (1997).

Bader SA, Fasching C, Brodeur GM, Stanbridge EJ: Dissociation of suppression of tumorigenicity and differentiation in vitro effected by transfer of single human chromosomes into human neuroblastoma cells. Cell Growth Differ 2:245–255 (1991).

Beheshti B, Braude I, Marrano P, Thorner P, Zielenska M, Squire JA: Chromosomal localization of DNA amplifications in neuroblastoma tumors using cDNA microarray comparative genomic hybridization. Neoplasia 5:53–62 (2003).

Bignell GR, Huang J, Greshock J, Watt S, Butler A, et al: High-resolution analysis of DNA copy number using oligonucleotide microarrays. Genome Res 14:287–295 (2004).

Boon K, Caron HN, van Asperen R, Valentijn L, Hermus MC, et al: N-myc enhances the expression of a large set of genes functioning in ribosome biogenesis and protein synthesis. EMBO J 20:1383–1393 (2001).

Bown N: Neuroblastoma tumour genetics: clinical and biological aspects. J Clin Pathol 54:897–910 (2001).

Bown N, Cotterill S, Lastowska M, O'Neill S, Pearson AD, et al: Gain of chromosome arm 17q and adverse outcome in patients with neuroblastoma. N Engl J Med 340:1954–1961 (1999).

Breen CJ, O'Meara A, McDermott M, Mullarkey M, Stallings RL: Coordinate deletion of chromosome 3p and 11q in neuroblastoma detected by comparative genomic hybridization. Cancer Genet Cytogenet 120:44–49 (2000).

Brinkschmidt C, Christiansen H, Terpe HJ, Simon R, Boecker W, et al: Comparative genomic hybridization (CGH) analysis of neuroblastomas – an important methodological approach in paediatric tumour pathology. J Pathol 181: 394–400 (1997).

Brinkschmidt C, Poremba C, Christiansen H, Simon R, Schafer KL, et al: Comparative genomic hybridization and telomerase activity analysis identify two biologically different groups of 4s neuroblastomas. Br J Cancer 77:2223–2229 (1998).

Brodeur GM: Neuroblastoma: biological insights into a clinical enigma. Nat Rev Cancer 3:203–216 (2003).

Brodeur GM, Fong CT: Molecular biology and genetics of human neuroblastoma. Cancer Genet Cytogenet 41:153–174 (1989).

Brodeur GM, Sekhon G, Goldstein MN: Chromosomal aberrations in human neuroblastomas. Cancer 40:2256–2263 (1977).

Brodeur GM, Seeger RC, Schwab M, Varmus HE, Bishop JM: Amplification of N-myc in untreated human neuroblastomas correlates with advanced disease stage. Science 224:1121–1124 (1984).

Cai WW, Mao JH, Chow CW, Damani S, Balmain A, Bradley A: Genome-wide detection of chromosomal imbalances in tumors using BAC microarrays. Nat Biotechnol 20:393–396 (2002).

Chen QR, Bilke S, Wei JS, Whiteford CC, Cenacchi N, et al: cDNA array-CGH profiling identifies genomic alterations specific to stage and MYCN-amplification in neuroblastoma. BMC Genomics 5:70 (2004).

Corvi R, Savelyeva L, Breit S, Wenzel A, Handgretinger R, et al: Non-syntenic amplification of MDM2 and MYCN in human neuroblastoma. Oncogene 10:1081–1086 (1995).

Cunsolo CL, Bicocchi MP, Petti AR, Tonini GP: Numerical and structural aberrations in advanced neuroblastoma tumours by CGH analysis; survival correlates with chromosome 17 status. Br J Cancer 83:1295–1300 (2000).

De Preter K, Pattyn F, Berx G, Strumane K, Menten B, et al: Combined subtractive cDNA cloning and array CGH: an efficient approach for identification of overexpressed genes in DNA amplicons. BMC Genomics 5:11 (2004).

De Preter K, Vandesompele J, Menten B, Carr P, Fiegler H, et al: Positional and functional mapping of a neuroblastoma differentiation gene on chromosome 11. BMC Genomics 6:11 (2005).

du Manoir S, Speicher MR, Joos S, Schrock E, Popp S, et al: Detection of complete and partial chromosome gains and losses by comparative genomic in situ hybridization. Hum Genet 90: 590–610 (1993).

Ejeskar K, Aburatani H, Abrahamsson J, Kogner P, Martinsson T: Loss of heterozygosity of 3p markers in neuroblastoma tumours implicate a tumour-suppressor locus distal to the FHIT gene. Br J Cancer 77:1787–1791 (1998).

Fiegler H, Carr P, Douglas EJ, Burford DC, Hunt S, et al: DNA microarrays for comparative genomic hybridization based on DOP-PCR amplification of BAC and PAC clones. Genes Chromosomes Cancer 36:361–374 (2003).

Fitzgibbon J, Smith LL, Raghavan M, Smith ML, Debernardi S, et al: Association between acquired uniparental disomy and homozygous gene mutation in acute myeloid leukemias. Cancer Res 65:9152–9154 (2005).

Fix A, Peter M, Pierron G, Aurias A, Delattre O, Janoueix-Lerosey I: High-resolution mapping of amplicons of the short arm of chromosome 1 in two neuroblastoma tumors by microarray-based comparative genomic hybridization. Genes Chromosomes Cancer 40:266–270 (2004).

Garnis C, Baldwin C, Zhang L, Rosin MP, Lam WL: Use of complete coverage array comparative genomic hybridization to define copy number alterations on chromosome 3p in oral squamous cell carcinomas. Cancer Res 63:8582–8585 (2003).

Gilbert F, Feder M, Balaban G, Brangman D, Lurie DK, et al: Human neuroblastomas and abnormalities of chromosomes 1 and 17. Cancer Res 44:5444–5449 (1984).

Greshock J, Naylor TL, Margolin A, Diskin S, Cleaver SH, et al: 1-Mb resolution array-based comparative genomic hybridization using a BAC clone set optimized for cancer gene analysis. Genome Res 14:179–187 (2004).

Guo C, White PS, Weiss MJ, Hogarty MD, Thompson PM, et al: Allelic deletion at 11q23 is common in *MYCN* single copy neuroblastomas. Oncogene 18:4948–4957 (1999).

Hallstensson K, Thulin S, Aburatani H, Hippo Y, Martinsson T: Representational difference analysis and loss of heterozygosity studies detect 3p deletions in neuroblastoma. Eur J Cancer 33:1966–1970 (1997).

Heiskanen MA, Bittner ML, Chen Y, Khan J, Adler KE, et al: Detection of gene amplification by genomic hybridization to cDNA microarrays. Cancer Res 60:799–802 (2000).

Hirai M, Yoshida S, Kashiwagi H, Kawamura T, Ishikawa T, et al: 1q23 gain is associated with progressive neuroblastoma resistant to aggressive treatment. Genes Chromosomes Cancer 25:261–269 (1999).

Hoebeeck J, Michels E, Menten B, Van Roy N, Eggert A, et al: High resolution deletion breakpoint mapping using tiling-path BAC arrays defines two small distinct critical regions at 3p21–p22 in neuroblastoma. Int J Cancer in press (2006).

Hoshi M, Otagiri N, Shiwaku HO, Asakawa S, Shimizu N: Detailed deletion mapping of chromosome band 14q32 in human neuroblastoma defines a 1.1-Mb region of common allelic loss. Br J Cancer 82:1801–1807 (2000a).

Hoshi M, Shiwaku HO, Hayashi Y, Kaneko Y, Horii A: Deletion mapping of 14q32 in human neuroblastoma defines an 1,100-kb region of common allelic loss. Med Pediatr Oncol 35:522–525 (2000b).

Iehara T, Hamazaki M, Sawada T: Cytogenetic analysis of infantile neuroblastomas by comparative genomic hybridization. Cancer Lett 178:83–89 (2002).

Ishkanian AS, Malloff CA, Watson SK, DeLeeuw RJ, Chi B, et al: A tiling resolution DNA microarray with complete coverage of the human genome. Nat Genet 36:299–303 (2004).

Jones TA, Flomen RH, Senger G, Nizetic D, Sheer D: The homeobox gene *MEIS1* is amplified in IMR-32 and highly expressed in other neuroblastoma cell lines. Eur J Cancer 36:2368–2374 (2000).

Kallioniemi A, Kallioniemi OP, Sudar D, Rutovitz D, Gray JW, et al: Comparative genomic hybridization for molecular cytogenetic analysis of solid tumors. Science 258:818–821 (1992).

Kaneko Y, Kanda N, Maseki N, Sakurai M, Tsuchida Y, et al: Different karyotypic patterns in early and advanced stage neuroblastomas. Cancer Res 47:311–318 (1987).

Kuroda H, White PS, Sulman EP, Manohar CF, Reiter JL, et al: Physical mapping of the *DDX1* gene to 340 kb 5′ of *MYCN*. Oncogene 13:1561–1565 (1996).

Lastowska M, Nacheva E, McGuckin A, Curtis A, Grace C, et al: Comparative genomic hybridization study of primary neuroblastoma tumors. United Kingdom Children's Cancer Study Group. Genes Chromosomes Cancer 18:162–169 (1997).

Look AT, Hayes FA, Nitschke R, McWilliams NB, Green AA: Cellular DNA content as a predictor of response to chemotherapy in infants with unresectable neuroblastoma. N Engl J Med 311:231–235 (1984).

Lucito R, Healy J, Alexander J, Reiner A, Esposito D, et al: Representational oligonucleotide microarray analysis: a high-resolution method to detect genome copy number variation. Genome Res 13:2291–2305 (2003).

Manohar CF, Salwen HR, Brodeur GM, Cohn SL: Co-amplification and concomitant high levels of expression of a DEAD box gene with *MYCN* in human neuroblastoma. Genes Chromosomes Cancer 14:196–203 (1995).

Maris JM, Matthay KK: Molecular biology of neuroblastoma. J Clin Oncol 17:2264–2279 (1999).

Maris JM, Weiss MJ, Guo C, Gerbing RB, Stram DO, et al: Loss of heterozygosity at 1p36 independently predicts for disease progression but not decreased overall survival probability in neuroblastoma patients: a Children's Cancer Group study. J Clin Oncol 18:1888–1899 (2000).

Molenaar JJ, van Sluis P, Boon K, Versteeg R, Caron HN: Rearrangements and increased expression of cyclin D1 (*CCND1*) in neuroblastoma. Genes Chromosomes Cancer 36:242–249 (2003).

Mosse Y, Greshock J, King A, Khazi D, Weber BL, Maris JM: Identification and high-resolution mapping of a constitutional 11q deletion in an infant with multifocal neuroblastoma. Lancet Oncol 4:769–771 (2003).

Mosse YP, Greshock J, Margolin A, Naylor T, Cole K, et al: High-resolution detection and mapping of genomic DNA alterations in neuroblastoma. Genes Chromosomes Cancer 43:390–403 (2005).

Plantaz D, Mohapatra G, Matthay KK, Pellarin M, Seeger RC, Feuerstein BG: Gain of chromosome 17 is the most frequent abnormality detected in neuroblastoma by comparative genomic hybridization. Am J Pathol 150:81–89 (1997).

Plantaz D, Vandesompele J, Van Roy N, Lastowska M, Bown N, et al: Comparative genomic hybridization (CGH) analysis of stage 4 neuroblastoma reveals high frequency of 11q deletion in tumors lacking *MYCN* amplification. Int J Cancer 91:680–686 (2001).

Raghavan M, Lillington DM, Skoulakis S, Debernardi S, Chaplin T, et al: Genome-wide single nucleotide polymorphism analysis reveals frequent partial uniparental disomy due to somatic recombination in acute myeloid leukemias. Cancer Res 65:375–378 (2005).

Reiter JL, Brodeur GM: High-resolution mapping of a 130-kb core region of the *MYCN* amplicon in neuroblastomas. Genomics 32:97–103 (1996).

Reiter JL, Brodeur GM: *MYCN* is the only highly expressed gene from the core amplified domain in human neuroblastomas. Genes Chromosomes Cancer 23:134–140 (1998).

Savelyeva L, Corvi R, Schwab M: Translocation involving 1p and 17q is a recurrent genetic alteration of human neuroblastoma cells. Am J Hum Genet 55:334–340 (1994).

Scaruffi P, Parodi S, Mazzocco K, Defferrari R, Fontana V, et al: Detection of *MYCN* amplification and chromosome 1p36 loss in neuroblastoma by cDNA microarray comparative genomic hybridization. Mol Diagn 8:93–100 (2004).

Schleiermacher G, Janoueix-Lerosey I, Combaret V, Derre J, Couturier J, et al: Combined 24-color karyotyping and comparative genomic hybridization analysis indicates predominant rearrangements of early replicating chromosome regions in neuroblastoma. Cancer Genet Cytogenet 141:32–42 (2003).

Schwab M: Oncogene amplification in solid tumors. Semin Cancer Biol 9:319–325 (1999).

Schwab M, Alitalo K, Klempnauer KH, Varmus HE, Bishop JM, et al: Amplified DNA with limited homology to *myc* cellular oncogene is shared by human neuroblastoma cell lines and a neuroblastoma tumour. Nature 305:245–248 (1983).

Seeger RC, Brodeur GM, Sather H, Dalton A, Siegel SE, et al: Association of multiple copies of the *N-myc* oncogene with rapid progression of neuroblastomas. N Engl J Med 313:1111–1116 (1985).

Selzer RR, Richmond TA, Pofahl NJ, Green RD, Eis PS, et al: Analysis of chromosome breakpoints in neuroblastoma at sub-kilobase resolution using fine-tiling oligonucleotide array CGH. Genes Chromosomes Cancer 44:305–319 (2005).

Shiloh Y, Shipley J, Brodeur GM, Bruns G, Korf B, et al: Differential amplification, assembly, and relocation of multiple DNA sequences in human neuroblastomas and neuroblastoma cell lines. Proc Natl Acad Sci USA 82:3761–3765 (1985).

Snijders AM, Nowak N, Segraves R, Blackwood S, Brown N, et al: Assembly of microarrays for genome-wide measurement of DNA copy number. Nat Genet 29:263–264 (2001).

Solinas-Toldo S, Lampel S, Stilgenbauer S, Nickolenko J, Benner A, et al: Matrix-based comparative genomic hybridization: biochips to screen for genomic imbalances. Genes Chromosomes Cancer 20:399–407 (1997).

Speicher MR, Gwyn Ballard S, Ward DC: Karyotyping human chromosomes by combinatorial multi-fluor FISH. Nat Genet 12:368–375 (1996).

Speleman F, Bown N: 17q gain in neuroblastoma, in Brodeur GM, Sawada T, Tsuchida Y, Voûte PA (eds): Neuroblastoma (Elsevier Science, Amsterdam, 2000).

Spieker N, van Sluis P, Beitsma M, Boon K, van Schaik BD, et al: The *MEIS1* oncogene is highly expressed in neuroblastoma and amplified in cell line IMR32. Genomics 71:214–221 (2001).

Stallings RL, Nair P, Maris JM, Catchpoole D, McDermott M, et al: High-resolution analysis of chromosomal breakpoints and genomic instability identifies *PTPRD* as a canidate tumor supressor gene in neuroblastoma. Cancer Res 66:3673–3680 (2006).

Su WT, Alaminos M, Mora J, Cheung NK, La Quaglia MP, Gerald WL: Positional gene expression analysis identifies 12q overexpression and amplification in a subset of neuroblastomas. Cancer Genet Cytogenet 154:131–137 (2004).

Takita J, Hayashi Y, Kohno T, Shiseki M, Yamaguchi N, et al: Allelotype of neuroblastoma. Oncogene 11:1829–1834 (1995).

Theobald M, Christiansen H, Schmidt A, Melekian B, Wolkewitz N, et al: Sublocalization of putative tumor suppressor gene loci on chromosome arm 14q in neuroblastoma. Genes Chromosomes Cancer 26:40–46 (1999).

Thompson PM, Seifried BA, Kyemba SK, Jensen SJ, Guo C, et al: Loss of heterozygosity for chromosome 14q in neuroblastoma. Med Pediatr Oncol 36:28–31 (2001).

van Duin M, van Marion R, Watson JE, Paris PL, Lapuk A, et al: Construction and application of a full-coverage, high-resolution, human chromosome 8q genomic microarray for comparative genomic hybridization. Cytometry A 63:10–19 (2005).

Van Gele M, Van Roy N, Jauch A, Laureys G, Benoit Y, et al: Sensitive and reliable detection of genomic imbalances in human neuroblastomas using comparative genomic hybridisation analysis. Eur J Cancer 33:1979–1982 (1997).

Van Roy N, Laureys G, Cheng NC, Willem P, Opde-nakker G, et al: 1;17 translocations and other chromosome 17 rearrangements in human primary neuroblastoma tumors and cell lines. Genes Chromosomes Cancer 10:103–114 (1994).

Van Roy N, Forus A, Myklebost O, Cheng NC, Versteeg R, Speleman F: Identification of two distinct chromosome 12-derived amplification units in neuroblastoma cell line NGP. Cancer Genet Cytogenet 82:151–154 (1995).

Van Roy N, Jauch A, Van Gele M, Laureys G, Versteeg R, et al: Comparative genomic hybridization analysis of human neuroblastomas: detection of distal 1p deletions and further molecular genetic characterization of neuroblastoma cell lines. Cancer Genet Cytogenet 97:139–142 (1997).

Van Roy N, Van Limbergen H, Vandesompele J, Van Gele M, Poppe B, et al: Combined M-FISH and CGH analysis allows comprehensive description of genetic alterations in neuroblastoma cell lines. Genes Chromosomes Cancer 32:126–135 (2001).

Van Roy N, Vandesompele J, Menten B, Nilsson H, De Smet E, et al: Translocation-excision-deletion-amplification mechanism leading to nonsyntenic coamplification of MYC and ATBF1. Genes Chromosomes Cancer 45:107–117 (2006).

Vandesompele J, Van Roy N, Van Gele M, Laureys G, Ambros P, et al: Genetic heterogeneity of neuroblastoma studied by comparative genomic hybridization. Genes Chromosomes Cancer 23:141–152 (1998).

Vandesompele J, Speleman F, Van Roy N, Laureys G, Brinskchmidt C, et al: Multicentre analysis of patterns of DNA gains and losses in 204 neuroblastoma tumors: how many genetic subgroups are there? Med Pediatr Oncol 36:5–10 (2001).

Vandesompele J, Baudis M, De Preter K, Van Roy N, Ambros P, et al: Unequivocal delineation of clinicogenetic subgroups and development of a new model for improved outcome prediction in neuroblastoma. J Clin Oncol 23:2280–2299 (2005).

Vettenranta K, Aalto Y, Wikstrom S, Knuutila S, Saarinen-Pihkala U: Comparative genomic hybridization reveals changes in DNA-copy number in poor-risk neuroblastoma. Cancer Genet Cytogenet 125:125–130 (2001).

Wessendorf S, Fritz B, Wrobel G, Nessling M, Lampel S, et al: Automated screening for genomic imbalances using matrix-based comparative genomic hybridization. Lab Invest 82:47–60 (2002).

White PS, Thompson PM, Gotoh T, Okawa ER, Igarashi J, et al: Definition and characterization of a region of 1p36.3 consistently deleted in neuroblastoma. Oncogene 24:2684–2694 (2005).

Zhao X, Li C, Paez JG, Chin K, Janne PA, et al: An integrated view of copy number and allelic alterations in the cancer genome using single nucleotide polymorphism arrays. Cancer Res 64:3060–3071 (2004).

Cytogenet Genome Res 115:283–288 (2006)
DOI: 10.1159/000095925

Gene copy number changes in dermatofibrosarcoma protuberans – a fine-resolution study using array comparative genomic hybridization

S. Kaur[a]   H. Vauhkonen[a]   T. Böhling[a]   F. Mertens[b]   N. Mandahl[b]
S. Knuutila[a]

[a]Department of Pathology, Haartman Institute and HUSLAB, University of Helsinki and Helsinki University Central Hospital, Helsinki (Finland)
[b]Department of Clinical Genetics, Lund University Hospital, Lund (Sweden)

Manuscript received 24 January 2006; accepted in revised form for publication by A. Geurts van Kessel, 5 May 2006.

Abstract. Dermatofibrosarcoma protuberans (DFSP) is a rare, slow-growing, low-grade dermal tumor. Cytogenetic and FISH studies have revealed that the chromosomal rearrangements characteristic of DFSP tumors involve both translocations and the formation of a supernumerary ring derived from chromosomes 17 and 22. The t(17;22)(q22;q13.1) translocation generates a gene fusion between COL1A1 and PDGFB, which serves as a diagnostic marker of DFSP. In the present study we performed array-CGH (aCGH) analysis on ten DFSP tumors. The COL1A1 region at 17q was gained in 71% (5/7) of the samples and the PDGFB region at 22q was gained in 43% (3/7) of the individual samples. In addition to the 17q and 22q gains, altogether 17 minimal common regions of gain and one region of loss were detected.

Copyright © 2006 S. Karger AG, Basel

Dermatofibrosarcoma protuberans (DFSP) is a rare cutaneous tumor of intermediate malignancy that is composed of spindle cells. The histological origin (fibroblastic, histiocytic or neural) of DFSP is still controversial (O'Brien et al., 1998; Sandberg and Bridge, 2003). Although this slowly but aggressively infiltrating tumor has a high tendency to recur, it seldom metastasizes or leads to tumor-related death. Thus, wide surgical excision is one of the main therapies. However, the tumor can transform into a high-grade fibrosarcomatous variant with an adverse clinical outcome (Domanski and Gustafson, 2002). DFSP is mainly seen on the trunk and proximal extremities of young to middle-aged adults. Strong CD34 immunopositivity differentiates DFSP from other spindle cell tumors, e.g., fibrosarcoma, synovial sarcoma, and malignant fibrous histiocytoma (Sonobe et al., 1999).

The distinct cytogenetic feature of DFSP is a reciprocal translocation involving chromosomes 17 and 22, t(17;22)(q22;q13), which fuses the collagen type I alpha 1 (COL1A1) gene on chromosome 17 with the platelet-derived growth factor B-chain (PDGFB) gene on chromosome 22 (Pedeutour et al., 1996; Simon et al., 2001). This characteristic gene fusion is also used in the diagnosis of DFSP (Sirvent et al., 2003). Sequences of 17q and 22q can be involved in the formation of a supernumerary ring chromosome (Pedeutour et al., 1994, 1995; Naeem et al., 1995), which has been reported to occur in close to 70% of DFSP tumors; most of the remaining cases show balanced or unbalanced translocations between chromosomes 17 and 22 (Mitelman Database of Chromosome Aberrations in Cancer, 2006). Whereas the breakpoint in the COL1A1 gene varies, the breakpoint in PDGFB is always in intron 1 (O'Brien et al., 1998). The COL1A1/PDGFB fusion preserves the PDGFB reading frame from exon 2 and results in aberrant expression of PDGFB. Thus, the PDGF receptor, a protein tyrosine kinase, is continuously activated through an autocrine mech-

Request reprints from Sakari Knuutila
  Department of Pathology, Haartman Institute, University of Helsinki
  POB 21 (Haartmaninkatu 3)
  FI–00014, Helsinki (Finland)
  telephone: +358 9 1912 6527; fax: +358 9 1912 6788
  e-mail: Sakari.Knuutila@helsinki.fi

Table 1. Clinical data and DNA copy number changes of dermatofibrosarcoma protuberans analyzed by metaphase CGH, G-banding and array-CGH. High-level amplifications by aCGH-smooth in boldface.

Case[a]	Age/Sex	DNA source[b]	Location/recurrence	Size (cm)/margins[c]	DNA copy number changes by metaphase CGH and G-banding	DNA copy number changes by array-CGH[d]
1	27/M	FFPE	Forearm/primary	2.8/wide	amp(17q,22q)	ND
2	46/M	FF	Groin/secondary	7/marginal	enh(7,12q,19p,17q21qter)	13K aCGH: +5q35.3,+17q23.2-qter, +18q21.1-q21.3, +19q12-pter, +21q22.3
3	28/M	FF	Chest/primary	2/marginal	amp(17q22qter)	13K aCGH: +3p21.31-p21.1, +8q24.3, +17q21.33-qter, +20q13.33, +22cen-q13.1
4	40/M	FF	Back/primary	6/wide	enh(5,8,11q13,5q12,18,19,20q), dim(13q21-q22), amp(17q,22q)	ND
5	52/M	FFPE	Scalp/primary	NA/marginal	amp(11,17q22qter,22q)	ND
6	36/F	FF	Back/primary	8/marginal	enh(1p35,1q,17q), amp(17q22qter)	13K aCGH: +1p35.3-pter, +1q21.2-qter, +17q21.31-q25.3/**17q24.1-q25.3**, +18q21.33-pter, +Xq28
P-1		Samples 1–6			amp(17q,22q)	13K aCGH: +1q32.1-q32.2, +8q24.3, +9q34.11, +11p15.5, +17q21.31-q21.33/**17q21.33-qter**, +22cen-q12.2/**22q12.2-q13.1** 44K aCGH: +1p35.1-p36.2, +1q21.2-qter, +17q21.33-qter, +22cen-q13.1
7	42/M	FF	Arm/secondary	7/wide	50, XY,+8,+18,+21,+22,der(22) t(17;22)(q22;q13)x2[11]/46,XY[7]	16K aCGH: +11p15.5, +17q23.2-qter, -22q13.2-qter
8	56/M	FF	Groin/primary	4/wide	87,XX,–Y,–Y,–3,–6,+8,–11,–14,–22,+r[17]/86,idem, –9[3]/46,XY[5]	16K aCGH: +17q24.2-qter
9	60/M	FF	Abdominal wall/primary	4/wide	46,XY[11]	16K aCGH: +6p21.2-p21.3, +17q21.2-qter, +19q13.1-q13.2, +19q13.42-q13.43, +22cen-q13.1
10	64/M	FF	Shoulder/primary	11/wide	46–52,XY,+5,+8,+18,+20,+1–2r[cp5]/46–53,XY, +1,del(3)(p21),+5,der(6)t(?5;6)(q15;q21),add(10) (q26), +15,–18,+20,+21,+r,+1–2mar[cp9]/46,XY[3]	16K aCGH:+8q24.2-q24.3,+13q34,+17q21.32-qter,+22cen-q13.1
P-2		Samples 7–10			amp(17q23qter, 22q11.22)	16K aCGH: +1p36.31-pter, +4p16.1-pter,+ 8q11.21-pter, +8q24.21-qter, +10q24.31-q25.1, +16p13.3-pter, +**17q21.33-qter**,+ 19q13.31-pter, +19q13.11-q13.12/**q13.12**, +20q13.33-qter, +21q22.3-qter, +**22cen-q13.1** 44K aCGH: +8q24.3, + 11p15.5, +17q21.33-qter, +19p13.11-pter, +19q13.2, +19q13.42, +22cen-q13.1, -22q13.2-qter
Control		Peripheral blood cells			No changes	13K aCGH, 16K aCGH, 44K aCGH: no changes

[a] Control = Self vs. self hybridization of normal male DNA.
[b] FFPE = Formaldehyde-fixed paraffin-embedded; FF = fresh-frozen.
[c] NA = Not available.
[d] ND = Not determined.

anism. FISH studies have shown that the DFSP-specific ring chromosomes contain sequences from 17q and 22q, which are gained at a low level, and include also the sequences of the *COL1A1/PDGFB* fusion gene (Pedeutour et al., 1995). Besides the specific t(17;22), other recurrent but less frequent aberrations, such as gains of chromosomes 5, 7 and 8, have been detected (Sirvent et al., 2003), indicating that additional molecular alterations can contribute to tumor development. DNA copy number changes in DFSP have been characterized previously by metaphase comparative genomic hybridization (CGH) (Nishio et al., 2001, 2002).

The present study was undertaken to gain further insight into the DNA copy number changes of DFSP. To observe aberrations not visible by low-resolution metaphase CGH, we used cDNA- and oligonucleotide-based array CGH.

Materials and methods

Tumor specimens

The DFSP samples were obtained from the orthopedic centers at the Helsinki University Central Hospital (cases 1–6) and the Lund University Hospital (cases 7–10). Archival formalin-fixed paraffin-embedded tumor tissue was analyzed from cases 1 and 5, while fresh-frozen tissue was available from all other tumors. The clinical characteristics of the samples are shown in Table 1. Cases 1–6 were used in Pool 1 (P-1) and cases 7–10 in Pool 2 (P-2). All tumors were re-evaluated histologically and the diagnosis was verified by positive immunohistochemistry using CD34 antibodies. DNA extraction from the fresh-frozen and formalin-fixed paraffin-embedded tissue samples was performed using standard methods. Reference male and female DNAs were extracted from pooled peripheral blood cells of healthy individuals.

Metaphase comparative genomic hybridization (mCGH)

mCGH on cases 1–6 was performed as described previously (El-Rifai et al., 1997). Briefly, tumor and reference DNA were labeled by nick translation with FITC-conjugated dCTP and dUTP (1:1; DuPont, Boston, Mass.), and Texas red-conjugated dCTP and dUTP (1:1; DuPont), respectively. Equal amounts of labeled tumor and reference DNA along with 20 μg of unlabeled human COT-1 DNA (Gibco BRL, Gaithersburg, Md.) were hybridized to metaphase spreads. After post-hybridization washes, the slides were analyzed using an Olympus fluorescence microscope and the ISIS digital image analysis system (Meta-Systems GmbH, Altlussheim, Germany).

Array comparative genomic hybridization (aCGH)

Array-CGH was performed using 13K Human 1 cDNA microarray slides (Agilent Technologies, Palo Alto, Calif.), a customized 16K cDNA microarray containing 16,000 annotated genes printed in duplicates (Finnish DNA Microarray Centre, Turku, Finland; http://microarrays.btk.fi) and Agilent's 60-mer oligonucleotide-based microarray (Human Genome CGH Microarray Kit 44B). CGH on the oligonucleotide array was performed according to the manufacturer's instructions (Agilent Technologies, Version 2). The protocol used for cDNA-based aCGH has been described previously (Pollack et al., 1999; Atiye et al., 2005). In brief, digested tumor and reference DNA (6 μg of each) were labeled with Cy5-dUTP and Cy3-dUTP (Amersham Biosciences Corp., Piscataway, N.J.), respectively, using the RadPrime DNA Labeling System kit (Gibco BRL). The 13K cDNA slides were hybridized and washed according to Monni et al. (2001) and Atiye et al. (2005). The customized 16K cDNA slides were hybridized for 17 h at 65°C in a water bath, with humidity maintained in the hybridization chamber by 3× SSC. The post-hybridization washes were performed at room temperature first in 0.5× SSC, 0.1% SDS to remove the coverslip (15 min), followed by 0.5× SSC, 0.1% SDS (15 min), 0.5× SSC, 0.01% SDS (15 min), 0.06× SSC (2 min) and 0.06× SSC (2 min). The slides were dried by centrifugation (400 g, 2 min) and scanned using a laser confocal scanner (Agilent Technologies). The data from the microarray images were extracted using Agilent's Feature Extraction software version 7.0.

Data analysis

Intensity-dependent normalization (Lowess) included in the Feature Extraction software package (Agilent Technologies) was used for normalization of the data. Data filtering, outlier removal and the linkage with genomic location were done using Genespring v4.2 (Silicon Genetics, Redwood City, Calif.). The genomic locations for the cDNA array features were retrieved from the UCSC database (http://genome.ucsc.edu/, April 2003 freeze for 13K slides and December 2004 freeze for 16K slides). Array-CGH data for Agilent 13K and customized 16K cDNA microarrays was analyzed using the aCGH-smooth program (http://www.few.vu.nl/~vumarray/) (Jong et al., 2004), as described previously (Vauhkonen et al., 2006). The aCGH-smooth software identifies copy number gains and losses using the maximum likelihood estimation in a local search algorithm. The software also categorizes the aberrations according to the copy number changes, i.e., 'loss', 'gain' and 'amplification'. In the present work, a minimum of five consecutive clones showing change was considered as a reliable change. The oligonucleotide microarrays were performed according to the manufacturer's protocols and analyzed using CGH Analytics v3.1 (Agilent Technologies) as described previously (Tyybäkinoja et al., 2006).

Results and discussion

The development of the microarray technology in the detection of copy number changes is proceeding rapidly. The present study of DNA copy number changes in dermatofibrosarcoma protuberans (DFSP) was started using Agilent 13K array-CGH (aCGH) platform with 13,000 cDNA clones and continued, due to the limited availability of the arrays, using customized 16K platform with 16,000 cDNA clones. When Agilent 44K oligonucleotide arrays with 44,000 oligonucleotide sequences of intra- and intergenic regions became available, we chose to analyze the remaining DNAs using this platform. Our earlier comparisons of results obtained using this high-resolution system and by 13K and 16K cDNA microarrays indicated superiority of the oligo system to detect small deletions and gains (Tyybäkinoja et al., 2006). Therefore we focus on the oligoarray results and consider the results by 13K and 16K cDNA arrays confirmatory. Because the amount of DNA was not sufficient to carry out the analysis and we had previously used pooled DNAs successfully for detection of recurrent primary changes in a certain tumor entity (Larramendy et al., 2006), we decided to conduct the analysis on pooled DNAs. Likewise, Kendziorski et al. (2005) identified biologically significant changes common to all samples from pools of limited material. The use of pooled genomic samples has also been shown to be highly accurate, for example in identification of relevant genomic regions by SNP microarrays (Craig et al., 2005). Finally, the effect of sample pooling in detecting gene expression changes by microarrays has recently been characterized quantitatively (Zhang and Gant, 2005). In the present work, the aCGH results of the pools resembled those of the individual samples included in the pools. However, a number of small changes occurring in single individual samples remained undetected in the pools.

The aCGH analysis was conducted on seven individual DFSP cases and on two sample pools. Cases 1–6 and the two sample pools, P-1 and P-2, were analyzed by metaphase-CGH (mCGH). The four samples included in P-2 were analyzed by G-banding. Copy number changes were detected in both pools and in all individual cases, except case 9 (Table 1). Three individual samples (2, 3 and 6) and P-1 were analyzed using Agilent's 13K Human 1 cDNA microarrays. Four individual samples (7–10) and P-2 were analyzed using custom-made 16K cDNA microarrays. Control self-versus-self hybridizations with male reference were used in the adjustment of the baseline copy number and parameters in the aCGH-smooth program. DNA copy number gains were seen in all cases, whereas amplifications (17q24.1→q25.3) and losses (22q13.2→qter), according to the aCGH-smooth program thresholds, were only seen in samples 6 and 7, respectively. P-1 was analyzed on the 13K array and P-2 on the 16K array (Table 1), and the results were confirmed using Agilent's 60-mer oligonucleotide microarrays. Both pools displayed the DFSP-characteristic gains in 17q and 22q that were not present in all of the individual samples. P-1 showed gains (17q21.31→q21.33 and 22cen→q12.2) and amplifications (17q21.33→qter and 22q12.2→q13.1) on the 13K cDNA arrays, whereas only gains (17q21.33→qter and 22cen→q13.1) were found using the oligonucleotide arrays. P-2 showed amplifications (17q21.33→qter and 22cen→q13.1) on the 16K cDNA microarray, whereas gains (17q21.33→qter and 22cen→q13.1) and loss (22q13.2→qter) were detected using the 44K oligonucleotide arrays. Both sample pools on the oligonucleotide arrays showed recurrent DNA copy number gains in 8q24.3, 17q21.33→qter, and 22cen→q13.1.

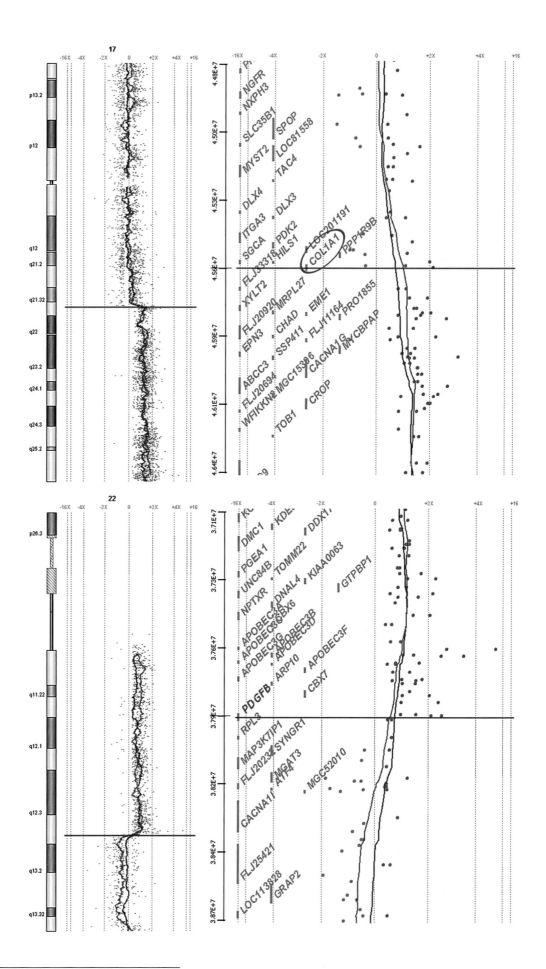

The presence of gains in 17q and 22q was observed in the individual samples and the pools both by mCGH and aCGH. The aCGH results were in accordance with the mCGH results. In addition, aCGH revealed changes not visible by mCGH. P-2 showed a copy number loss at 22q13.2→qter. The only case showing loss of distal 22q had an unbalanced t(17;22), a well-known variant from previous cytogenetic analyses. The loss that was observed in the pool suggests that several individual cases contained this change, even when cDNA-based aCGH only showed it in one of the individual cases. The cytogenetic subgroups of DFSP are characterized by supernumerary rings, balanced t(17;22) and unbalanced t(17;22). Because none of the cases in P-1 were cytogenetically analyzed, it was not possible to classify them with certainty, but the mCGH results showed that they were not balanced translocation cases.

Both the *COL1A1* and *PDGFB* genes were gained in sample 3, P-1 (on the 13K array) and P-2 (on the oligonucleotide array). Gain of the genes was always associated with gains of the corresponding 17q and 22q regions. However, *COL1A1* was not spotted on the custom-made 16K cDNA arrays, on which samples 7–10 were analyzed. Because the oligonucleotide platform contains only 60 nucleotides of the sequence, no sequences of the actual gained region of *COL1A1* in P-1 were represented on the microarray, that thus yielded an apparently neutral copy number result. The analysis of the sample pools on oligonucleotide arrays enabled the detection of breakpoints for gains in chromosomes 17 and 22. The translocation breakpoints were found at the *PDGFB* gene in 22q13.1 and at the *COL1A1* gene in 17q21.33 (Fig. 1). As expected, *PDGFB* was gained in both pools on oligonucleotide arrays; however, *COL1A1* was gained in P-2 but not in P-1. Our findings support previous reports of a constant breakpoint at *PDGFB*, located in intron 1, and a variable breakpoint at *COL1A1*, which shifts within the alpha-helical domain region (O'Brien et al., 1998). A complete list of the

genes detected in the gained 17q and 22q regions (343 and 244 genes represented on the oligoarrays, respectively) is included in Appendix 1 available at www.helsinki.fi/cmg/microarray_data.

Previous mCGH studies have reported gains at 8q11.2→qter, 17q21→qter, and 22q11.2→q13 (Nishio et al., 2001, 2002). In addition, recurrent copy number changes in chromosomes 1, 5, 8, 12, 17 and 22 have been reported in 11 cases of DFSP (Kiuru-Kuhlefelt et al., 2001). Array-CGH analysis using a cDNA platform revealed chromosomal aberrations in addition to 17q and 22q regions, e.g., gains of chromosomes 5, 7, 8, 18 and 21, and loss of large parts of chromosome 19 (Linn et al., 2003). In the present work, 21 different regions of DNA copy number gain were found by aCGH, in addition to the 17q and 22q regions, whereas losses were only seen at 22q, as discussed above. Supplementary data in Appendix 1 (www.helsinki.fi/cmg/microarray_data) shows a complete list of the genes with copy number alterations. In P-1, 1p35.1→p36.2, 1q21.2→qter, 17q21.33→qter and 22cen→q13.1 were gained. Gains of 8q24.3, 11p15.5, 17q21.33→qter, 19q13.2, 19q13.42 and 22cen→q13.1, and loss of 22q13.2→qter were found in P-2. Because the reference DNA used in the hybridizations was not from the same individual as the sample DNA, the apparent gains may also be caused by polymorphisms. For example, the gained regions on chromosome 19 are known to show frequent copy number variation among individuals (http://projects.tcag.ca/variation/).

In short, we report cDNA- and oligonucleotide-based microarray CGH results on seven individual cases and two pools of DFSP. In addition to the 17q and 22q gains characteristic of DFSP, we found DNA copy number changes that have not been reported previously. Additional studies are needed to assess the significance that gene amplifications and losses in the altered regions may have in the tumorigenesis and progression of DFSP.

References

Atiye J, Wolf M, Kaur S, Monni O, Böhling T, et al: Gene amplifications in osteosarcoma-CGH microarray analysis. Genes Chromosomes Cancer 42:158–163 (2005).

Craig DW, Huentelman MJ, Hu-Lince D, Zismann VL, Kruer MC, et al: Identification of disease causing loci using an array-based genotyping approach on pooled DNA. BMC Genomics 6:138 (2005).

Domanski HA, Gustafson P: Cytologic features of primary, recurrent, and metastatic dermatofibrosarcoma protuberans. Cancer 96:351–361 (2002).

El-Rifai W, Larramendy ML, Bjorkqvist AM, Hemmer S, Knuutila S: Optimization of comparative genomic hybridization using fluorochrome conjugated to dCTP and dUTP nucleotides. Lab Invest 77:699–700 (1997).

Jong K, Marchiori E, Meijer G, Vaart AV, Ylstra B: Breakpoint identification and smoothing of array comparative genomic hybridization data. Bioinformatics 200:3636–3637 (2004).

Kendziorski C, Irizarry RA, Chen KS, Haag JD, Gould MN: On the utility of pooling biological samples in microarray experiments. Proc Natl Acad Sci USA 102:4252–4257 (2005).

Kiuru-Kuhlefelt S, El-Rifai W, Fanburg-Smith J, Kere J, Miettinen M, Knuutila S: Concomitant DNA copy number amplification at 17q and 22q in dermatofibrosarcoma protuberans. Cytogenet Cell Genet 92:192–195 (2001).

Larramendy ML, Kaur S, Svarvar C, Böhling T, Knuutila S: Gene copy number profiling of soft tissue leiomyosarcoma by array-CGH. Cancer Genet Cytogenet 169:94–101 (2006).

Linn SC, West RB, Pollack JR, Zhu S, Hernandez-Boussard T, et al: Gene expression patterns and gene copy number changes in dermatofibrosarcoma protuberans. Am J Pathol 163:2383–2395 (2003).

Mitelman Database of Chromosome Aberrations in Cancer. Mitelman F, Johansson B, Mertens F (eds.). http://cgap.nci.nih.gov/Chromosomes/Mitelman (2006).

Monni O, Barlund M, Mousses S, Kononen J, Sauter G, et al: Comprehensive copy number and gene expression profiling of the 17q23 amplicon in human breast cancer. Proc Natl Acad Sci USA 98:5711–5716 (2001).

Naeem R, Lux ML, Huang SF, Naber SP, Corson JM, Fletcher JA: Ring chromosomes in dermatofibrosarcoma protuberans are composed of interspersed sequences from chromosomes 17 and 22. Am J Pathol 147:1553–1558 (1995).

Fig. 1. Translocation breakpoint regions in chromosomes 17 and 22 shown by oligonucleotide array-CGH. DNA copy number changes involving chromosome arms 17q and 22q in DFSP pools P-1 (blue) and P-2 (red), and the translocation breakpoints, *COL1A1* on 17q and *PDGFB* on 22q.

Nishio J, Iwasaki H, Ohjimi Y, Ishiguro M, Isayama T, et al: Supernumerary ring chromosomes in dermatofibrosarcoma protuberans may contain sequences from 8q11.2-qter and 17q21-qter: A combined cytogenetic and comparative genomic hybridization study. Cancer Genet Cytogenet 129:102–106 (2001).

Nishio J, Iwasaki H, Ohjimi Y, Ishiguro M, Isayama T, et al: Overrepresentation of 17q22-qter and 22q13 in dermatofibrosarcoma protuberans but not in dermatofibroma: A comparative genomic hybridization study. Cancer Genet Cytogenet 132:102–108 (2002).

O'Brien KP, Seroussi E, Dal Cin P, Sciot R, Mandahl N, et al: Various regions within the alpha-helical domain of the COL1A1 gene are fused to the second exon of the PDGFB gene in dermatofibrosarcomas and giant-cell fibroblastomas. Genes Chromosomes Cancer 23:187–193 (1998).

Pedeutour F, Coindre JM, Sozzi G, Nicolo G, Leroux A, et al: Supernumerary ring chromosomes containing chromosome 17 sequences. A specific feature of dermatofibrosarcoma protuberans? Cancer Genet Cytogenet 76:1–9 (1994).

Pedeutour F, Simon MP, Minoletti F, Sozzi G, Pierotti MA, et al: Ring 22 chromosomes in dermatofibrosarcoma protuberans are low-level amplifiers of chromosome 17 and 22 sequences. Cancer Res 55:2400–2403 (1995).

Pedeutour F, Simon MP, Minoletti F, Barcelo G, Terrier-Lacombe MJ, et al: Translocation, t(17;22)(q22;q13), in dermatofibrosarcoma protuberans: A new tumor-associated chromosome rearrangement. Cytogenet Cell Genet 72:171–174 (1996).

Pollack JR, Perou CM, Alizadeh AA, Eisen MB, Pergamenschikov A, et al: Genome-wide analysis of DNA copy-number changes using cDNA microarrays. Nat Genet 23:41–46 (1999).

Sandberg AA, Bridge JA: Updates on the cytogenetics and molecular genetics of bone and soft tissue tumors. Dermatofibrosarcoma protuberans and giant cell fibroblastoma. Cancer Genet Cytogenet 140:1–12 (2003).

Simon MP, Navarro M, Roux D, Pouyssegur J: Structural and functional analysis of a chimeric protein COL1A1-PDGFB generated by the translocation t(17;22)(q22;q13.1) in dermatofibrosarcoma protuberans (DP). Oncogene 20:2965–2975 (2001).

Sirvent N, Maire G, Pedeutour F: Genetics of dermatofibrosarcoma protuberans family of tumors: From ring chromosomes to tyrosine kinase inhibitor treatment. Genes Chromosomes Cancer 37:1–19 (2003).

Sonobe H, Furihata M, Iwata J, Ohtsuki Y, Chikazawa M, et al: Dermatofibrosarcoma protuberans harboring t(9;22)(q32;q12.2). Cancer Genet Cytogenet 110:14–18 (1999).

Tyybäkinoja A, Saarinen-Pihkala U, Elonen E, Knuutila S: Amplified, lost, and fused genes in 11q23–25 amplicon in acute myeloid leukemia, an array-CGH study. Genes Chromosomes Cancer 45:257–264 (2006).

Vauhkonen H, Vauhkonen M, Sajantila A, Sipponen P, Knuutila S: DNA copy number aberrations in intestinal-type gastric cancer revealed by array-based comparative genomic hybridization. Cancer Genet Cytogenet 167:150–154 (2006).

Zhang SD, Gant TW: Effect of pooling samples on the efficiency of comparative studies using microarrays. Bioinformatics 21:4378–4383 (2005).

Cytogenet Genome Res 115:289–297 (2006)
DOI: 10.1159/000095926

Molecular parameters associated with insulinoma progression: chromosomal instability versus p53 and CK19 status

Y.M.H. Jonkers[a] S.M.H. Claessen[a] J.A. Veltman[b] A. Geurts van Kessel[b]
W.N.M. Dinjens[c] B. Skogseid[d] F.C.S. Ramaekers[a] E.-J.M. Speel[a]

[a]Department of Molecular Cell Biology, Research Institute Growth and Development, University of Maastricht, Maastricht; [b]Department of Human Genetics, Radboud University Medical Centre Nijmegen, Nijmegen
[c]Department of Pathology, University Medical Center Rotterdam, Rotterdam (The Netherlands)
[d]Department of Medical Sciences, University Hospital Uppsala, Uppsala (Sweden)

Manuscript received 3 February 2006; accepted in revised form for publication by M. Schmid, 2 May 2006.

Abstract. Insulinomas represent the predominant syndromic subtype of endocrine pancreatic tumors (EPTs). Their metastatic potential cannot be predicted reliably using histopathological criteria. In the past few years, several attempts have been made to identify prognostic markers, among them *TP53* mutations and immunostaining of p53 and recently cytokeratin 19 (CK19). In a previous study using conventional comparative genomic hybridization (CGH) we have shown that chromosomal instability (CIN) is associated with metastatic disease in insulinomas. It was our aim to evaluate these potential parameters in a single study. For the determination of CIN, we applied CGH to microarrays because it allows a high-resolution detection of DNA copy number changes in comparison with conventional CGH as well as the analysis of chromosomal regions close to the centromeres and telomeres, and at 1pter→p32, 16p, 19 and 22. These regions are usually excluded from conventional CGH analysis, because they may show DNA gains in negative control hybridizations. Array CGH analysis of 30 insulinomas (15 tumors of benign, eight tumors of uncertain and seven tumors of malignant behavior) revealed that ≥20 chromosomal alterations and ≥6 telomeric losses were the best predictors of malignant progression. A subset of 22 insulinomas was further investigated for *TP53* exon 5–8 gene mutations, and p53 and CK19 expression. Only one malignant tumor was shown to harbor an arginine 273 serine mutation and immunopositivity for p53. CK19 immunopositivity was detected in three malignant tumors and one tumor with uncertain behavior. In conclusion, our results indicate that CIN as well as telomeric loss are very powerful indicators for malignant progression in sporadic insulinomas. Our data do not support a critical role for p53 and CK19 as molecular parameters for this purpose.

Copyright © 2006 S. Karger AG, Basel

This study was supported by the Netherlands Foundations Vanderes and Sacha Swarttouw-Hijmans, and the Association for International Cancer Research (AICR), St. Andrews (UK) and in part by the National Science Foundation (31-618845.0), Swiss Cancer Research Foundation (997-02-2000).

Request reprints from Yvonne Jonkers
  Department of Molecular Cell Biology (box 17)
University of Maastricht, P.O. Box 616
NL–6200 MD Maastricht (The Netherlands)
telephone: +31 43 388 1365; fax: +31 43 388 4151
e-mail: Y.Jonkers@MOLCELB.unimaas.nl

We declare that there is no conflict of interest that would prejudice the impartiality of the study.

Chromosomal instability (CIN) is a feature of most human cancers. CIN refers to an increased rate of losing or gaining whole or large parts of chromosomes during cell division (Draviam et al., 2004; Michor et al., 2005). It is known that critically short telomeres, in the setting of abrogated DNA damage checkpoints, cause CIN due to end-to-end chromosomal fusions, subsequent breakage, and rearrangement, resulting in an increased cancer incidence in animal models (Meeker et al., 2002). The role of telomeres in preventing chromosome fusion has led to the proposal that loss of telomere function is a mechanism for CIN in cancer (Murnane and Sabatier, 2004). In addition, defects in mitotic segregation seem to cause CIN (Rajagopalan and Lengauer, 2004). A crucial question of cancer biology is whether CIN is an early event resulting in gene mutations that drive tumorigenesis, or a late event in tumor progression as a consequence of alterations in oncogenes and tumor suppressor genes (TSGs) (Duesberg and Rasnick, 2000; Michor et al., 2005). In many neuroendocrine tumor types, including pheochromocytomas, adrenocortical tumors, and different endocrine pancreatic tumor (EPT) subtypes, CIN has been detected as a late event in tumor progression (Kjellman et al., 1996; Speel et al., 1999; Zhao et al., 1999; Dannenberg et al., 2000).

Insulinomas are the most frequently detected functioning EPTs. They show evidence of beta-cell differentiation and clinical symptoms of hypoglycemia due to uncontrolled insulin production. Insulinomas clearly differ from other EPT subtypes with respect to their clinical behavior and low MEN1 mutation frequency. According to the most recent WHO classification, the only feature that separates benign from malignant disease is organ and/or lymph node infiltration or distant metastases (Komminoth et al., 2004). When only a primary lesion is identified, however, no reliable markers for malignancy are available. Tumors with parameters such as a tumor diameter ≥2 cm, an increased mitotic index and/or necrosis are classified as tumors with uncertain behavior, having an increased risk for malignant outgrowth compared to benign tumors (Hochwald et al., 2002). Interestingly, by using conventional comparative genomic hybridization (CGH) we observed significant differences in the number of genomic alterations per tumor between benign and malignant insulinomas. CIN was a more powerful predictor of malignancy than a tumor diameter >2 cm or a proliferative index ≥2% (Jonkers et al., 2005).

Besides chromosomal alterations, a number of immunomarkers have been indicated that predict the prognosis of insulinomas, including the alpha chain of human chorionic gonadotropin (HCG-α), p53 and cytokeratin 19 (CK19). HCG-α is expressed by approximately 65% of malignant functioning EPTs. Because it is also expressed in benign tumors, this marker is considered to be of limited value (Heitz et al., 1987; Graeme-Cook et al., 1990). The TP53 TSG is mutated in more than 50% of all human neoplasms (Hollstein et al., 1991). If the remaining wildtype TP53 gene is inactivated (predominantly by deletion), these mutations abrogate the negative growth regulatory functions of p53 and are often associated with CIN. Immunohistochemical detection of p53 is associated with the presence of a TP53 mutation in most cases. Controversy exists with respect to the p53 status in EPTs. Lee suggested no role for p53, whereas Pavelic et al. identified p53 overexpression in three out of three cases of malignant insulinomas (Pavelic et al., 1995; Lee, 1996). Mutations of TP53 have only been found in a few isolated EPT cases (Bartz et al., 1996; Lin et al., 1997). Cytokeratin 19 (CK19) is widely expressed in (pre)malignant cells of epithelial origin (Kwaspen et al., 1997). Its presence

in normal cells has been related to functional growth, keeping post-stem cells in a flexible state of differentiation. In the normal pancreas, it is only expressed in the exocrine ducts (Bouwens, 1998). CK19 has recently been proposed as a predictor of survival in EPTs, including insulinomas (Deshpande et al., 2004). Recently, La Rosa et al. confirmed these findings with the restriction that CK19 expression should be detected with the RCK108 antibody (La Rosa et al., 2005). Albarello et al. however demonstrated a low specificity for CK19 immunostaining, already showing expression in 57% of EPTs with benign and uncertain behavior (Albarello et al., 2004).

The aim of this study was to evaluate CIN and the p53 and CK19 status as prognostic parameters in insulinomas. For this purpose we analyzed a group of 30 insulinomas with CGH to genomic microarrays containing 3,700 FISH-verified bacterial artificial chromosome (BAC) clones. Array CGH was used because of its higher resolution compared to conventional CGH and to allow a more reliable analysis of DNA copy number changes at regions close to the centromeres and telomeres, and at chromosomes 1pter→p32, 16p, 19, and 22. These regions are usually excluded in conventional CGH, because they often show gains in negative control hybridizations. A subgroup of 22 tumors was subsequently examined for mutations of TP53 and immunoreactivity for p53 and CK19.

Materials and methods

Tumor material and patient data
36 cases of insulinoma (19 females, mean age 51.4 ± 17.5 years and 17 males, mean age 50.9 ± 12.8 years) were selected from the archives of the Departments of Pathology of the University Hospital Zurich, Switzerland and the University Medical Centers Rotterdam, Utrecht and Nijmegen (The Netherlands). From all cases paraffin-embedded material was available. Frozen material was present from 30 of these cases. They were all sporadic tumors and not associated with the inherited MEN1 (multiple endocrine neoplasia) syndrome. The tumors were classified according to the most recent WHO classification (Komminoth et al., 2004). The samples included 17 benign tumors, nine tumors of uncertain behavior, and ten malignant tumors. All insulinomas exhibited hyperinsulinism followed by a hypoglycemia syndrome. The study protocol was approved by the institutional ethical committee, and all of the patients gave informed consent.

The 30 insulinomas of which frozen material was available were analyzed by array CGH. A subgroup of 22 insulinomas was analyzed for TP53 mutations and p53 and CK19 expression by immunohistochemistry on paraffin tissue sections.

DNA extraction
Genomic DNA, isolated from blood lymphocytes of four cytogenetically normal, healthy individuals (two males and two females), was used for array validation and as normal reference DNA. Genomic DNA from frozen insulinoma samples was extracted by homogenizing approximately 5 mm^3 of each sample prior to proteinase K treatment and purification using the QIAamp DNA mini kit (Qiagen, Hilden, Germany) (Jonkers et al., 2005).

Array CGH analysis
Array CGH was performed on microarrays containing 3,700 FISH-verified bacterial artificial chromosome (BAC) clones in triplicate, including ~3,200 clones selected through an international collaboration to cover the genome with a 1-Mb resolution, and clones specifically

Table 1. P53 exon 5–8 PCR primer information

Primer	Forward/reverse	Sequence	Product size (bp)
P53 exon 5/1	F	CCT GAC TTT CAA CTC TTG CTC	158
	R	ACT GCT TGT AGA TGG CCA TG	
P53 exon 5/2	F	CAG CTG TGG GTT GAT TCC AC	176
	R	CTG GGG ACC CTG GGC AAC	
P53 exon 6/1	F	AGG CCT CTG ATT CCT CAC TG	127
	R	GCA CCA CCA CAC TAT GTC GA	
P53 exon 6/2	F	CTC CTC AGC ATC TTA TCC GA	159
	R	CCA CTG ACA ACC ACC CTT	
P53 exon 7/1	F	AGG CGC ACT GGC CTC ATC TT	141
	R	TCC AGT GTG ATG ATG GTG AGG	
P53 exon 7/2	F	CAT GTG TAA CAG TTC CTG CAT G	135
	R	GCG GCA AGC AGA GGC TGG	
P53 exon 8/1	F	CCT TAC TGC CTC TTG CTT CTC	130
	R	CTT GCG GAG ATT CTC TTC CTC	
P53 exon 8/2	F	TTG TGC CTG TCC TGG GAG AG	127
	R	CTC CAC CGC TTC TTG TCC T	

selected for previous studies. Array preparation, labeling, hybridization, and scanning procedures were performed as described elsewhere (Vissers et al., 2003). In brief, tumor and reference DNA were labeled by random priming in a total volume of 80 μl. For labeling, 500 ng DNA was dissolved in a mixture containing 50 mM Tris-HCl (pH 6.8), 5 mM MgCl$_2$, 10 mM 2-mercaptoethanol, and 300 μg/ml random octamers (Bioprime DNA labeling system; 1× random primers solution, Invitrogen) and denatured for 10 min at 100°C. After cooling to 4°C tumor DNA was incubated with 4 nmol Cy3-dUTP, and control DNA with 4 nmol Cy5-dUTP (Amersham Pharmacia Biotech), in combination with 2 mM dGTP, 2 mM dCTP, 2 mM dATP, 1 mM dTTP and 64 U of Klenow enzyme (Invitrogen). Labeling was performed overnight at 37°C. The labeled probes were purified over a QIAquick column (Qiagen) to remove unincorporated fluorescent nucleotides. Cy3- and Cy5-labeled probes were mixed together with 120 μg Cot-1 DNA (Roche) and co-precipitated for at least 2 h at –20°C. Pellets were air dried and dissolved in a total volume of 130 μl hybridization solution, containing 50% formamide, 10% dextran sulphate, 4% SDS, 100 μg yeast tRNA, and 2× saline sodium citrate (SSC). This probe mixture was denatured for 15 min at 70°C and pre-annealed for 30 min at 37°C. After pre-annealing the sample was applied to a pretreated and denatured microarray (Vissers et al., 2003). Hybridization and post-hybridization washing procedures were performed using a GeneTac hybridization station (Genomic Solutions, Cambridgeshire, UK) according to the manufacturer's instructions.

Image analysis and evaluation
Fluorescence images of microarray slides were acquired by using an Affymetrix 428 scanner and analyzed using GenePix Pro 6.0 software (Axon Instruments Inc., Foster City, Calif.), as described elsewhere (Vissers et al., 2003). To obtain a genomic copy number ratio for each spot, the median local background was subtracted from the median pixel intensity of both dyes. Data normalization was performed by using the software package SAS version 8.0 (SAS institute, Cary, N.C.) for each array sub-grid, by applying loess curve fitting with a smoothing factor of 0.3 to predict the log$_2$-transformed test-over-reference values. This smoothing factor was shown to result in the lowest percentage of false-positive results while not increasing the amount of false-negative results in the validation experiments. To utilize the spatial coherence between nearby clones, we used an unsupervised Hidden Markov Models (HMM) approach (Fridlyand et al., 2004). The clones are partitioned into the states which represent the underlying copy number of the group of clones. Chromosomal aberrations ≥10 Mb were counted as a measure for CIN. Furthermore, telomeric loss was counted when at least two clones at the chromosomal end were deleted. All mapping information regarding clone locations, cytogenetic bands, and genomic content were retrieved from the UCSC genome browser (May 2004 freeze).

Single-Strand Conformation Polymorphism (SSCP) and sequence analysis of p53 exons 5–8
Exons 5–8 of the *TP53* gene were investigated by SSCP analysis in 22 insulinoma samples. Each exon was amplified in two overlapping fragments. All primers used are listed in Table 1. DNA was amplified by a radioactive 15-μl Polymerase Chain Reaction (PCR). The PCR mix per sample consisted of 10 μl distilled H$_2$O, 1.5 μl goldbuffer, 1.5 μl 25-mM MgCl$_2$ solution, 0.3 μl 10-mM dGTP, dTTP, dCTP, 0.3 μl 1-mM dATP, 0.9 Units (5 U/μl × 0.18 μl) Amplitaq polymerase (Perkin-Elmer, Wellesley, Mass., USA), 30 ng (0.1 μg/μl × 0.3 μl) of forward and reverse primer, 0.075 μl αP^{32}-dATP (Amersham, Buckinghamshire, UK) and 1 μl DNA sample. Before amplification the PCR-mix was heated at 95°C for 5 min to activate the Amplitaq polymerase. The temperatures for amplification were 95°C for 30 s, 55°C for 45 s and 72°C for 45 s. These steps were repeated for 35 cycles followed by a final extension at 72°C for 10 min.

PCR products were diluted with 14 μl loading buffer (95% formamide, 10 mM EDTA pH 8, 0.05% bromophenol blue and 0.05% xylene cyanol) and denatured at 95°C for 5 min. Solutions were chilled on ice and, per sample, 4 μl was loaded on a 15% polyacrylamide gel (acrylamide to bisacrylamide 49:1) containing 10% of glycerol. Electrophoresis was performed at 8 W (15.8 V/cm) overnight at room temperature. The gels were vacuum dried at 80°C and exposed to X-ray films. Films were evaluated by visual inspection.

TP53 mutations indicated by SSCP analysis were identified by direct sequencing. PCR products were used for cycle sequencing using a Dye Terminator Cycle Sequencing Ready Reaction and analyzed on an ABI Prism 3100 genetic analyzer according to the instructions of the manufacturer (PE Biosystems, Foster City, Calif.).

Immunostaining of p53 and CK19
p53 and CK19 antigen staining was performed on 4-μm-thick paraffin-embedded tissue sections of 22 insulinomas (seven benign, five of unknown behavior and ten malignant) as described previously (Hafkamp et al., 2003). Briefly, sections were deparaffinized and treated with 10 mM citrate buffer (pH 6.0) in a microwave oven at 600 W for 15 min (antigen retrieval). Endogenous peroxidase was inactivated by treatment with 2% H$_2$O$_2$ in methanol, followed by incubation in 3% BSA/PBS to block non-specific binding of antibody conjugates. The sections were incubated for 1 h at room temperature either with mouse monoclonal antibody directed against human CK19 (RCK108, Mubio,

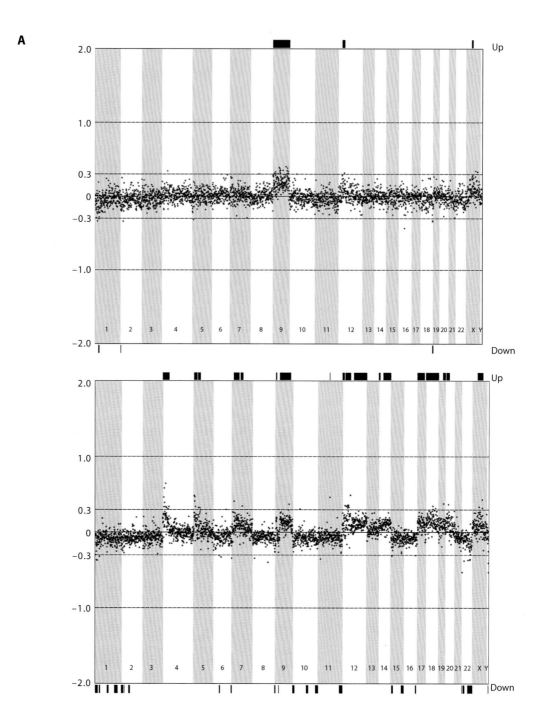

A

B

Chromosomal aberrations ≥ 10 Mb

Losses ≥ 2 clones at chromosomal ends

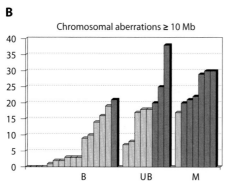

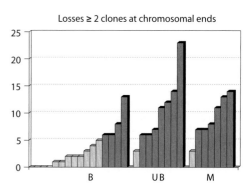

Maastricht, the Netherlands) at a 1:200 dilution in 1% bovine serum albumin (BSA)/PBS, or with mouse monoclonal antibody DO7 against p53 protein (Dako, Glostrup, Denmark) at a 1:50 dilution in 1% BSA/PBS. Primary antibodies were detected using biotin-labeled horse anti-mouse antibody at a 1:200 dilution in 1% BSA/PBS, and avidin-biotinylated peroxidase complex (Vector Laboratories, Burlingame, Calif.) at a 1:50 dilution in 4× SSC. Peroxidase activity was visualized using diaminobenzidine (DAB)/H_2O_2 (Sigma Chemical Co., St Louis, Mo.) and sections were counterstained with hematoxylin and mounted in Entellan (Merck, Darmstadt, Germany).

Although the DO-7 antibody binds to both normal and mutant p53 protein, in general normal levels of wild-type p53 protein are too low to detect by immunohistochemistry. A premalignant laryngeal specimen was used as a positive control, showing nuclear p53 staining above the threshold level of ≥30% of cells (Hafkamp et al., 2003). All tumor cases with cytoplasmic staining for CK19 in ≥10% of tumor cells were considered positive in this study. Ductal cells of the normal exocrine pancreas expressing CK19 in the cytoplasm served as a positive control in the tissue sections. Three observers independently evaluated all immunostained slides.

Results

DNA copy number alterations detected by array CGH

Genomic DNA extracted from 30 frozen insulinoma specimens was analyzed by array CGH for the presence of chromosomal alterations. In the benign group, the average number of large chromosomal changes per tumor (≥10 Mb) was 6.6 ± 7.2, whereas the tumors with uncertain behavior and malignant behavior showed an average number of 19.1 ± 9.7 and 24.1 ± 5.4, respectively. Representative examples of an array CGH profile of a benign and a malignant tumor are shown in Fig. 1A. The most optimal discrimination between benign and malignant tumors (when excluding the tumors with uncertain behavior) could be made by classification of the tumors according to the presence of more or less than 20 chromosomal aberrations of ≥10 Mb (Fig. 1B; left graph). More than 20 alterations (CIN) were detected in one out of 15 benign tumors, three out of eight tumors with uncertain behavior, and six out of seven malignant tumors. Based on this classification, the insulinomas with uncertain behavior comprise both tumors that most likely belong to the benign group and tumors that rather belong to the malignant group. Comparison of the benign with the malignant tumors showed that CIN is a very sensitive marker for malignancy (OR = 84), which is in agreement with our previous conventional CGH data. Both the specificity and sensitivity of this parameter were further improved by the use

of array CGH (93 and 86% vs. 82 and 83% with conventional CGH) (Table 2).

In order to identify the chromosomal regions most frequently involved in CIN, we determined those regions that encompass at least three adjacent BAC clones, and occur in insulinomas with CIN at a frequency of ≥25% higher than in tumors without CIN. Only those regions that are significantly different in frequency between those two groups are listed in Table 2. Furthermore, the percentage of malignant tumors with the aberration, defined as sensitivity, and the percentage of benign tumors without the aberration, defined as specificity, and their odds ratios were calculated. The regions 22q11.21→13.31 and 7p21.1→11.2 were the best classifying markers for malignant behavior according to their sensitivity in univariate analysis (71% each). Discrimination on basis of more or less than 20 aberrations per tumor however showed to be more sensitive (86%).

Loss of telomeric regions

The loss of telomeric regions, defined as a deletion of at least two clones at the chromosomal end, was subsequently determined. The average number of telomeric losses per tumor were significantly higher in the tumors with CIN than without CIN (10.0 ± 5.6 vs. 4.9 ± 4.5; $P = 0.01$). The best classification between benign and malignant tumors could be achieved by using a threshold of six telomeric losses (OR = 39; see Table 2), which approaches the discriminating value of CIN. Figure 1B (right graph) shows the number of telomeric losses per tumor in insulinomas with benign, uncertain and malignant behavior. At least six telomeric losses were detected in four out of 15 benign tumors, seven out of eight tumors with uncertain behavior and six out of seven malignant tumors. In addition, in insulinomas with uncertain behavior telomeric losses were more frequently observed than CIN.

TP53 mutation analysis and immunohistochemistry

A subgroup of 22 insulinomas, including five cases of which only paraffin embedded material was available, was analyzed for *TP53* mutations. The results are shown in Table 3. Only one hotspot mutation in exon 8 (arginine 273 serine) was detected in a malignant insulinoma (Fig. 2B and C). This mutation coincided with loss of chromosome 17 as detected by array CGH, indicating deletion of the wild-type locus. This insulinoma was the only tumor with less than 20 chromosomal aberrations in the malignant group. p53 immunostaining was positive in this tumor only. The results are shown in Table 3. Figure 2D and E show the presence and absence of nuclear p53 expression in tumor case 20 and tumor case 16.

CK19 immunohistochemistry

Consecutive tissue sections of the 22 insulinomas were also analyzed for CK19 immunoreactivity. Table 3 shows that only four tumors expressed cytoplasmic CK19, i.e. three out of ten malignant insulinomas and one out of five tumors with uncertain behavior (Fig. 2F). Ductal cells of the normal pancreas expressing cytokeratin 19 in the cyto-

Fig. 1. (**A**) Representative examples of an array CGH profile of a benign (above) and a malignant tumor (below). Bars above the figure are chromosomal gains detected by Hidden Markov analysis. Bars below are losses. Clones are ordered from chromosome 1 to 22 and X,Y (X-axis). On the Y-axis the $\log_2$-transformed test over reference values are indicated. (**B**) Graphs representing the number of chromosomal aberrations of ≥10 Mb (left side), and the number of telomeric losses (loss of at least two BAC clones at the chromosomal ends) (right side) in tumors with benign (B), uncertain (UB) and malignant (M) behavior. Each bar represents one tumor. The dark grey bars are used in the left graph for ≥20 chromosomal aberrations (CIN) and in the right graph for ≥6 telomeric losses per tumor.

Table 2. Chromosomal aberrations associated with chromosomal instability

Chromosomal region of loss	bp position[a]	Candidate genes	Size (Mb)	No CIN[b]	CIN[b]	P value[b]	Sens.[c]	Spec.[c]	OR >1[c]
1p36.33–34.1	294,060	APITD1	45	13	58	0.03	57	87	9
1p31.1–22.1	82,255,496		9	0	30	0.03	0	93	
1p12	117,527,043		2	5	40	0.031	29	93	
1q43–44	239,198,790	AKT3	3	17	60	0.03	57	87	9
2q11.2–12.2	99,888,629		7	5	40	0.031	43	100	>11
3p25.3–21.31	9,204,214	PPARG	37	2	42	0.008	43	93	11
6p21.32–21.1	33,032,994	VEGF	10	4	44	0.031	43	93	11
6q24.3–27	148,731,560		19	0	41	0.008	43	100	>11
8p23.3–23.2	384,739		3	0	30	0.03	14	100	
10p15.3–14	290,388		9	2	40	0.008	43	93	11
10q21.3	64,873,350		4	1	32	0.03	29	100	
10q22.2–23.33	77,323,046	FAS	17	0	50	0.002	43	100	>11
10q25.2–26.11	113,549,135		6	0	30	0.03	29	100	
10q26.13–26.3	124,043,135	BCCIP	11	4	50	0.009	43	93	11
15q12–14	23,790,070	TRPM1	12	4	42	0.031	29	87	3
22q11.21–13.31	19,910,708	NF2	25	32	73	0.056	71	73	7

Chromosomal region of gain	bp position[a]	Candidate genes	Size (Mb)	No CIN[b]	CIN[b]	P value[b]	Sens.[c]	Spec.[c]	OR[c]
4p16.2–q35.2	5,000,272	MAD2L1, CDC4	178	4	43	0.031	43	100	>11
7p21.1–11.2	17,428,379	GCK	37	14	60	0.03	71	87	16
7q11.22–31.32	69,645,684		52	8	47	0.026	43	93	11
7q33–35	134,622,057	BRAF	10	6	46	0.009	43	93	11
12p13.31–13.2	9,155,207		1	6	48	0.009	57	100	>19
12p12.1–11.23	23,984,770	KRAS	3	6	40	0.031	43	100	>11
12q12–24.33	39,747,507	KNTC1	90	0	51	0.002	43	93	11
13q21.1–33.1	57,539,975		45	2	36	0.008	29	93	6
14q11.2–32.2	20,145,562		80	6	51	0.009	43	100	>11
17p13.1–q25.3	8,282,767	CK19, BRCA1	67	1	36	0.008	43	100	>11
18p11.32–11.31	2,222,012		4	0	30	0.03	43	100	>11
18q11.2–12.1	19,366,416		5	0	30	0.03	43	100	>11
18q12.3	36,066,444		3	0	30	0.03	43	100	>11
18q21.32–22.2	56,872,706	BCL2	8	0	30	0.03	43	100	>11
20p13–11.23	467,506		19	18	65	0.015	57	80	5

CIN							86	93	84
Telomeric loss[d]							86	87	39
P53							14	100	
CK19							14	100	

[a] Map positions and cytogenetic locations are based on data available through the University of California Santa Cruz genome browser (May 2004 freeze).

[b] Percentage of tumors with the aberration in the CIN group (≥ 20 aberrations of at least 10 Mb; n = 10) and the No CIN group (<20 aberrations of at least 10 Mb; n = 20). This percentage is the mean of the percentages per clone in that region. Regions contain at least five clones with a maximum of two intermediate clones without the aberration.

[c] Sens.: sensitivity, the percentage of malignant tumors with the aberration. Spec.: specificity, the percentage of benign tumors without the aberration; OR, Odds Ratio. Only OR >1 are indicated.

[d] Telomeric loss as defined by at least six telomeric losses (two BAC clones lost at the chromosomal ends).

plasm served as positive control in the tissue sections (Fig. 2G). Although no benign tumors showed immunopositivity, the sensitivity of this parameter is insufficient to serve as a reliable predictor of malignancy.

Discussion

We performed a genome-wide array-based CGH analysis on a series of 30 human sporadic insulinomas with the goal of identifying powerful genomic parameters that can pre-

dict malignant progression. In addition, a subset of tumors was analyzed for TP53 mutations and expression of p53 and CK19 by immunohistochemistry, which have been indicated as prognostic markers in EPTs. Particularly a high number of chromosomal alterations and loss of telomeric ends were strongly associated with metastatic disease. p53 and CK19 status proved to be of little value for this purpose, because only rare, isolated cases showed a TP53 mutation or detectable amounts of protein.

In many cancers, alterations in the number of chromosomes are detected, which are believed to be caused by CIN.

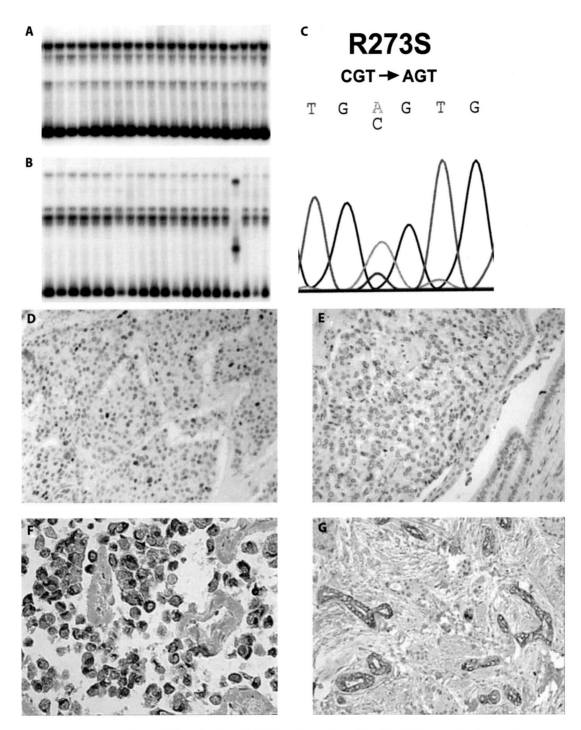

Fig. 2. Mutation analysis of *TP53*, showing (**A**) SSCP analysis of exon 7/1 of the *TP53* gene, showing no aberrations, (**B**) SSCP analysis of exon 8/1 of the *TP53* gene, showing one tumor with an aberrant SSCP pattern (tumor 20, Table 3), and (**C**) sequence profile of tumor 20 with the *TP53* mutation, arginine 273 serine. Immunohistochemistry for nuclear p53 and cytoplasmic CK19 expression, showing (**D**) a p53 positive insulinoma (tumor 20), (**E**) a p53-negative insulinoma (tumor 16), (**F**) a CK19-positive insulinoma (tumor 19), and (**G**) a CK19-negative insulinoma with positive staining in ductal cells (tumor 2).

Mutations in genes playing a role in mitotic segregation as well as loss of telomeric ends have been recognized as molecular mechanisms underlying this phenomenon (Gisselsson et al., 2001; Draviam et al., 2004; Murnane and Sabatier, 2004; Rajagopalan and Lengauer, 2004). On the basis of the number of alterations per tumor as identified by array CGH in this study, a marked distinction between benign and malignant insulinomas could be made. The most potential indicators for malignant progression are ≥20 chromosomal alterations of ≥10 Mb and ≥6 telomeric losses per tumor.

Table 3. Results of mutation analysis *(TP53)* and immunohistochemistry (p53 and CK19)

Tumor	Classification[a]	Regions ≥ 10 Mb	*TP53* m.a.[b]	p53 IHC[c]	CK19 IHC[c]
1	Benign		–	–	–
2	Benign	3	–	–	–
3	Benign		–	–	–
4	Benign	3	–	–	–
5	Benign		–	–	–
6	Benign	16	–	–	–
7	Benign	10	–	–	–
8	UB	18	–	–	–
9	UB	18	–	–	–
10	UB	38	–	–	–
11	UB	20	–	–	–
12	UB	8	–	–	+
13	Malignant	30	–	–	–
14	Malignant	30	–	–	–
15	Malignant		–	–	–
16	Malignant		–	–	–
17	Malignant	22	–	–	–
18	Malignant	21	–	–	–
19	Malignant	20	–	–	+
20	Malignant	17	+	+	+
21	Malignant	29	–	–	–
22	Malignant		–	–	+

[a] UB = Uncertain behavior.
[b] *TP53* m.a. = *TP53* mutation analysis.
[c] IHC = Immunohistochemistry.

It is tempting to speculate that the tumors with uncertain behavior and undetectable metastases can be classified as benign or malignant according to these genomic parameters. Since this group shows evident heterogeneity in the number of genomic alterations per tumor. The clinical follow-up data of patients required to evaluate such a classification are currently being collected. Interestingly, seven out of eight insulinomas with uncertain behavior harbored ≥6 telomeric losses per tumor, whereas only three of these cases contained ≥20 chromosomal aberrations. This suggests that telomeric loss occurs prior to and is causative for CIN during insulinoma tumorigenesis.

Besides genomic parameters, we examined the value of *TP53* exon 5–8 mutations and the expression of nuclear p53 for predicting metastatic disease in insulinomas. Only one malignant insulinoma proved to exhibit a hot-spot mutation in exon 8 of the *TP53* gene, i.e. A273S. Interestingly, this tumor also showed a different genomic profile compared to the other malignant tumors. First, it revealed loss of chromosome 17, indicating deletion of the remaining wild-type allele, whereas chromosome 17 was gained in four out of seven malignant insulinomas. Second, it was the only malignant tumor with <20 aberrations. The fact that only one malignant tumor showed a *TP53* mutation indicates that this gene does not play an important role in insulinoma progression. This finding is in agreement with earlier studies describing only rare EPT cases with a *TP53* mutation (Bartz et al., 1996; Lin et al., 1997). Immunopositivity for p53 was only found in the tumor with the mutation, further underscoring the little value of p53 in predicting malignant progression. Nevertheless, if a *TP53* mutation is identified, the insulinoma is most likely malignant.

CK19 is expressed in many types of simple and non-keratinizing normal and neoplastic epithelia, including pancreatic ductal cells. Normal endocrine pancreatic cells are negative for this marker. Deshpande et al. have recently reported that CK19 immunostaining is a powerful predictor of survival in EPTs and that four out of 20 insulinomas expressed CK19, two of which occurred in patients with advanced disease (Deshpande et al., 2004). It was unclear which CK19 monoclonal antibody (clone BA17 and RCK108, both from Dako) was used in this study. It was recently found that CK19 expression only when tested with the RCK108 antibody correlates with prognosis in EPTs and especially in insulinomas (La Rosa et al., 2005). Therefore, we have used the RCK108 antibody in this study for critical evaluation of its predictive value in malignant insulinoma progression. CK19 immunoreactivity was detected in three tumors with malignant and one with uncertain behavior, whereas the exocrine duct cells stained strongly positive in many CK19-negative tumor cases. Our study thus does not support the use of CK19 immunopositivity as a strong predictor for insulinoma progression. Because we are in the process of collecting the clinical patient data, we were unable to determine the role of CK19 as a parameter associated with patient survival.

Our previous molecular studies have shown that gain of chromosome 9q, rather than mutations in the multiple endocrine neoplasia type 1 *(MEN1)* gene at 11q13, is an early event in insulinoma development (Speel et al., 2001; Jonkers et al., 2005). Besides CIN and telomeric losses, as described above, we searched for chromosomal regions which are most often involved in the tumors with malignant behavior and therefore may contain candidate genes involved in tumor progression. The regions 7p21.1→p11.2 and 22q11.21→q13.31 were the best classifying markers for malignant behavior according to their sensitivity in univariate analysis. A putative candidate gene in the 7p region is the glucokinase *(GCK)* gene. Glucokinase is a key regulatory enzyme in the pancreatic β-cell. It plays a crucial role in the regulation of insulin secretion and has been termed the pancreatic β-cell sensor. Mutations in this gene have been reported to cause both hyperglycemia and hypoglycemia (Gloyn, 2003), and thus can be considered an interesting candidate gene in insulinoma tumorigenesis. However, because hypoglycemia can already be detected in patients with small benign insulinomas, a relation with malignant progression is disputable. Losses of 22q loci have also been found by Wild et al., who excluded a putative role of the *hSNF5/INI1* gene in insulinomas (Wild et al., 2001). A candidate gene in the 22q11.21→q13.31 region identified by array CGH is the *NF2* gene, which is often deleted in sporadic and neurofibromatosis type 2 (NF2)-related meningiomas, schwannomas and ependymomas (Gutmann, 2001). A gene involved in various tumors with CIN is *BRCA1* (Hartman and Ford, 2003), which is localized on the 17p13.1→q25.3 region, often detected in insulinomas with CIN. Mutations of this gene are usually seen in combination with loss of this locus. In our series we detect predominantly gain of this region. Therefore, the intriguing finding that duplication/amplification of mutated alleles may also lead to tumorigenesis (Zhuang et al., 1998) should be examined in this respect. A role for these genes in insulinoma progression remains to be elucidated.

In conclusion, the presented findings indicate that CIN as well as telomeric loss are very powerful indicators for malignant progression in sporadic insulinomas. Our data do not support a critical role for p53 and CK19 as molecular parameters for this purpose. Furthermore, the chromosomal regions identified in tumors with CIN may harbor candidate cancer genes important in insulinoma progression.

Acknowledgements

We thank J.L.M. Uytdewilligen and H.F.B.M. Sleddens (Department of Pathology, UMC Rotterdam, the Netherlands) and M. Halin (Department of Medical Sciences, University Hospital Uppsala, Sweden) for expert technical assistance, and Dr. A. Perren (Department of Pathology, University Hospital Zurich, Switzerland), Prof. Dr. P. Komminoth (Department of Pathology, Hospital Baden, Switzerland), Prof. Dr. A. de Bruïne (Department of Pathology, UMC Maastricht, the Netherlands), Dr. A.A. Verhofstad (Department of Pathology, RUNMC Nijmegen, the Netherlands), Dr. L.J. Hofland (Department of Internal Medicine, UMC Rotterdam, the Netherlands), Dr. R.R. de Krijger (Department of Pathology, UMC Rotterdam, the Netherlands), and Prof. Dr. P.J. Slootweg (Department of Pathology, RUNMC Nijmegen, the Netherlands) for the collection of samples and helpful discussions.

References

Albarello L, Capitanio V, Zerbi A, Di Carlo V, Doglioni C: Cytokeratin 19 expression in pancreatic endocrine tumors. J Pancreas 6 (5 suppl):514 (2004).

Bartz C, Ziske C, Wiedenmann B, Moelling K: p53 tumor suppressor gene expression in pancreatic neuroendocrine tumor cells. Gut 38:403–409 (1996).

Bouwens L: Cytokeratins and cell differentiation in the pancreas. J Pathol 184:234–239 (1998).

Dannenberg H, Speel EJ, Zhao J, Saremaslani P, van Der Harst E, et al: Losses of chromosomes 1p and 3q are early genetic events in the development of sporadic pheochromocytomas. Am J Pathol 157:353–359 (2000).

Deshpande V, Fernandez-del Castillo C, Muzikansky A, Deshpande A, Zukerberg L, et al: Cytokeratin 19 is a powerfull predictor of survival in pancreatic endocrine tumors. Am J Surg Pathol 28:1145–1153 (2004).

Draviam VM, Xie S, Sorger PK: Chromosome segregation and genomic stability. Curr Opin Genet Dev 14:120–125 (2004).

Duesberg P, Rasnick D: Aneuploidy, the somatic mutation that makes cancer a species of its own. Cell Motil Cytoskeleton 47:81–107 (2000).

Fridlyand J, Snijders AM, Pinkel D, Albertson DG, Jain AN: Hidden markov models approach to the analysis of array CGH data. J Multivariate Analysis 90:132–153 (2004).

Gisselsson D, Jonson T, Petersen A, Strombeck B, Dal Cin P, et al: Telomere dysfunction triggers extensive DNA fragmentation and evolution of complex chromosome abnormalities in human malignant tumors. Proc Natl Acad Sci USA 98:12683–12688 (2001).

Gloyn AL: Glucokinase (GCK) mutations in hyper- and hypoglycemia: maturity-onset diabetes of the young, permanent neonatal diabetes, and hyperinsulinemia of infancy. Hum Mutat 22:353–362 (2003).

Graeme-Cook F, Nardi G, Compton CC: Immunocytochemical staining for human chorionic gonadotropin subunits does not predict malignancy in insulinomas. Am J Clin Pathol 93:273–276 (1990).

Gutmann DH: The neurofibromatosis: when less is more. Hum Mol Genet 10:747–755 (2001).

Hafkamp HC, Speel EJM, Haesevoets A, Bot FJ, Dinjens WNM, et al: A subset of head and neck squamous cell carcinomas exhibits integration of HPV 16/18 DNA and overexpression of p16^{INK4A} and p53 in the absence of mutations in p53 exons 5–8. Int J Cancer 107:394–400 (2003).

Hartman AR, Ford JM: BRCA1 and p53: compensatory roles in DNA repair. J Mol Med 81:700–707 (2003).

Heitz PU, von Herbay G, Kloppel G, Komminoth P, Kasper M, et al: The expression of subunits of human chorionic gonadotropin (hCG) by non-trophoblastic, nonendocrine, and endocrine tumors. Am J Clin Pathol 88:467–472 (1987).

Hochwald SN, Zee S, Conlon KC, Colleoni R, Louie O, et al: Prognostic factors in pancreatic endocrine neoplasms: an analysis of 136 cases with a proposal for low-grade and intermediate-grade groups. J Clin Oncol 20:2633–2642 (2002).

Hollstein M, Sidransky D, Vogelstein B, Harris CC: P53 mutations in human cancers. Science 253:49–53 (1991).

Jonkers YMH, Claessen SMH, Perren A, Schmid S, Komminoth P, et al: Chromosomal instability predicts metastatic disease in patients with insulinomas. ERC 12:435–447 (2005).

Kjellman M, Kallioniemi OP, Karhu R, Hoog A, Farnebo LO, et al: Genetic aberrations in adrenocortical tumors detected using comparative genomic hybridization correlate with tumor size and malignancy. Cancer Res 56:4219–4223 (1996).

Komminoth P, Perren A, Öberg K, Rindi G, Heitz PU, Klöppel G: Insulinoma, in DeLellis RA, Lloyd RV, Heitz PU, Eng C (eds): Pathology & Genetics. Tumours of endocrine organs, pp 183–186 (IARC Press, Lyon 2004).

Kwaspen FHL, Smedts FMM, Broos A, Bulten H, Debie WMH, Ramaekers FCS: Reproducible and highly sensitive detection of the broad spectrum epithelial marker keratin 19 in routine cancer diagnosis. Histopathology 31:503–516 (1997).

La Rosa S, Bianchi V, Rigoli E, Uccella S, Capella C: The prognostic significance of cytokeratin 19 expression in pancreatic endocrine tumors (PETs). Virchows Arch 447:188 (2005).

Lee CS: Lack of p53 immunoreactivity in pancreatic endocrine tumors. Pathology 28:139–141 (1996).

Lin HJ, French SW, Reichenbach D, Wan YY, Passaro E, Sawicki MP: Novel p53 mutation in a malignant tumor secreting vasoactive intestinal peptide. Arch Pathol Lab Med 121:125–128 (1997).

Meeker AK, Hicks JL, Platz EA, March GE, Bennett CJ, et al: Telomere shortening is an early somatic DNA alteration in human prostate tumorigenesis. Cancer Res 62:6405–6409 (2002).

Michor F, Iwasa Y, Vogelstein B, Lengauer C, Nowak MA: Can chromosomal instability initiate tumorigenesis? Sem Cancer Biol 15:43–49 (2005).

Murnane JP, Sabatier L: Chromosome rearrangements resulting from telomere dysfunction and their role in cancer. BioEssays 26:1164–1174 (2004).

Pavelic K, Hrascan R, Kapitanovic S, Karapandza N, Vranes Z, et al: Multiple genetic alterations in malignant metastatic insulinomas. J Pathol 177:395–400 (1995).

Rajagopalan H, Lengauer C: Aneuploidy and cancer. Nature 432:338–341 (2004).

Speel EJM, Richter J, Moch H, Egenter C, Saremaslani P, et al: Genetic differences in endocrine pancreatic tumor subtypes detected by comparative genomic hybridization. Am J Pathol 155:1787–1794 (1999).

Speel EJ, Scheidweiler AF, Zhao J, Matter C, Saremaslani P, et al: Genetic evidence for early divergence of small functioning and nonfunctioning endocrine pancreatic tumors: gain of 9q34 is an early event in insulinomas. Cancer Res 61:5186–5192 (2001).

Vissers LELM, de Vries BBA, Osoegawa K, Janssen IM, Feuth T, et al: Array-based comparative genomic hybridization for the genomewide detection of submicroscopic chromosomal abnormalities. Am J Hum Genet 73:1261–1270 (2003).

Wild A, Langer P, Ramaswamy A, Chaloupka B, Bartsch DK: A novel insulinoma tumor suppressor gene locus on chromosome 22q with potential prognostic implications. J Clin Endocrinol Metab 86:5782–5787 (2001).

Zhao J, Speel EJM, Muletta-Feurer S, Rütimann K, Saremaslani P, et al: Analysis of genomic alterations in sporadic adrenocortical lesions. Am J Pathol 155:1039–1045 (1999).

Zhuang Z, Park WS, Pack S, Schmidt L, Vortmeyer AO, et al: Trisomy 7-harbouring non-random duplication of the mutant MET allele in hereditary papillary renal carcinoma. Nat Genet 20:66–69 (1998).

Cytogenet Genome Res 115:298–302 (2006)
DOI: 10.1159/000095927

Lung cancer genetics and pharmacogenomics

V.A. Joshi[a–c]   R. Kucherlapati[a, c]

[a]Harvard Medical School-Partners, Healthcare Center for Genetics and Genomics, Cambridge
[b]Department of Pathology, Massachusetts General Hospital, [c]Harvard Medical School, Boston, MA (USA)

Manuscript received 8 March 2006; accepted in revised form for publication by A. Geurts van Kessel, 1 May 2006.

Abstract. Epidermal growth factor receptor (EGFR)-targeted therapies have demonstrated remarkable success in a small subset of non-small cell lung cancer patients. The mechanism of response has been an area of active research, with somatic mutation in a number of genes in the *EGFR* signal transduction pathway and copy number alterations of genes of the *EGFR* family as candidates contributing towards response. Continuing studies should help determine an appropriate biomarker or combination of biomarkers that can be used to predict response to this class of therapy.

Copyright © 2006 S. Karger AG, Basel

Lung cancer is the leading cause of death from cancer in both men and women, with over 180,000 new diagnoses and 150,000 deaths annually in the US (Edwards et al., 2005). There are two types of lung cancer: small cell lung cancer and non-small cell lung cancer (NSCLC), of which NSCLC comprises 80% of cases. NSCLC is further divided into three types: adenocarcinoma, large cell carcinoma and squamous cell carcinoma. Bronchioloalveolar carcinoma (BAC) is a subtype of adenocarcinoma. Although progress has been made in developing more successful treatment regimens, prognosis remains grim, as the 1-year life expectancy for individuals treated with chemotherapy is only about 33% (Schiller et al., 2002). Novel therapies targeting the specific molecular aberrations in lung tumor cells have been developed with varying degrees of success (Raben et al., 2004). This review will discuss some of the molecular aberrations observed in lung tumor cells, targeted therapies, and the identification of individuals likely to respond to these therapies.

The epidermal growth factor receptor

The epidermal growth factor receptor (EGFR) family, also known as ERBB or HER, consists of four receptor tyrosine kinases: EGFR, HER2/neu, ERBB3, and ERBB4. These proteins are located on the surface of epithelial cells and consist of an extracellular ligand binding domain, a transmembrane domain, and an intracellular kinase domain. Upon ligand binding, EGFR proteins homo- or heterodimerize, inducing receptor internalization and autophosphorylation of the intracellular kinase domain. Phosphorylation activates both the mitogen-activated protein kinase (MAPK) and the phosphatidylinositol-3-kinase PI3K/AKT and STAT signaling pathways to stimulate cell cycle progression, promote cell motility, adhesion, invasion, angiogenesis, and/or inhibit apoptosis. The MAPK kinase pathway is activated when GTP is exchanged for GDP on RAS, and signal transduction occurs through RAF, MEK, and ERK. ERKs activate transcription factors, such as c-Myc, that promote cell growth. AKT is an inhibitor of apoptosis, and PTEN is a negative regulator of the PI3/AKT pathway (for review see Herbst, 2004; Raben et al., 2004).

Because of their known role in cell proliferation, and because amplification and/or over-expression of *EGFR* family members has been observed in many solid epithelial tumors, much effort has been directed towards developing

Request reprints from Victoria A. Joshi, PhD
65 Landsdowne Street, Cambridge, MA 02139 (USA)
telephone: +1 617 768 8324; fax: +1 617 768 8513
e-mail: vjoshi@partners.org

KARGER

Fax +41 61 306 12 34
E-Mail karger@karger.ch
www.karger.com

© 2006 S. Karger AG, Basel
1424–8581/06/1154–0298$23.50/0

Accessible online at:
www.karger.com/cgr

Table 1. Many retrospective studies of individuals treated with gefitinib and erlotinib have been conducted to determine whether individuals with somatic *EGFR* kinase domain mutations are more likely to respond to these EGFR-TKIs. In these studies, 80.8% of EGFR-TKI-responsive individuals have somatic *EGFR* mutations and 8.2% of non-responders have mutations.

	Responders, n	Responders with *EGFR* mutations, n/%	Non-responders, n	Non-responders with *EGFR* mutations, N/%
GEFITINIB				
Paez et al., 2004	5	5/100	4	0/0
Pao et al., 2004	10	7/70	8	0/0
Lynch et al., 2004	9	8/88	7	0/0
Huang et al., 2004	9	7/78	7	1/14.3
Taron et al., 2005	24	16/67	43	1/2.3
Takano et al., 2005	35	32/91	31	7/22.6
Total GEFITINIB	92	75/81.5	100	9/9
ERLOTINIB				
Pao et al., 2004	7	5	10	0/0
Total GEFITINIB + ERLOTINIB	99	80/80.8	110	9/8.2

therapeutic compounds that specifically target and inactivate these proteins. Two classes of *EGFR* inhibitors have been developed: monoclonal antibodies targeting the extracellular domain of the receptors and small molecule inhibitors of the receptors. Gefitinib (Iressa) and erlotinib (Tarceva) are two such small molecule inhibitors, referred to as EGFR tyrosine kinase inhibitors (EGFR-TKIs), as their mechanism of action is to block EGFR signal transduction through competitive inhibition with ATP in the tyrosine kinase domain (Hynes and Lane, 2005).

Phase II clinical trials of gefitinib and erlotinib revealed a clinical response in a subset of NSCLC patients, with an overall response rate between 8 and 27.5% (Fukuoka et al., 2003; Kris et al., 2003; Perez-Soler et al., 2004; Shepherd et al., 2005; Tsao et al., 2005), and erlotinib was shown to prolong survival by at least two months in a placebo-controlled trial (Shepherd et al., 2005). Responders tend to have adenocarcinoma histology, female gender, non-smoking status, and Asian ethnicity (Fukuoka et al., 2003; Kris et al., 2003; Janne et al., 2004; Shepherd et al., 2005). However, four large clinical trials with similar designs comparing chemotherapy alone versus chemotherapy plus either gefitinib or erlotinib failed to show a clinical benefit, as measured by response rate, time to progression, or survival (Giaccone et al., 2004; Herbst et al., 2004, 2005). It is possible that if a patent stratification strategy utilizing an appropriate set of EGFR-TKI 'responsive' biomarkers were used, a different outcome may have resulted.

EGFR mutations and response

Although it was recognized that the EGFR-TKIs are highly effective in a subset of lung cancer patients, the reasons why certain patients responded and others did not was not known. Two groups investigated the role of somatic mutations in certain genes on the response of the tumors. Both groups examined the status of EGFR in tumor cells and identified somatic activating mutations in the EGFR kinase domain in 13 of 14 (93%) individuals with a dramatic clinical response. These mutations were either point mutations or small in-frame deletions in exon 19 that increase EGF-dependent receptor activation (Lynch et al., 2004; Paez et al., 2004). A third class of mutations consisting of in-frame insertions or duplications in exon 20 has subsequently been described; these may also be predictive of an EGFR-TKI response (Huang et al., 2004; Shigematsu et al., 2005a). However, in vitro studies indicate that cell lines transformed by this class of EGFR mutation are resistant to gefitinib and erlotinib (Greulich et al., 2005). EGFR kinase domain mutations are found in approximately 10% of individuals with adenocarcinoma in the North American population, and up to 55% of individuals with adenocarcinoma in Asian populations (Huang et al., 2004). The clinical characteristics predictive of EGFR-TKI response, that is, adenocarcinoma histology, female gender, non-smoking status, and Asian ethnicity, were identical to the clinical characteristics predictive of EGFR mutations (Lynch et al., 2004; Paez et al., 2004; Shigematsu et al., 2005a).

Many subsequent retrospective studies of individuals treated with gefitinib and erlotinib have supported the idea that individuals with *EGFR* kinase domain mutations are more likely to respond to EGFR-TKIs (Huang et al., 2004; Pao et al., 2004; Eberhard et al., 2005; Takano et al., 2005; Taron et al., 2005). In these studies, 80.8% of EGFR-TKI-responsive individuals have somatic *EGFR* mutations and 8.2% of non-responders have mutations (Table 1). However, other studies have not found a significant correlation between mutation status and response (Cappuzzo et al., 2005a; Tsao et al., 2005). In a study of 89 NSCLC patients treated with gefitinib, 6/15 (40%) patients with mutations had progressive disease (Cappuzzo et al., 2005a). In the BR.21 clinical trial of erlotinib versus placebo in NSCLC patients, *EGFR* mutations were identified in 40 individuals (22%). Only three (16%) of these individuals had a response to erlotinib. Although this was nearly double the response rate in individuals with wild type *EGFR*, it was not statistically significant. It is important to note that 53% of the mutations identified in this study had not been previously described (Tsao et al., 2005).

There are a number of potential explanations for the observation that some individuals with *EGFR* mutations have progressive disease when treated with EGFR-TKIs and that some responders do not have mutations. Variables in data interpretation, false negative and false positive results, as well as other genetic factors, could affect the correlation of mutations with response.

Mutation detection in *EGFR* from tumor tissue involves isolation of tumor cells from formalin-fixed paraffin embedded (FFPE) or frozen sections of tumor tissue and isolation of genomic DNA followed by DNA sequencing. Tissue insufficiency, lack of sensitivity of mutation detection, and lack of reproducibility are significant problems in the DNA sequencing of FFPE tumor biopsies. Tumors are often a complex mix of tumor and normal tissue and many samples require microdissection to obtain a sufficient number of tumor cells. A typical DNA sequencing protocol is limited in its sensitivity of mutation detection, such that a mutation will only be detected if it represents at least 20% of the overall signal; therefore, false negative results are inevitable (Janne et al., 2006). In addition, non-reproducible, presumably artifactual mutations could account for up to 8% of all mutations detected (Bell et al., 2005). Some studies have confirmed positive test results by repeating PCR and sequencing whereas others have not. Unconfirmed results, especially of novel mutations not previously described, should be interpreted with caution, as the mutation could be spurious, and could lead to a dilution of the association of mutations with response.

All mutations may not contribute equally towards survival or response. Studies suggest that compared to individuals without mutations, individuals with exon 19 deletions have poorer survival, whereas individuals with an L858R mutation have better survival (Shigematsu et al., 2005a; Jackman et al., 2006). Multiple mutations have been detected in the same individual, yet the effect of combinations of *EGFR* mutations has not been closely examined in most cases. More individuals with subsets of mutations will need to be examined to further delineate genotype/phenotype correlations.

Acquired resistance to initially successful treatment has been observed with targeted therapies, most notably in individuals with chronic myeloid leukemia (CML) and gastrointestinal stromal tumors (GISTs) treated with imatinib (Gleevec), a molecule that targets the kinase important in the biology of the disease (Branford et al., 2002; Antonescu et al., 2005). Not surprisingly, in NSCLC patients that initially show response to EGFR-TKIs, progressive disease eventually ensues. Four individuals with NSCLC have been described that initially had single activating mutations in

EGFR and were responsive to either gefitinib or erlotinib. DNA sequencing of biopsies collected upon relapse indicated that these individuals all had acquired an identical secondary mutation, T790M, in exon 20 of *EGFR* (Kobayashi et al., 2005; Pao et al., 2005a). Interestingly, the T790 amino acid of EGFR corresponds to the T315 of the ABL tyrosine kinase domain affected in CML patients, which has been shown to be mutated to isoleucine in some instances of acquired imatinib resistance (Gorre et al., 2001; Kobayashi et al., 2005).

Copy number change and response

High polysomy or gene amplification of *EGFR*, as defined as ≥ 3 copies per cell, has been observed in 7–45% of NSCLC cases (Bell et al., 2005; Cappuzzo et al., 2005a; Hirsch et al., 2005; Takano et al., 2005; Tsao et al., 2005). *EGFR* amplification is associated with poorer prognosis (Hirsch et al., 2003). A positive correlation between increased *EGFR* copy number and response to EGFR-TKIs, increased time to progression, and increased survival in patients enrolled in clinical trials of either gefitinib or erlotinib has been found (Cappuzzo et al., 2005a; Hirsch et al., 2005; Takano et al., 2005; Tsao et al., 2005).

It is important to recognize that amplification of both the normal and mutant *EGFR* allele occur, although not all studies have directly examined the mutation status of the amplified allele (Bell et al., 2005; Takano et al., 2005). Cappuzzo et al. (2005) noted an association between amplification status and the presence of a mutation, whereas Takano et al. (2005) found that the amplified allele was mutant in 18/29 cases. Amplification of the mutant allele could contribute to greater sensitivity of the tumor to EGFR-TKIs, whereas amplification of the normal allele could serve as a mechanism for acquired resistance in an individual with a sensitizing somatic mutation. As of yet, only one gefitinib-sensitive individual with amplification of the normal *EGFR* allele has been described (Bell et al., 2005). Fluorescence in situ hybridization (FISH) may prove to be a reliable indicator of either prognosis or response, but the genotype of the amplified allele may be necessary for accurate interpretation of the effect of amplification. Continuing studies and prospective clinical trials will more completely elucidate the predictive value of somatic *EGFR* mutations and *EGFR* amplification towards EGFR-TKI response.

Other *EGFR* family members are commonly amplified in solid tumors, and are logical candidates for an involvement in EGFR-TKI response. *ERBB2* (alias *HER2*) overexpression may be present in up to 38% of cases of lung adenocarcinoma, and, as in breast cancer, a meta-analysis revealed an association between overexpression and poorer survival (Slamon et al., 1987; Nakamura et al., 2005). Gene amplification of *ERBB2* may also have predictive value for EGFR-TKI response, as a study of 102 NSCLC patients revealed that increased *ERBB2* copy number was significantly associated with a better response to gefitinib, time to progression, and longer survival (Cappuzzo et al., 2005c). *ERBB3* (alias *HER3*) amplification, present in up to 26.8% of NSCLC tumors, does not appear to be a marker for EGFR-TKI response or resistance (Cappuzzo et al., 2005b).

Related biomarkers and response

Mutation of downstream effectors of EGFR could contribute to either EGFR-TKI sensitivity or primary or acquired resistance. As many as 38% of individuals with NSCLC have specific activating mutations in codons 12, 13, and 61 of *KRAS* (Ahrendt et al., 2001). As opposed to *EGFR* mutations that are found more commonly in non-smokers, *KRAS* mutations are more often associated with smoking status (Ahrendt et al., 2001). Mutations in *EGFR* and *KRAS* have proven to be mutually exclusive, suggesting independent mechanisms of growth advantage for tumor cells (Kondo et al., 2005; Shigematsu et al., 2005b). In 60 individuals with lung adenocarcinoma, *KRAS* mutations were associated with a primary lack of sensitivity to either erlotinib or gefitinib (Pao et al., 2005b). In a molecular analysis of four large international clinical trials of gefitinib, no mutations in *KRAS* or *PTEN* in either responsive (n = 5) or non-responsive (n = 3) *EGFR* mutant tumors were found, and loss of *PTEN* expression was not associated with response. *TP53* mutations were found in 2/6 gefitinib responders and 1/7 non-responders with *EGFR* mutations (Bell et al., 2005). The number of individuals in these studies was small; these and other candidate genes should be continuously examined to help elucidate the molecular mechanisms of response.

Somatic in-frame insertions in exon 20 of *ERBB2* may be present in up to 10% of individuals with lung adenocarcinoma, and, like *EGFR* mutations, are more common in females, non-smokers, and Asians (Stephens et al., 2004; Shigematsu et al., 2005b). The effect of these mutations on prognosis, responsiveness to EGFR-TKIs, or responsiveness to other therapies such as the anti-HER2 monoclonal antibody trastuzumab, has not yet been determined.

In a genome-wide cDNA microarray analysis of 33 biopsies of NSCLC patients treated with gefitinib, 51 genes were differentially expressed in responders and non-responders. Using an expression profile of 12 genes with the most significant difference between responders and non-responders, EGFR-TKI response was accurately predicted in additional NSCLC patients (Kakiuchi et al., 2004).

Several academic and commercial laboratories have developed diagnostic tests that are in use by physicians to predict patient response to EGFR-TKIs. It is not yet clear which biomarkers, or combinations of biomarkers, are best used to predict which patients will benefit most from these drugs. NSCLCs with similar histology can have very different molecular profiles, and these different tumor subtypes will inevitably have differing responses to targeted therapies. It is quite possible that rather than a single optimal diagnostic assay, a panel of markers involving both genotyping and assessment of amplification of a number of chromosomal loci may be required to most accurately predict response. This story illustrates the future of molecular pathology, oncology and diagnostics, where an individual's genetic makeup will contribute towards the choice of appropriate healthcare.

References

Ahrendt SA, Decker PA, Alawi EA, Zhu Yr YR, Sanchez-Cespedes M, et al: Cigarette smoking is strongly associated with mutation of the *K-ras* gene in patients with primary adenocarcinoma of the lung. Cancer 92:1525–1530 (2001).

Antonescu CR, Besmer P, Guo T, Arkun K, Hom G, et al: Acquired resistance to imatinib in gastrointestinal stromal tumor occurs through secondary gene mutation. Clin Cancer Res 11:4182–4190 (2005).

Bell DW, Lynch TJ, Haserlat SM, Harris PL, Okimoto RA, et al: Epidermal growth factor receptor mutations and gene amplification in non-small-cell lung cancer: molecular analysis of the IDEAL/INTACT gefitinib trials. J Clin Oncol 23:8081–8092 (2005).

Branford S, Rudzki Z, Walsh S, Grigg A, Arthur C, et al: High frequency of point mutations clustered within the adenosine triphosphate-binding region of BCR/ABL in patients with chronic myeloid leukemia or Ph-positive acute lymphoblastic leukemia who develop imatinib (STI571) resistance. Blood 99:3472–3475 (2002).

Cappuzzo F, Hirsch FR, Rossi E, Bartolini S, Ceresoli GL, et al: Epidermal growth factor receptor gene and protein and gefitinib sensitivity in non-small-cell lung cancer. J Natl Cancer Inst 97:643–655 (2005a).

Cappuzzo F, Toschi L, Domenichini I, Bartolini S, Ceresoli GL, et al: HER3 genomic gain and sensitivity to gefitinib in advanced non-small-cell lung cancer patients. Br J Cancer 93:1334–1340 (2005b).

Cappuzzo F, Varella-Garcia M, Shigematsu H, Domenichini I, Bartolini S, et al: Increased *HER2* gene copy number is associated with response to gefitinib therapy in epidermal growth factor receptor-positive non-small-cell lung cancer patients. J Clin Oncol 23:5007–5018 (2005c).

Eberhard DA, Johnson BE, Amler LC, Goddard AD, Heldens SL, et al: Mutations in the epidermal growth factor receptor and in KRAS are predictive and prognostic indicators in patients with non-small-cell lung cancer treated with chemotherapy alone and in combination with erlotinib. J Clin Oncol 23:5900–5909 (2005).

Edwards BK, Brown ML, Wingo PA, Howe HL, Ward E, et al: Annual report to the nation on the status of cancer, 1975–2002, featuring population-based trends in cancer treatment. J Natl Cancer Inst 97:1407–1427 (2005).

Fukuoka M, Yano S, Giaccone G, Tamura T, Nakagawa K, et al: Multi-institutional randomized phase II trial of gefitinib for previously treated patients with advanced non-small-cell lung cancer (The IDEAL 1 Trial) [corrected]. J Clin Oncol 21:2237–2246 (2003).

Giaccone G, Herbst RS, Manegold C, Scagliotti G, Rosell R, et al: Gefitinib in combination with gemcitabine and cisplatin in advanced non-small-cell lung cancer: a phase III trial–INTACT 1. J Clin Oncol 22:777–784 (2004).

Gorre ME, Mohammed M, Ellwood K, Hsu N, Paquette R, et al: Clinical resistance to STI-571 cancer therapy caused by BCR-ABL gene mutation or amplification. Science 293:876–880 (2001).

Greulich H, Chen TH, Feng W, Janne PA, Alvarez JV, et al: Oncogenetic transformation by inhibitor-sensitive and -resistant EGFR mutants. PloS Med 2:e313 (2005).

Herbst RS: Review of epidermal growth factor receptor biology. Int J Radiat Oncol Biol Phys 59:21–26 (2004).

Herbst RS, Giaccone G, Schiller JH, Natale RB, Miller V, et al: Gefitinib in combination with paclitaxel and carboplatin in advanced non-small-cell lung cancer: a phase III trial–INTACT 2. J Clin Oncol 22:785–794 (2004).

Herbst RS, Prager D, Hermann R, Fehrenbacher L, Johnson BE, et al: TRIBUTE: a phase III trial of erlotinib hydrochloride (OSI-774) combined with carboplatin and paclitaxel chemotherapy in advanced non-small-cell lung cancer. J Clin Oncol 23:5892–5899 (2005).

Hirsch FR, Varella-Garcia M, Bunn PA Jr, Di Maria MV, Veve R, et al: Epidermal growth factor receptor in non-small-cell lung carcinomas: correlation between gene copy number and protein expression and impact on prognosis. J Clin Oncol 21:3798–3807 (2003).

Hirsch FR, Varella-Garcia M, McCoy J, West H, Xavier AC, et al: Increased epidermal growth factor receptor gene copy number detected by fluorescence in situ hybridization associates with increased sensitivity to gefitinib in patients with bronchioloalveolar carcinoma subtypes: a Southwest Oncology Group Study. J Clin Oncol 23:6838–6845 (2005).

Huang SF, Liu HP, Li LH, Ku YC, Fu YN, et al: High frequency of epidermal growth factor receptor mutations with complex patterns in non-small cell lung cancers related to gefitinib responsiveness in Taiwan. Clin Cancer Res 10:8195–8203 (2004).

Hynes NE, Lane HA: ERBB receptors and cancer: the complexity of targeted inhibitors. Nat Rev Cancer 5:341–354 (2005).

Jackman DM, Yeap BY, Sequist LV, Lindeman N, Holmes AJ, et al: Exon 19 deletion mutations of epidermal growth factor receptor are associated with prolonged survival in non-small cell lung cancer patients treated with gefitinib and erlotinib. Clin Cancer Res 12:3908–3914 (2006).

Janne PA, Gurubhagavatula S, Yeap BY, Lucca J, Ostler P, et al: Outcomes of patients with advanced non-small cell lung cancer treated with gefitinib (ZD1839 'Iressa') on an expanded access study. Lung Cancer 44:221–230 (2004).

Janne PA, Borras AM, Kuang Y, Rogeers AM, Joshi VA, et al: A rapid and sensitive enzymatic method for EGFR mutation screening. Clin Cancer Res 12:751–758 (2006).

Kakiuchi S, Daigo Y, Ishikawa N, Furukawa C, Tsunoda T, et al: Prediction of sensitivity of advanced non-small cell lung cancers to gefitinib (Iressa ZD1839). Hum Mol Genet 13:3029–3043 (2004).

Kobayashi S, Boggon TJ, Dayaram T, Janne PA, Kocher O, et al: EGFR mutation and resistance of non-small-cell lung cancer to gefitinib. N Engl J Med 352:786–792 (2005).

Kondo M, Yokoyama T, Fukui T, Yoshioka H, Yokoi K, et al: Mutations of epidermal growth factor receptor of non-small cell lung cancer were associated with sensitivity to gefitinib in recurrence after surgery. Lung Cancer 50:385–391 (2005).

Kris MG, Natale RB, Herbst RS, Lynch TJ Jr, Prager D, et al: Efficacy of gefitinib, an inhibitor of the epidermal growth factor receptor tyrosine kinase in symptomatic patients with non-small cell lung cancer: a randomized trial. JAMA 290:2149–2158 (2003).

Lynch TJ, Bell DW, Sordella R, Gurubhagavatula S, Okimoto RA, et al: Activating mutations in the epidermal growth factor receptor underlying responsiveness of non-small-cell lung cancer to gefitinib. N Engl J Med 350:2129–2139 (2004).

Nakamura H, Kawasaki N, Taguchi M, Kabasawa K: Association of HER-2 overexpression with prognosis in nonsmall cell lung carcinoma: a metaanalysis. Cancer 103:1865–1873 (2005).

Paez JG, Janne PA, Lee JC, Tracy S, Greulich H, et al: EGFR mutations in lung cancer: correlation with clinical response to gefitinib therapy. Science 304:1497–1500 (2004).

Pao W, Miller V, Zakowski M, Doherty J, Politi K, et al: EGF receptor gene mutations are common in lung cancers from 'never smokers' and are associated with sensitivity of tumors to gefitinib and erlotinib. Proc Natl Acad Sci USA 101:13306–13311 (2004).

Pao W, Miller VA, Politi KA, Riely GJ, Somwar R, et al: Acquired resistance of lung adenocarcinomas to gefitinib or erlotinib is associated with a second mutation in the EGFR kinase domain. PLoS Med 2:e73 (2005a).

Pao W, Wang TY, Riely GJ, Miller VA, Pan Q, et al: KRAS mutations and primary resistance of lung adenocarcinomas to gefitinib or erlotinib. PLoS Med 2:e17 (2005b).

Perez-Soler R, Chachoua A, Hammond LA, Rowinsky EK, Huberman M, et al: Determinants of tumor response and survival with erlotinib in patients with non-small-cell lung cancer. J Clin Oncol 22:3238–3247 (2004).

Raben D, Helfrich B, Bunn PA Jr: Targeted therapies for non-small-cell lung cancer: biology rationale and preclinical results from a radiation oncology perspective. Int J Radiat Oncol Biol Phys 59:27–38 (2004).

Schiller JH, Harrington D, Belani CP, Langer C, Sandler A, et al: Comparison of four chemotherapy regimens for advanced non-small-cell lung cancer. N Engl J Med 346:92–98 (2002).

Shepherd FA, Rodrigues Pereira J, Ciuleanu T, Tan EH, Hirsh V, et al: Erlotinib in previously treated non-small-cell lung cancer. N Engl J Med 353:123–132 (2005).

Shigematsu H, Lin L, Takahashi T, Nomura M, Suzuki M, et al: Clinical and biological features associated with epidermal growth factor receptor gene mutations in lung cancers. J Natl Cancer Inst 97:339–346 (2005a).

Shigematsu H, Takahashi T, Nomura M, Majmudar K, Suzuki M, et al: Somatic mutations of the HER2 kinase domain in lung adenocarcinomas. Cancer Res 65:1642–1646 (2005b).

Slamon DJ, Clark GM, Wong SG, Levin WJ, Ullrich A, McGuire WL: Human breast cancer: correlation of relapse and survival with amplification of the HER-2/neu oncogene. Science 235:177–182 (1987).

Stephens P, Hunter C, Bignell G, Edkins S, Davies H, et al: Lung cancer: intragenic ERBB2 kinase mutations in tumours. Nature 431:525–526 (2004).

Takano T, Ohe Y, Sakamoto H, Tsuta K, Matsuno Y, et al: Epidermal growth factor receptor gene mutations and increased copy numbers predict gefitinib sensitivity in patients with recurrent non-small-cell lung cancer. J Clin Oncol 23:6829–6837 (2005).

Taron M, Ichinose Y, Rosell R, Mok T, Massuti B, et al: Activating mutations in the tyrosine kinase domain of the epidermal growth factor receptor are associated with improved survival in gefitinib-treated chemorefractory lung adenocarcinomas. Clin Cancer Res 11:5878–5885 (2005).

Tsao MS, Sakurada A, Cutz JC, Zhu CQ, Kamel-Reid S, et al: Erlotinib in lung cancer – molecular and clinical predictors of outcome. N Engl J Med 353:133–144 (2005).

Cytogenet Genome Res 115:303–309 (2006)
DOI: 10.1159/000095928

Medical applications of array CGH and the transformation of clinical cytogenetics

L.G. Shaffer   B.A. Bejjani

Signature Genomic Laboratories, LLC, Spokane, WA (USA)

Manuscript received 23 April 2006; accepted in original form for publication by A. Geurts van Kessel, 2 May 2006.

Abstract. Microarray-based comparative genomic hybridization (array CGH) merges molecular diagnostics with traditional chromosome analysis and is transforming the field of cytogenetics. Prospective studies of individuals with developmental delay and dysmorphic features have demonstrated that array CGH has the ability to detect any genomic imbalance including deletions, duplications, aneuploidies and amplifications. Detection rates for chromosome abnormalities with array CGH range from 5–17% in individuals with normal results from prior routine cytogenetic testing.

In addition, copy number variants (CNVs) were identified in all studies. These CNVs may include large-scale variation and can confound the diagnostic interpretations. Although cytogeneticists will require additional training and laboratories must become appropriately equipped, array CGH holds the promise of being the initial diagnostic tool in the identification of visible and submicroscopic chromosome abnormalities in mental retardation and other developmental disabilities.

Copyright © 2006 S. Karger AG, Basel

Large-scale variation in the human genome has been known for decades to those devoted to the study of chromosomes. As identified by the examination of banded chromosomes, variation can be normal or abnormal. Normal variation includes rearrangements or visible differences that are seen in the general population without clinical significance. These include the common pericentric inversion of chromosome 9 and the morphological and staining differences between homologues of the acrocentric short arms, the pericentromeric heterochromatin – mainly in the long arms of chromosomes 1, 9 and 16 – and the distal long arm of the Y chromosome. Abnormal variation includes balanced rearrangements such as inversions, reciprocal translocations, and Robertsonian translocations and unbalanced rearrangements such as derivative chromosomes and supernumerary marker chromosomes. Thus, the traditional study of human chromosomes with banding techniques has revealed large-scale genomic changes, typically referred to as chromosome abnormalities, for over 30 years. Once an esoteric field, clinical cytogenetics has evolved into an indispensable diagnostic discipline for the identification of chromosome abnormalities.

The purpose of this review is to present the use of microarray technologies in the identification and delineation of chromosome abnormalities. In addition, we will present some of the issues relevant to the use of this new technology in clinical medicine.

Clinical cytogenetics

Cytogenetics is an important part of the investigation of causes of fetal anomalies and demise, children with birth defects, developmental delay or other developmental dis-

Request reprints from Lisa G. Shaffer, PhD
    Signature Genomic Laboratories, LLC, 44 W 6th Ave, Suite 202
    Spokane, WA 99204 (USA)
    telephone: +1 509 474 6840; fax: +1 509 474 6839
    e-mail: Shaffer@signaturegenomics.com

abilities, and individuals suspected to have hematologic malignancy or for the evaluation of solid tumors. The type of tissue studied may differ depending on the reason for investigation, but the characteristic banding patterns indicative of specific chromosomes define us as human beings. Large-scale variation must be recognized and understood for the proper interpretation of any chromosomal banding pattern that deviates from 'normal'.

Given that the majority of first-trimester spontaneous abortions have an aneuploidy, that ~3.7% of children with global developmental delay have a cytogenetic aberration (Shevell et al., 2003), and that most cancers demonstrate diagnostic chromosome abnormalities or chromosome instability, cytogenetics will remain part of the diagnostic evaluation in many medical specialties. Reasons for referral for a chromosome analysis may include mental retardation, developmental delay, seizures and other developmental disabilities, physical birth defects, infertility, multiple miscarriages, and various cancers. The identification of a chromosome abnormality is important for clinical management of the condition, critical for anticipating potential medical problems, essential for understanding recurrence risks for offspring or other family members and, most importantly, instrumental in providing a diagnosis for those individuals affected with a cytogenetic disorder.

Although many aberrations are revealed through cytogenetic studies, conventional cytogenetic analysis cannot reliably detect rearrangements of genomic segments smaller than 3–5 million base pairs (Mb). Furthermore, microscopic examination of the chromosomes may not reveal the chromosomal origin of small supernumerary chromosomes (marker chromosomes) because their limited size is insufficient to provide a recognizable characteristic banding pattern, may not identify subtle rearrangements of the subtelomeric regions (Flint and Knight, 2003; Knight and Flint, 2004), and may not elucidate the complexity of some rearrangements, especially in solid tumors and leukemias.

Molecular cytogenetics

The introduction of fluorescence in situ hybridization (FISH) circumvented all these limitations. FISH has become an integral part of a comprehensive cytogenetic evaluation. It permits the determination of the number and location of specific DNA sequences both in metaphase chromosomes and in interphase nuclei, thus substantially simplifying the preparation and evaluation of samples. The applications of FISH include aneuploidy screening in prenatal specimens and certain suspected malignancies, evaluation for gene rearrangements (fusion chromosomes) in leukemias and lymphomas, microdeletions in contiguous gene syndromes, and rearrangements of the subtelomeric regions. Typically, most of these rearrangements are difficult or impossible to visualize with conventional banding technologies for a variety of reasons including small size, lack of staining intensity, and deficiency of banding patterns of the altered segments.

FISH can use a variety of probe types to interrogate particular segments of the genome. For example, repetitive sequence probes that are unique to each centromere are used to identify the copy number of particular chromosomes or identify the chromosomal origin of marker chromosomes; whole-chromosome painting probes are helpful for delineating translocations; and unique sequence probes (single-copy probes) are used to identify deletions associated with contiguous gene syndromes or other microdeletion syndromes. However, FISH usually requires that the patient either exhibits features consistent with a well-defined syndrome with a known chromosomal etiology or demonstrates an abnormal karyotype that requires further molecular characterization (e.g. marker chromosome). This is because single FISH probes reveal gains, losses, or rearrangement of only the segments being interrogated and do not provide information about the rest of the genome. Thus, a centromeric repetitive probe may demonstrate the chromosomal origin of a marker chromosome but cannot delineate the extent of euchromatin on the marker. Likewise, subtelomere probes may identify an unbalanced translocation, but the amount of chromatin that is gained or lost cannot be determined using these single FISH assays. Thus, most FISH analyses will not reveal abnormalities distinct from the genomic segments for which probes have been designed and used. Furthermore, the clinical cytogenetics laboratory must rely heavily on the clinical directive from the physician evaluating the patient. In many cases, the physician's clinical judgment will influence or directly determine the laboratory's choice of probes for establishing a diagnosis. Finally, another limitation to FISH is the number of probes that can be applied in a simultaneous assay (Ligon et al., 1997). This limitation is based on the number of fluorochromes that are available for labeling DNA probes and on the difficulty of obtaining uniform simultaneous hybridization for heterogeneous segments of the genome.

One type of FISH that has the potential to reveal imbalances across the genome is comparative genomic hybridization (CGH). In CGH, DNA is extracted from an individual with a known, usually normal, karyotype (control) and from an individual with an unknown karyotype or a known abnormal karyotype that requires further characterization. These two DNA specimens are differentially labeled with two different fluorochromes and applied to metaphase chromosomes prepared from a karyotypically normal individual. Differences between the fluorescent intensities along the length of any given chromosome will reveal gains or losses of genomic segments (Levy et al., 1998). The limitations to this technology include many of the same limitations found in conventional cytogenetics, mainly because the substrate for analysis is the metaphase cell. Thus, like traditional cytogenetic techniques, the resolution of CGH has been limited to that of metaphase chromosomes, 5–10 Mb for most clinical applications (Kirchhoff et al., 1998, 2001; Lichter et al., 2000).

In addition to the limitations described above, the regions interrogated by some FISH probes can show population variants, which may hinder the interpretation of such segments. These include polymorphisms of the centromeric regions (Verma and Luke, 1992; Stergianou et al., 1993; Bossuyt et al., 1995; Verma et al., 1997; Lo et al., 1999) and polymorphisms in the subtelomeric regions (Shaffer et al., 1999; Ballif et al., 2000). As with chromosomal variants, the laboratory should be able to recognize such variation, but often parental studies are needed to distinguish FISH variants from clinically relevant abnormalities (Ballif et al., 2000). In one study of 154 individuals referred for subtelomere testing, 73% of the abnormalities identified were found to be familial variants (Ballif et al., 2000). Because of the desire to interrogate the genome at a higher resolution than that provided by banded metaphase chromosomes and to examine loci commonly involved in rearrangements not evident by the light microscope, methods were developed that achieve both of these goals (Pinkel et al., 1998).

Array-based comparative genomic hybridization (array CGH)

To achieve the simultaneous examination of multiple loci at a higher resolution than that achieved by conventional cytogenetics, CGH was applied to an array of targets fixed to a solid support. Like CGH on metaphase chromosomes, array CGH directly compares DNA content between two differentially labeled genomes. The two genomes (a test or patient and a reference or control) are labeled and co-hybridized onto a solid support (usually a glass microscope slide) upon which cloned DNA segments have been immobilized. Arrays have been constructed with a variety of DNA targets ranging from oligonucleotides (25–85 bp) (Lucito et al., 2003; Ylstra et al., 2006) to bacterial artificial chromosomes (BACs; 80–200 kb) (Bejjani et al., 2005). The main advantage of array CGH is the ability to detect aneuploidy, deletion, duplication or amplification of any locus represented on the array. In contrast, multi-FISH analysis on metaphase chromosomes will detect aneuploidy and may detect microdeletions, but it has limited ability to detect duplications. Indeed, duplications involving segments smaller than 3–5 Mb may be routinely missed even by FISH of interphase nuclei. Microarray analysis can identify any segmental imbalance (aneuploidy, deletion, duplication) of the loci represented on the microarray with the resolution being limited only by the size of the insert used and the distance between clones.

Whereas most research applications require dense coverage of the genome with a resolution as high as possible, clinical applications present unique and distinct challenges to the design, validation and use of such arrays. Microarrays constructed with oligonucleotides (Lucito et al., 2003; Jobanputra et al., 2005) have the advantage of detecting gains or losses of very short genomic segments. However, the clinical significance of such alterations may not always be apparent. Initial studies using these methods have shown great promise; however, given the background 'noise' and the unclear significance of most alterations less than 1 Mb, these types of microarrays are not yet ready for clinical use.

Furthermore, the independent confirmation of results from oligonucleotide arrays may not be easily achieved in the clinical laboratory, because it would require the generation of FISH probes or the PCR amplification of the patient's alteration, which in this latter example is difficult in the presence of the normal homologue and would require the identification of a junction fragment or another similar novel alteration in the patient. Multiplex ligation-dependent probe amplification (MLPA) may be used to confirm DNA dosage difference at specific loci (Schouten et al., 2002; Koolen et al., 2004; Hochstenbach et al., 2005; Kirchhoff et al., 2005), but this technology requires pre-designed primers and is not used routinely in most clinical cytogenetic laboratories. Finally, although published literature clearly demonstrates the ability of oligonucleotide arrays to detect chromosome abnormalities, the difficulty lies in determining whether a normal result is truly normal. Very small segments of perhaps one or two oligonucleotides that lie outside the established ranges for normal results would necessitate further investigation and may likely turn each diagnostic case into its own research project.

Microarrays assembled from BACs have been constructed at varying densities including whole-genome tiling path arrays (Vissers et al., 2003; Ishkanian et al., 2004), arrays with some arbitrary coverage – such as one BAC placed every 1 Mb (Snijders et al., 2001; Greshock et al., 2004; Shaw-Smith et al., 2004) – and targeted arrays, which utilize the knowledge of clinical cytogenetics to construct useful and meaningful arrays for diagnostics (Bejjani et al., 2005; Cheung et al., 2005). Although whole-genome arrays are important for the discovery of new chromosomal syndromes (Vissers et al., 2004), the finding of copy number polymorphisms/variants (CNV) (large-scale genomic variation) in the human genome (Iafrate et al., 2004; Sebat et al., 2004) will make the use of these types of arrays prohibitive in the clinical setting until all variants are identified, catalogued, and understood. Even if this were to occur, care must be exercised in interpreting such variation, even if identified in the general population, because there is no circumstance that would preclude the region that contains CNVs to be involved in cytogenetic abnormalities. For example, if an array covered a small region that contained a CNV and a gain or loss were identified at this location, the laboratory may interpret that abnormality as normal variation when in fact it may be a larger deletion or duplication that simply encompasses a CNV and is clinically relevant in that individual.

It is generally accepted that a targeted array that covers specific areas of the genome of known clinical significance provides significant advantages. A well-designed targeted microarray should achieve an optimal balance between maximizing the detection of clinically relevant chromosome imbalances and minimizing the number of confirmatory FISH tests needed to evaluate for possible CNVs. Although this diagnostic field is continuing to evolve, it is anticipated that, because of their high yield in detecting chromosomal abnormalities in the patient suspected of having a cytogenetic imbalance, microarrays will become the

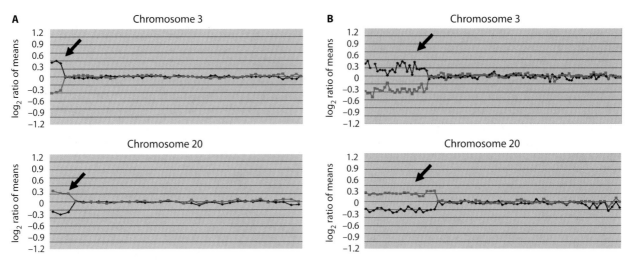

Fig. 1. Comparison of two targeted microarrays with different densities of DNA targets. For each plot, clones are arranged along the x-axis according to their location on the chromosome with the most distal telomeric short arm clones on the left and the most distal/telomeric long-arm clones on the right. The dark blue line represents the control: patient fluorescence intensity ratios, whereas the pink line represents the fluorescence intensity ratios obtained from a second hybridization in which the dyes have been reversed (patient:control). (**A**) A microarray was constructed using three overlapping BAC clones to each of the subtelomere regions (SignatureChip, Version 3). The top plot shows a deletion of these three BAC clones at the subtelomere region of the short arm of chromosome 3. The bottom plot shows the gain of the three overlapping BAC clones to the distal short arm of chromosome 20. This result is consistent with an unbalanced translocation. (**B**) A microarray was constructed using three-clone contigs spaced every 0.5 Mb over a 5.0-Mb region at each subtelomere (SignatureChip, Version 4). The top plot shows a >5.7-Mb deletion of the distal short arm of chromosome 3. The bottom plot shows a 4.7-Mb gain of the distal short arm of chromosome 20. This increased resolution allowed for the sizing of the segment duplicated from 20p. The size of the deletion from 3p could not be precisely delineated but is determined to be larger than the region represented on the microarray (>5.7 Mb).

initial diagnostic approach for the identification of chromosomal abnormalities in the future. Indeed, recent publications illustrate the high yield of array CGH in the clinical cytogenetics laboratory (Shaffer et al., 2006).

Array CGH in the diagnostic laboratory and clinical medicine

Although only a few studies have reported the prospective clinical yield of array CGH, these studies illustrate the anticipated impact on the field of clinical cytogenetics. Vissers et al. (2003) reported the study of 20 patients with mental retardation and dysmorphic features by array CGH using a genome-wide array with an average coverage of one clone per Mb across the genome. Seven de novo alterations were identified (14%; six deletions and one duplication). Shaw-Smith et al. (2004) reported the study of 50 patients with learning disabilities and dysmorphic features using a genome-wide array with an average coverage similar to that of Vissers et al. (2003). Two deletions were identified and shown to be de novo (10%). In both of these studies utilizing arrays with an average coverage of 1 Mb, additional alterations were identified in ~25% of subjects. These were also found in a clinically normal parent and, thus, were likely to be CNVs.

In a more recent prospective study, 100 patients with unexplained MR were analyzed using a tiling-resolution genome-wide microarray. Ten percent of cases showed altera-

tions of clinical relevance (de Vries et al., 2005). However, of the 97 patients with reproducible copy-number changes, the majority had alterations inherited from phenotypically normal parents and were, therefore, likely CNVs. Recently, Miyake et al. (2006) screened 30 subjects with idiopathic mental retardation with a 1.4-Mb resolution BAC array and found chromosome abnormalities in 17%. Most patients also showed CNVs. Thus, the use of genome-wide arrays in a clinical setting will uncover these variants and may confound the interpretation of such cases, especially in the absence of parental samples. However, of greater importance than the identification of CNVs, these studies support the role of array CGH in identifying cytogenetic abnormalities, perhaps in as many as 10–17% of cases in a carefully selected population with mental retardation or developmental delay.

In contrast, in the largest published study to date of a heterogeneous population, we reported the use of a targeted array (SignatureChip®, Signature Genomic Laboratories, LLC, Spokane, Wash.) in the identification of chromosome abnormalities in 1,500 consecutive patient samples sent to our clinical laboratory for a variety of developmental problems (Shaffer et al., 2006). These cases were in an unselected population that illustrates the types of cases typically referred for cytogenetic evaluation. In this group of consecutive cases, 5.6% showed clinically relevant abnormalities. Most patients were referred by geneticists and neurologists for a variety of medical problems and most had a previously determined normal karyotype. Many had also had

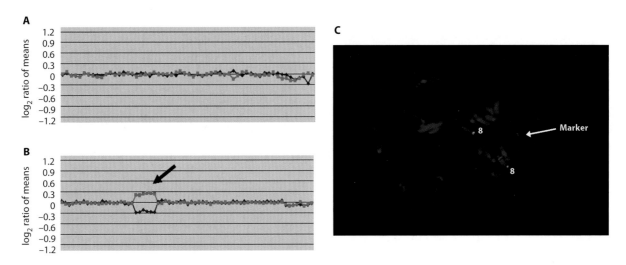

Fig. 2. Results from a marker chromosome 8. For each chromosome 8 plot, the clones are arranged as described in the legend for Fig. 1. (**A**) A normal result for chromosome 8. (**B**) A plot showing a gain of a three-clone contig from the 8p pericentromeric region and a gain of a three-clone contig from the 8q pericentromeric region. (**C**) FISH analysis using a BAC clone from the 8q pericentromeric region demonstrated a marker chromosome.

subtelomere FISH and molecular diagnostic testing. Interestingly, known microdeletion syndromes were among the most common abnormalities identified, which may indicate that the phenotypic spectrum of presentation varies more than previously anticipated by the clinical community (Shaffer et al., 2006). As expected based on published literature (Knight et al., 1999), subtelomeric abnormalities were common among the patients (Fig. 1). In addition, cases of trisomy mosaicism and marker chromosomes (Fig. 2) were identified by array CGH, even in cases with previous purportedly normal cytogenetic studies (Shaffer et al., 2006). These results suggest that trisomy mosaicism or marker chromosomes may be missed by traditional cytogenetic techniques either because low-level mosaicism may not be detected in the limited number of cells analyzed in routine cytogenetics, or because some aneuploidies may not be evident in the T-cells that are stimulated by phytohemagglutinin to progress through mitosis to metaphase in routine culturing of peripheral blood. Whatever the reason, mosaicism will likely be detected by array CGH if present in the peripheral blood or tissue used for analysis because DNA is extracted from the whole specimen, free of any culturing biases.

Among these 1,500 cases, 2.4% showed DNA copy-number changes that were found to be familial or population variants (Fig. 3). Thus, even after stringent criteria for clone selection and inclusion (Bejjani et al., 2005), our targeted array still showed regions of CNV (Shaffer et al., 2006). Because of the abundance of these CNVs in the human genome, complete avoidance on a clinical microarray may not be possible because, as discussed above, these CNVs can also be involved in or encompassed by clinically relevant chromosome abnormalities. However, if a microarray is constructed expressly for clinical cytogenetic applications with knowledge of the potential of CNVs, this tool can be used efficiently to identify unbalanced subtelomeric rearrangements, microdeletions, reciprocal duplications, marker chromosomes, and aneuploidy, including low-level mosaicism.

In this review, we have already shown that in several studies, the detection of array CGH is at least double that of routine cytogenetic testing (3.7%; Shevell et al., 2003). However, array CGH will not identify balanced rearrangements (Robertsonian translocations, reciprocal translocations, balanced insertions, and inversions) or single-gene mutations, other than small deletions that approximate the size of the clone or DNA target. Given these considerations, we examined the potential of array CGH to replace clinical cytogenetics. We reviewed the potential yield of array CGH to detect cytogenetic abnormalities as detected by routine chromosome analysis and targeted FISH studies by examining the abnormalities identified in a clinical cytogenetics laboratory (Shaffer, unpublished data). Of all abnormalities examined, 95% would have been identified by our original targeted microarray (Bejjani et al., 2005). Of the 5% that would not have been detected, ~36% of these were either balanced Robertsonian translocations or balanced reciprocal translocations and ~38% were inversions. As stated above, these balanced rearrangements would not be detected by array CGH, regardless of density of coverage of the genome. About 26% of these undetectable cases (1.1% of all abnormal cases examined) were either interstitial deletions or duplications of regions not represented on the array and therefore would not have been detected. Even with these results, a well-constructed targeted array has the potential to detect all visible unbalanced karyotypes and all DNA gains and losses resulting from submicroscopic chromosome abnormalities. Thus, given this potential, we anticipate array CGH to be the initial diagnostic approach for the identification of chromosomal abnormalities in the future.

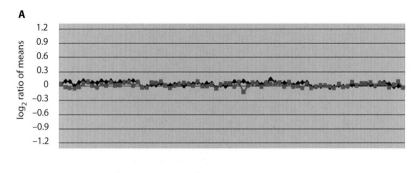

A

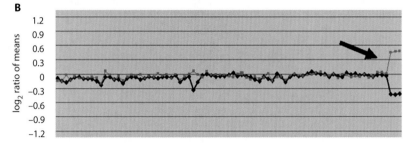

B

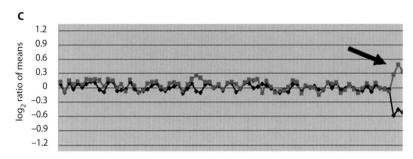

C

Fig. 3. Copy number variation found in a child and parent. For each plot, the clones for chromosome 1 are arranged as described in the legend to Fig. 1. (**A**) A normal result for chromosome 1. (**B**) A plot showing a gain of a three-clone contig in the subtelomeric region of the distal long arm of chromosome 1 in a child with developmental delay. (**C**) A plot from the clinically normal parent of the patient shown in **B**. This parent also shows the gain of the same three-clone contig. Because this individual is clinically normal, this gain likely represents a CNV. Note that this three-clone alteration is similar in appearance to the de novo alterations seen in Fig. 1A and illustrates the need for parental studies for clarification and interpretation of most alterations seen by array CGH.

Final considerations

The development of array CGH represents the latest advancement in molecular cytogenetics. This new technology has resulted in technical convergence between molecular diagnostics and clinical cytogenetics, two disciplines that have been distinct historically. This technical overlap may tempt non-cytogeneticists to offer array CGH diagnostic testing in their laboratories. Although the technical elements may be well-understood and mastered by non-cytogeneticists, the accurate analyses of these tests not only retain the existing high complexity of cytogenetic interpretation but also have added another layer of convolution due to the inevitable CNVs.

It is critical that cytogeneticists refine and advance their understanding of these new technologies to keep abreast of their rapidly evolving field. It is imperative that cytogeneticists obtain the necessary training to utilize this new technology. These changes will require the establishment of new training programs to prepare emerging cytogeneticists to face the future challenges of this exciting field.

Similar to what happened following the advent of FISH in the early 1990s, the evolution of the cytogenetic laboratory is inevitable. The expectations of clinical cytogenetics from the medical community have been raised even higher as array CGH becomes part of the cytogeneticist's tools to examine chromosomes at an unprecedented resolution. The cytogenetic laboratory of the future may have fewer microscopes than that of today. The scrupulous band-by-band analysis of metaphase chromosomes may become a historical curiosity as scanners and computers assist technologists in their evaluations of chromosomal abnormalities. This transformation of clinical cytogenetics into an automated and objective discipline will allow for higher through-put, increased diagnostic yield, and the identification of chromosome abnormalities at an unprecedented resolution.

Acknowledgements

We thank Aaron Theisen for his expert editing of the manuscript and Emily Rorem, Kyle Sundin and Kelly White (Signature Genomic Laboratories, LLC) for their assistance in preparing the figures for the manuscript.

References

Ballif BC, Kashork CD, Shaffer LG: The promise and pitfalls of telomere region-specific probes. Am J Hum Genet 67:1356–1359 (2000).

Bejjani BA, Saleki R, Ballif BC, Rorem EA, Sundin K, et al: Use of targeted array-based CGH for the clinical diagnosis of chromosomal imbalance: Is less more? Am J Med Genet A 134:259–267 (2005).

Bossuyt PJ, Van Tienen MN, De Gruyter L, Smets V, Dumon J, Wauters JG: Incidence of low-fluorescence alpha satellite region on chromosome 21 escaping detection of aneuploidy at interphase by FISH. Cytogenet Cell Genet 68:203–206 (1995).

Cheung SW, Shaw CA, Yu W, Li J, Ou Z, et al: Development and validation of a CGH microarray for clinical cytogenetic diagnosis. Genet Med 7:422–432 (2005).

de Vries BB, Pfundt R, Leisink M, Koolen DA, Vissers LE, et al: Diagnostic genome profiling in mental retardation. Am J Hum Genet 77:606–616 (2005).

Flint J, Knight S: The use of telomere probes to investigate submicroscopic rearrangements associated with mental retardation. Curr Opin Genet Dev 13:310–316 (2003).

Greshock J, Naylor TL, Margolin A, Diskin S, Cleaver SH, et al: 1-Mb resolution array-based comparative genomic hybridization using a BAC clone set optimized for cancer gene analysis. Genome Res 14:179–187 (2004).

Hochstenbach R, Meijer J, van de Brug J, Vossebeld-Hoff I, Jansen R, et al: Rapid detection of chromosomal aneuploidies in uncultured amniocytes by multiplex ligation-dependent probe amplification (MLPA). Prenat Diagn 25:1032–1039 (2005).

Iafrate AJ, Feuk L, Rivera MN, Listewnik ML, Donahoe PK, et al: Detection of large-scale variation in the human genome. Nat Genet 36:949–951 (2004).

Ishkanian AS, Malloff CA, Watson SK, DeLeeuw RJ, Chi B, et al: A tiling resolution DNA microarray with complete coverage of the human genome. Nat Genet 36:299–303 (2004).

Jobanputra V, Sebat J, Troge J, Chung W, Anyane-Yeboa K, et al: Application of ROMA (representational oligonucleotide microarray analysis) to patients with cytogenetic rearrangements. Genet Med 7:111–118 (2005).

Kirchhoff M, Gerdes T, Rose H, Maahr J, Ottesen AM, Lundsteen C: Detection of chromosomal gains and losses in comparative genomic hybridization analysis based on standard reference intervals. Cytometry 31:163–173 (1998).

Kirchhoff M, Rose H, Lundsteen C: High resolution comparative genomic hybridisation in clinical cytogenetics. J Med Genet 38:740–744 (2001).

Kirchhoff M, Gerdes T, Brunebjerg S, Bryndorf T: Investigation of patients with mental retardation and dysmorphic features using comparative genomic hybridization and subtelomeric multiplex ligation dependent probe amplification. Am J Med Genet A 139:231–233 (2005).

Knight SJ, Flint J: The use of subtelomeric probes to study mental retardation. Methods Cell Biol 75:799–831 (2004).

Knight SJ, Regan R, Nicod A, Horsley SW, Kearney L, et al: Subtle chromosomal rearrangements in children with unexplained mental retardation. Lancet 354:1676–1681 (1999).

Koolen DA, Nillesen WM, Versteeg MH, Merkx GF, Knoers NV, et al: Screening for subtelomeric rearrangements in 210 patients with unexplained mental retardation using multiplex ligation dependent probe amplification (MLPA). J Med Genet 41:892–899 (2004).

Levy B, Dunn TM, Kaffe S, Kardon N, Hirschhorn K: Clinical applications of comparative genomic hybridization. Genet Med 1:4–12 (1998).

Lichter P, Joos S, Bentz M, Lampel S: Comparative genomic hybridization: uses and limitations. Semin Hematol 37:348–357 (2000).

Ligon AH, Beaudet AL, Shaffer LG: Simultaneous, multilocus FISH analysis for detection of microdeletions in the diagnostic evaluation of developmental delay and mental retardation. Am J Hum Genet 61:51–59 (1997).

Lo AW, Liao GC, Rocchi M, Choo KH: Extreme reduction of chromosome-specific alpha-satellite array is unusually common in human chromosome 21. Genome Res 9:895–908 (1999).

Lucito R, Healy J, Alexander J, Reiner A, Esposito D, et al: Representational oligonucleotide microarray analysis: a high-resolution method to detect genome copy number variation. Genome Res 13:2291–2305 (2003).

Miyake N, Shimokawa O, Harada N, Sosonkina N, Okubo A, et al: BAC array CGH reveals genomic aberrations in idiopathic mental retardation. Am J Med Genet A 140:205–211 (2006).

Pinkel D, Segraves R, Sudar D, Clark S, Poole I, et al: High resolution analysis of DNA copy number variation using comparative genomic hybridization to microarrays. Nat Genet 20:207–211 (1998).

Schouten JP, McElgunn CJ, Waaijer R, Zwijnenburg D, Diepvens F, Pals G: Relative quantification of 40 nucleic acid sequences by multiplex ligation-dependent probe amplification. Nucleic Acids Res 30:e57 (2002).

Sebat J, Lakshmi B, Troge J, Alexander J, Young J, et al: Large-scale copy number polymorphism in the human genome. Science 305:525–528 (2004).

Shaffer LG, Kashork CD, Bacino CA, Benke PJ: Caution: telomere crossing. Am J Med Genet 87:278–280 (1999).

Shaffer LG, Kashork CD, Saleki R, Rorem E, Sundin K, et al: Targeted genomic microarray analysis for identification of chromosome abnormalities in 1,500 consecutive clinical cases. J Pediatr 49:98–102 (2006).

Shaw-Smith C, Redon R, Rickman L, Rio M, Willatt L, et al: Microarray based comparative genomic hybridisation (array-CGH) detects submicroscopic chromosomal deletions and duplications in patients with learning disability/mental retardation and dysmorphic features. J Med Genet 41:241–248 (2004).

Shevell M, Ashwal S, Donley D, Flint J, Gingold M, et al: Practice parameter: evaluation of the child with global developmental delay: report of the Quality Standards Subcommittee of the American Academy of Neurology and The Practice Committee of the Child Neurology Society. Neurology 60:367–380 (2003).

Snijders AM, Nowak N, Segraves R, Blackwood S, Brown N, et al: Assembly of microarrays for genome-wide measurement of DNA copy number. Nat Genet 29:263–264 (2001).

Stergianou K, Gould CP, Waters JJ, Hulten MA: A DA/DAPI positive human 14p heteromorphism defined by fluorescence in-situ hybridisation using chromosome 15-specific probes D15Z1 (satellite III) and p-TRA-25 (alphoid). Hereditas 119:105–110 (1993).

Verma RS, Luke S: Variations in alphoid DNA sequences escape detection of aneuploidy at interphase by FISH technique. Genomics 14:113–116 (1992).

Verma RS, Batish SD, Gogineni SK, Kleyman SM, Stetka DG: Centromeric alphoid DNA heteromorphisms of chromosome 21 revealed by FISH-technique. Clin Genet 51:91–93 (1997).

Vissers LE, de Vries BB, Osoegawa K, Janssen IM, Feuth T, et al: Array-based comparative genomic hybridization for the genomewide detection of submicroscopic chromosomal abnormalities. Am J Hum Genet 73:1261–1270 (2003).

Vissers LE, van Ravenswaaij CM, Admiraal R, Hurst JA, de Vries BB, et al: Mutations in a new member of the chromodomain gene family cause CHARGE syndrome. Nat Genet 36:955–957 (2004).

Ylstra B, van den Ijssel P, Carvalho B, Brakenhoff RH, Meijer GA: BAC to the future! or oligonucleotides: a perspective for micro array comparative genomic hybridization (array CGH). Nucleic Acids Res 34:445–450 (2006).

Author Index

KARGER

Fax +41 61 306 12 34
E-Mail karger@karger.ch
www.karger.com

© 2006 S. Karger AG, Basel

Accessible online at:
www.karger.com/cgr